Indian Veterinary Drug Refresher 2010

Dr. Rakesh Kumar Shukla
Veterinary Officer
UP Animal Husbandry Department
Gorakhpur - 273 001 (UP) India

Dr. M.K. Shukla
Assistant Professor (Animal Reproduction)
Veterinary College
(Jawaharlal Nehru Krishi Vishwavidyalaya)
Rewa, Madhya Pradesh

ibdc publishers

Published by

ibdc publishers

Khushnuma Complex Basement
7, Meerabai Marg (Behind Jawahar Bhawan)
Lucknow 226 001 U.P. (INDIA)
Tel. : 91-522-2209542, 2209543, 2209544, 2209545
Fax : 0522-4045308
E-Mail : word-press@hotmail.com

First Edition 2010

ISBN 978-81-8189-484-7

Composed & Designed at :
Panacea Computers
3rd Floor, Agrawal Sabha Bhawan
Subhash Mohal, Sadar Cantt. Lucknow-226 002
Tel. : 0522-2483312, 9335927082, 9452295008
E-mail : prasgupt@rediffmail.com

Printed at:
Salasar Imaging Systems
C-7/5, Lawrence Road Industrial Area
Delhi - 110 035
Tel. : 011-27185653, 9810064311

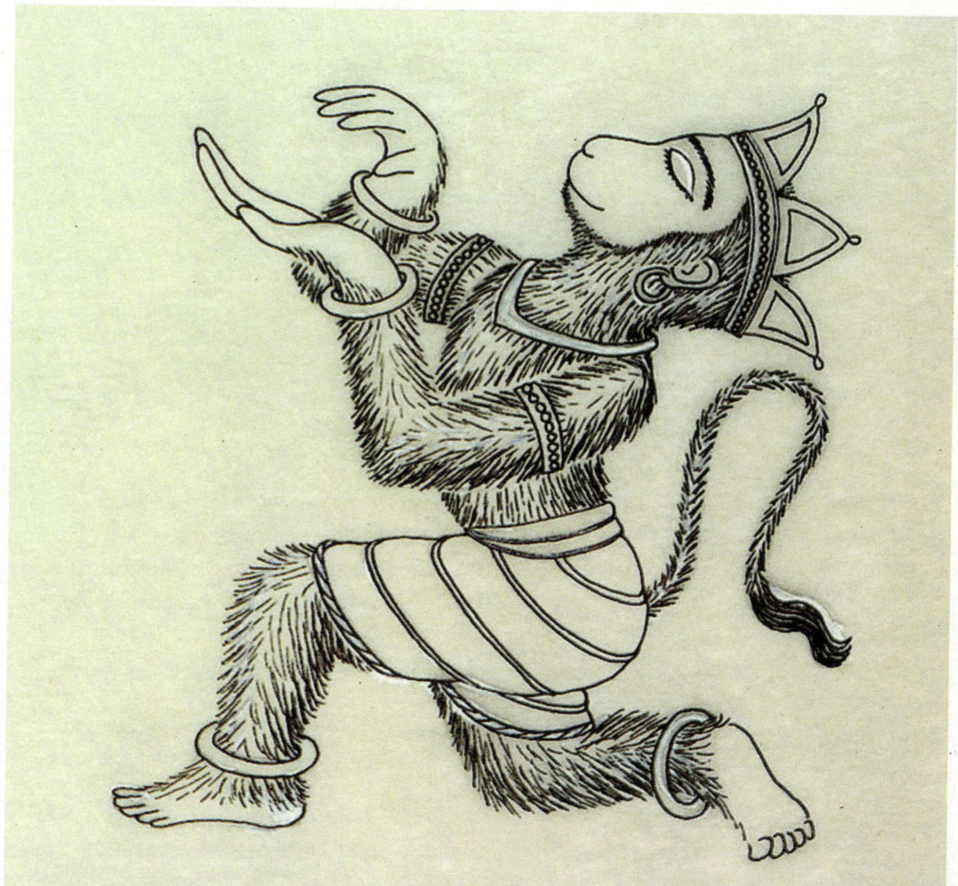

Dedicated to
Hanumanji

Preface

It is a matter of pride that veterinary sector is growing at appreciable rate resulting simultaneous demand for veterinary pharmaceuticals. Increasing demand for livestock products by rapidly growing population lead to maintain supply of these product from healthy livestock, which requires new research based products to maintain health and production of precious livestock, poultry and pets. Therefore, in order to fulfill growing need of informations about veterinary drugs, we present "Indian Veterinary Drug Refresher 2010" in service of dear veterinarians, energetic veterinary students and all those who want to be updated. Information is the key power for fast growth and development of individual and nation. We have tried our best to compile latest information about drugs and related fields of veterinary sector in a best possible manner. We will welcome suggestions and comments about the manuscript.

Dr. Rakesh Kumar Shukla
(rakesh22440@gmail.com)
Dr. M.K. Shukla
(manish15@gmail.com)

Contents

Chapter 1

Recent Advances in Veterinary Science

ADVANCES IN VETERINARY IMAGING DIAGNOSTICS

MRI IN EQUINES

MRI has for many years been the imaging modality of choice in human medicine for soft tissue, making it the gold standard for diagnosing pathology in orthopaedic and oncology studies. Hallmarq's EQ2 system brings the same diagnostic capability to the equine clinical practice. When tissue is placed in a strong magnetic field and a short pulse of radio waves is applied, a weak signal echoes back and is used to create an image. The tissue examined must be completely inside the magnet, limiting MRI to limbs (standing) and heads (in large, anesthesia only machines). Because MRI transmits and receives radio signals, scanning must take place in a screened room MRI uses no ionising radiation and has no known hazardous biological effects

What do MR images look like ?

The images appear as black-and-white slices through the tissue. The position of the slice is chosen by the scanner operator.

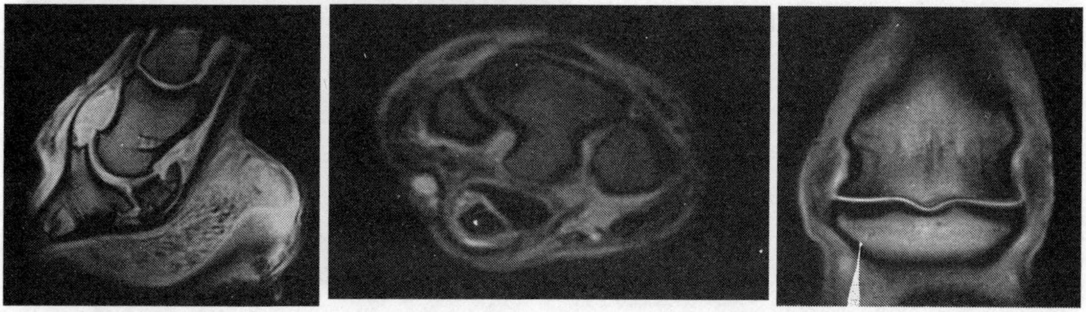

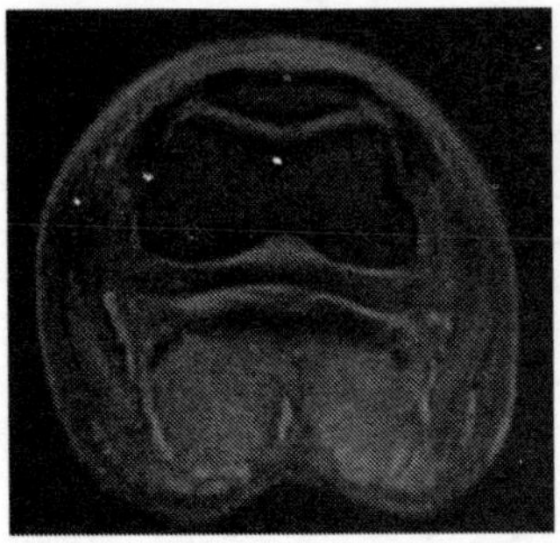

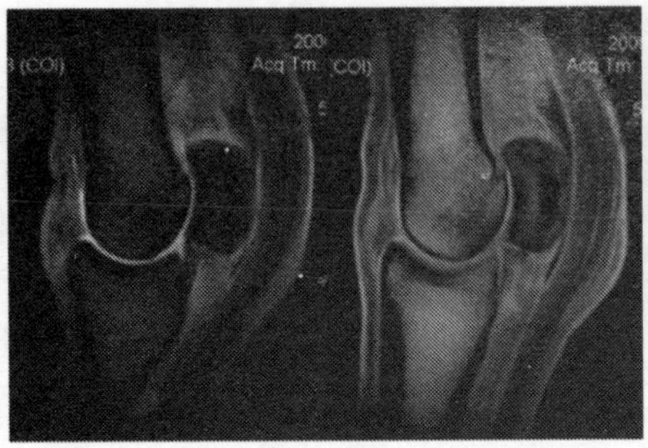

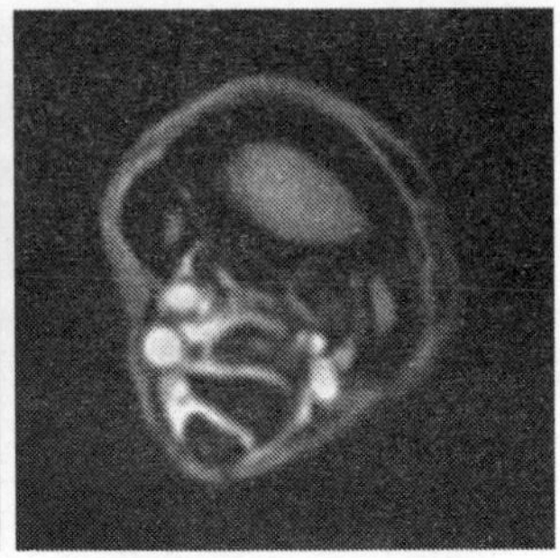

Sequence types

The exact appearance of an MR image is determined by the timing of the various radiofrequency and magnetic field gradient pulses used to collect the data, collectively known as the imaging sequence. Different sequences generate images that show fat (eg in bone) and water (eg edema) at different brightnesses

A full range of sequences is available using the Hallmarq system, including T1 and T2 weighted gradient echo and fast spin echo images, and fat suppressed STIR images. All sequence types are available with motion detection and correction to assist scanning the higher joints.

T1 Weighted Sequence

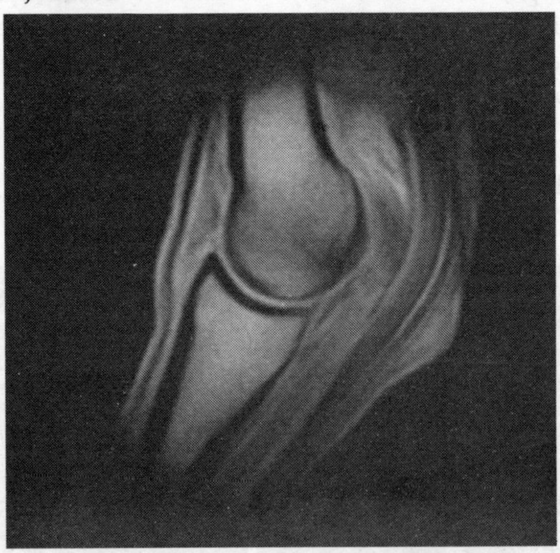

- Optimised for visualisation of anatomical structures
- Typical Tissue Appearances
  - Cartilage / Blood Vessels - Bright white
  - Fat / Bone / Fibrous Tissues - Light
  - Water / Synovial Fluids - Grey
  - Tendon / Ligaments - Dark grey
  - Cortical Bone - Black

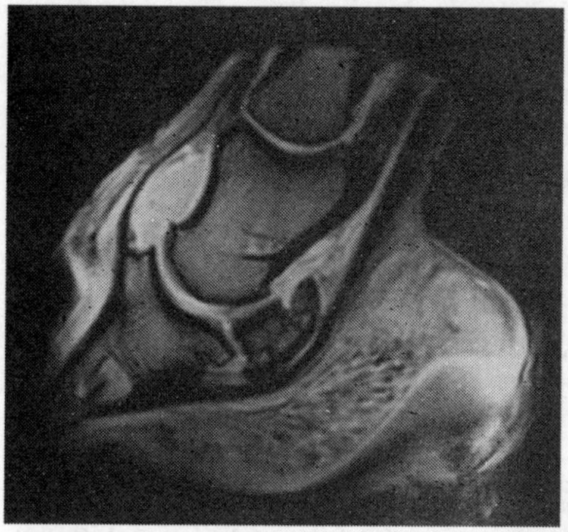

T2 weighted sequence

- Optimised for visualisation of inflammation in soft tissues
- Typical Tissue Appearances
  - Cartilage / Synovial fluid - Bright
  - Fat / Bone / Fibrous Tissues - Light Grey
  - Ligaments - Grey
  - Tendon - Dark grey
  - Cortical bone - Dark

STIR sequence

- Optimised for visualisation of inflammation in bone
- Typical Tissue Appearances
  - Synovial fluid / Water - Bright
  - Fibrous Tissues - Light grey
  - Fat - Dark grey
  - Ligaments - Grey
  - Tendon / Cortical bone — Dark grey

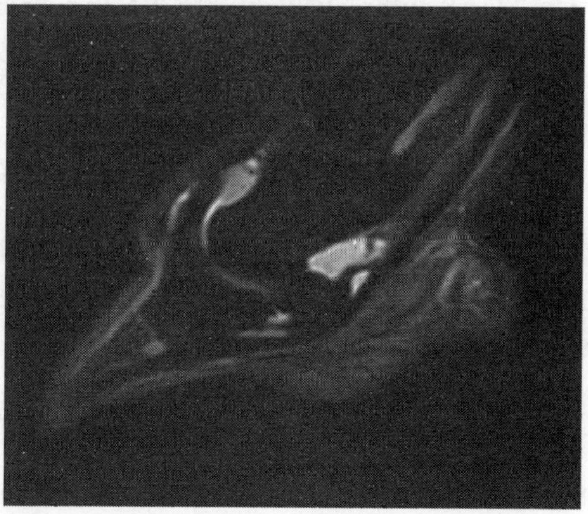

BIRD FLU: AN UPDATE (AVIAN INFLUENZA-HIGHLY PATHOGENIC (HPAI), FOWL PLAGUE)

Recently (2009), the latest outbreak of the birdflu in poultry in India was reported in West Bengal and Sikkim. This viral disease can cause exceptionally high mortality, especially in turkeys. It was **first identified** in **Italy** in the early **1900s** and is now known to exist worldwide. Strains of avian influenza virus may infect various types of animals, including birds, pigs, horses, seals, whales and humans. However, wild fowl act as natural asymptomatic carriers, spreading it to more susceptible domestic stocks. Avian influenza virus spreads in the air and in manure and there is no evidence that the virus can survive in well cooked meat.

In addition official control measures disrupt trade in poultry products from affected areas. The cause is a virus, Orthomyxovirus type A, its pathogenicity is variable, and isolates are designated sero-type/ species/location/reference number/year/subtype designation (H/N). Highly pathogenic forms are usually of the H groups 5 and 7 and may now be identified (if H5 or H7) by the presence of a sequence at the haemagglutinin cleavage site that codes for multiple basic amino acids. The virus infects chickens, turkeys, ducks, partridges, pheasants, quail, pigeons, and ostriches. Effectively all birds are considered to be at risk of infection. Apathogenic and mildly pathogenic influenza A viruses occur worldwide.

Outbreak of Avian Influenza in India

- First outbreak (Feb. 2006): Nandurbar district of Maharashtra and Surat district of Gujarat.
- Second outbreak (March-April, 2006) Jalgaon, Maharashtra; Burhanpur district of Madhya Pradesh.
- Third outbreak: village chingmeirong, near Imphal east Imphal district, Manipur (25-07- 2007)
- Outbreak during 2008: Assam, West Bengal
- Outbreak during 2009: West Bengal, Sikkim

Highly pathogenic avian influenza A (HPAI) viruses of the H5 and H7 HA subtypes have been isolated occasionally from free-living birds. Outbreaks due to HPAI were recorded in the Pennsylvania area, USA, in the years 1983-84. More recently outbreaks have occurred in Australia, Pakistan, India, Mexico and, from December 1999, in northern Italy. A serious outbreak occurred in The Netherlands in 2003 with a few linked cases in Belgium and one in Germany. H5 viruses of low pathogenicity may become highly pathogenic usually after circulating in poultry flocks for a time (Pennsylvania, Italy). Because of this, and the high mortality that 'low-path' AI can cause in turkeys, OIE and other bodies are currently examining ways to improve control of LPAI. See current OIE records for up to date information on distribution of HPAI. Morbidity is high but mortality usually relatively low, 5-50%.

The route of infection is probably oral initially, but possibly by the conjunctival or respiratory route and the incubation period is 3-5 days. Transmission is by direct contact with secretions from infected birds, especially faeces, waterfowl, equipment, clothing, drinking water. The virus replicates mainly in respiratory tissues of chickens and turkeys but in the intestinal tract of clinically normal waterfowl. Avirulent in one species may be virulent in others. Broken contaminated eggs may infect chicks in the incubator simulating vertical transmission. The virus is moderately resistant, can survive 4 days in water at 22°C, over 30 days at 0°C. It is inactivated by a temperature of 56°C in 3 hours and 60°C in 30 min, by acid pH, by oxidising agent and by formalin and iodine compounds. It can remain viable for long periods in tissues. Infections with other pathogens (e.g. Pasteurella) may increase mortality, even with 'low pathogenicity' strains.

Avian Influenza is a potential zoonosis. It can result in inapparent infection, conjunctivitis or severe pneumonia. The small number of human deaths associated with HPAI appear to have resulted from direct exposure to infected birds on farm or in markets.

Signs

- Sudden death.
- Marked loss of appetite, reduced feed consumption.
- Cessation of normal flock vocalisation.
- Drops in egg production.
- Depression.
- Coughing.
- Nasal and ocular discharge.
- Swollen face.
- Cyanosis of comb/wattles.
- Diarrhoea (often green).
- Nervous signs such as paralysis.

Post-mortem lesions

- Inflammation of sinuses, trachea, air sacs and conjunctiva.
- Ovarian regression or haemorrhage.
- Necrosis of skin of comb and wattles.
- Subcutaneous oedema of head and neck.
- Dehydration.
- Muscles congested.
- Haemorrhage in proventricular and gizzard mucosae and lymphoid tissue of intestinal tract.

> ➢ Turkey lesions tend to be less marked than those of chickens, while ducks may be symptomless, lesionless carriers of highly pathogenic virus.

Diagnosis

A presumptive diagnosis may be made on history and post-mortem lesions. Confirmation is by viral isolation in chick embryo, HA+, NDV-, DID+. Commercial Elisa test kits are now available. However, as with many such tests occasional false positive reactions can occur. The agar gel precipitation test is non-group-specific and is used to confirm any positives. **Differentiate** from Newcastle disease, fowl cholera, infectious laryngotracheitis, other respiratory infections, bacterial sinusitis in ducks.

How to Recognise Avian Influenza

What to look for

- Ruffled feathers
- Soft-shelled eggs
- Depression and droopiness
- Sudden drop in egg production
- Loss of appetite
- Cyanosis (purplish-blue coloring) of wattles and comb
- Edema and swelling of head, eyelids, comb, wattles, and hocks
- Green diarrhea
- Blood-tinged discharge from nostrils
- Incoordination, including loss of ability to walk and stand
- Pin-point hemorrhages (most easily seen on the feet and shanks)
- Respiratory distress
- Increased death losses in a flock
- Sudden death
- Nasal discharges

Treatment

None, but good husbandry, nutrition and antibiotics may reduce losses. Eradication by slaughter is usual in chickens and turkeys.

Prevention

- ➢ Hygiene, quarantine, all-in/all-out production, etc.
- ➢ Minimise contact with wild birds, controlled marketing of recovered birds.

- Vaccination is not normally recommended because, although it may reduce losses initially, vaccinated birds may remain carriers if exposed to the infection. Vaccines have been used in recent outbreaks in Mexico and Pakistan. To be effective inactivated vaccines must be the right subtype for the particular situation (H5 will not protect against H7 and vice versa).
- In outbreaks a regime of slaughter, correct disposal of carcasses, cleaning, disinfection, isolation, 21-day interval to re-stocking should be followed. Survivors can be expected to have a high degree of immunity but may harbour virulent virus.

Advantages of Vaccination

- Vaccination reduces susceptibility to infection.
- A higher dose of virus is necessary to infect the vaccinated birds.
- Vaccinated birds shed less virus resulting decreased contamination of the environment and decreased risk of human infection.
- Used strategically vaccination compliments a stamping out strategy by slowing/stopping the spread of the virus

EMERGENCY HOUSEHOLD MEDICATIONS

PRODUCT	COMMON USAGE	CANINE DOSAGE
Buffered Aspirin	Pain relief, anti-inflammatory	10 mg per Kg every 12 hrs
Vitamin B	Used as an appetite stimulant	1/2 to 2 ml subcutaneously, every 24 hrs
Benadryl	Treats allergies, itching, insect stings, bites	1 mg per Kg every 8 hrs, maximum 2 mg per/lb
Dimenhydrinate	Reduces motion sickness	Up to 50 mg every 8 hrs
Hydrogen Peroxide 3%	Used to induce vomiting after accidental ingestion of poison	10 ml by mouth every 15 min
Epinephrine 1:1000	Used to treat reactions to medications, insect stings, bites	1/10 to 1/2 ml intramuscular or subcutaneously
Bismuth subsalicylate preparation	For diarrhoea, vomiting and anti-gas	2 tsp per 5 kg every 6 hrs
Di Gel Liquid	Antacid and anti-gas	Up to 4 tablespoon every 8 hrs
Mineral Oil	Eliminates constipation	Up to 4 tablespoon daily
Kaopectate	Relieves diarrhoea	2 ml per kg every 2 hrs

ETHNOVETERINARY MEDICINES

Scientific name, (botanical family)	Local name	Part(s) used	Ethnoveterinary use
Achillea millefolium L. (Asteraceae)	yarrow	Aerial parts	Mastitis, wounds, sternal abscess
Achlys triphylla (Berberidaceae)	Vanilla leaf	leaves	flies
Alchemilla vulgaris L. (Rosaceae)	Lady's mantle	aerial parts	Retained placenta
Allium cepa L. (Alliaceae)	onion	Skins	endoparasites
Allium sativum L. (Amaryllidaceae)	garlic	minced cloves	Endoparasites, respiratory tonic
Althaea officinalis L. (Malvaceae)	marshmall ow	Aerial parts	Diarrhea, scours
Anethum graveolens L. (Apiaceae)	Dill	seed	Diarrhea, scours, milk production
Apium graveolens L. (Apiaceae)	celery	Aerial parts	endoparasites
Arctium lappa L. (Asteraceae)	Burdock	root	mastitis
Arnica sp. (Asteraceae)	Wild arnica	Leaves or flowers	wounds
Artemisia sp. (Compositae)	wormwoo d	leaves	endoparasites
Artemisia vulgaris L. (Asteraceae)	mugwort	plant	Zinc deficiency
Azadirachta indica A. Juss.	neem	powder	lice
Berberis aquifolium Pursh. Mahonia aquifolium (Berberidaceae)	Oregon grape	roots	wounds
Blechnum spicant (L.) Roth (Polypodiaceae)	Deer fern	Aerial parts	Magnesium imbalance
Bovista pila, Bovista plumbea Pers. (Lycoperdaceae)	puffball	Spore mass	Disbudding, cuts, wounds, sternal abscess
Calendula officinalis L. (Asteraceae)	calendula	Flower oil	Cuts, scratches, diarrhea, sore stomachs
Capsella bursa-pastoris (L.) Medic. (Brassicaceae)	shepherd's purse	leaves	wounds

Cinnamomum zeylanicum Blume (Lauraceae)	cinnamon	Inner bark	Diarrhea, scours
Curcuma longa L. (Zingiberaceae)	turmeric	rhizome	Caprine arthritis encephalitis palliative, proud flesh
Cymbopogon nardus (L.) Rendle (Poaceae)	citronella	oil	flies
Daucus carota L. (Apiaceae)	carrots	Roots & tops	endoparasites
Echinacea purpurea (L.) Moench (Asteraceae)	Echinacea	root	abscess, Pre-show protection, wounds, respiratory tonic
Epilobium augustifolium L. (Onagraceae)	fireweed	Fresh or dry plant	Appetite stimulant
Eugenia caryophyllata Thunb (Myrtaceae)	cloves	Essential oil	flies
Euphrasia officinalis agg. (Scrophulariaceae)	eyebright	Aerial parts	Eye problems
Galium aparine L. (Rubiaceae)	cleavers	Aerial parts	mastitis
Gaultheria shallon Pursh. (Ericaceae)	salal	Aerial parts	Rumen tonic, ketosis
Hedera helix L. (Araliaceae)	English ivy	leaves	Retained placenta
Helianthus annuus L. (Asteraceae)	sunflower	seeds	endoparasites
Hypericum perforatum L. (Hypericaceae)	St. John's Wort	Infused oil of flowers	Proud flesh, wounds
Juniperus communis L. (Cupressaceae)	juniper	branches	Endoparasites, liver fluke
Lavandula officinalis L. (Labiatae)	lavender	Essential oil	Flies, proud flesh
Mahonia nervosa (Pursh) Nutt (Berberidaceae)	Oregon grape	Root decoction	Abscess, Respiratory tonic
Malva sylvestris (Malvaceae)	mallow	plant	wounds
Matricaria chamomilla L. (Compositae)	chamomile	flower	eye problems
Medicago sativa L. (Leguminosae)	alfalfa	Pellets from high-selenium regions, aerial parts	Selenium deficiency, nutrition after calving
Melaleuca alternifolia L. (Myrtaceae)	Tea tree oil	drops	endoparasites

Mentha piperita L. (Lamiaceae)	peppermin t	Essential oil	flies
Mentha pulegium L. (Lamiaceae)	pennyroyal	Aerial parts	Flies, lice
Nepeta cataria L. (Lamiaceae)	catnip	Aerial parts	Pain killer
Pastinaca sativa L. (Apiaceae)	parsnip	tops	endoparasites
Petroselinum crispum L. (Apiaceae)	parsley	Aerial parts	endoparasites
Pinus ponderosa Douglas ex Lawson (Pinaceae)	long needle yellow pine	branches	Diarrhea grey pasty young animals, endoparasites
Plantago lanceolata L. (Plantaginaceae)	plantain	leaves	diarrhea
Polystichum munitum (Kaulf.) Presl. (Polypodiaceae)	Sword fern	Aerial parts	Stimulate digestion
Portulaca oleracea L. Portulacaceae	purslane	shoot	Zinc deficiency
Potentilla rectaL. (Rosaceae)	cinquefoil	Aerial parts	Appetite stimulant, diarrhea, scours
Prunella vulgaris L. (Lamiaceae)	self heal	plant	wounds
Pseudotsuga menziesii (Mirbel) Franco (Pinaceae)	Douglas fir	Top branches	Appetite stimulant, coccidiosis, endoparasites
Quercus alba L. (Fagaceae)	White oak	shoot	Zinc deficiency
Rubus sp. (Rosaceae)	thornless raspberry	leaves	Milk production
Rubus ursinus L. and Rubus laciniatus Willd. (Rosaceae)	blackberry	leaves	Unknown illness
Ruta graveolens L. (Rutaceae)	rue	leaves	flies
Salix alba L. var. sericea Gaudin (Salicaceae)	White willow	bark	Diarrhea, scours, mastitis, pain, unknown illness
Salix scouleriana Barratt ex Hook, Salix lucida Muhl. ssp. lasiandra (Benth.) E. Murr. (Salicaceae)	Scoulers willow, Pacific willow	Branches	Caprine arthritis encephalitis palliative
Salvia officinalis L. (Lamiaceae)	Garden sage	leaves	Drying off
Senna sp. (Fabaceae)	senna	pod	Diarrhea, scours
Symphoricarpos albusvar. laevigatus (Caprifoliaceae)	snowberry	branches	endoparasites

Symphytum officinale L. (Boraginaceae)	comfrey	Leaves fresh/dry	Abscess, wounds, diarrhea, flystrike, proudflesh
Symphytum officinale L. (Boraginaceae)	comfrey	Aerial parts	Increase butterfat; laxative, ketosis, udder edema
Syzygium aromaticum (L.) (Myrtaceae)	cloves	bud	coccidia
Taraxacum officinale (L.) (Asteraceae)	dandelions	leaves	Udder edema
Teucrium scorodonia L. (Labiatae)	woodsage	Tincture	mastitis
Thuja plicata Donn ex D. Don (Cupressaceae)	cedar	Bark shavings	lice
Thuja plicata Donn ex D. Don (Cupressaceae)	Red cedar	branches	Copper deficiency, endoparasites
Ulmus fulva Michx. (Ulmaceae)	Slippery elm	Bark powder	Blood in stool
Ulmus fulva Michx. (Ulmaceae)	Slippery elm	Inner bark	Diarrhea, scours
Urtica dioica L. (Urticaceae)	nettle	Ground seeds	endoparasites
Urtica dioica L. (Urticaceae)	nettles	Aerial parts	Pre-show protection, zinc deficiency, diarrhea
Usnea longissima Ach. (Parmeliaceae)	usnea	Aerial parts	Dehorning adults, foot rot, sternal abscess
Vaccinium parvifolium Sm. (Ericaceae)	huckleberr y	plant	ketosis
Valeriana officinalis L. (Valerianaceae)	valerian	roots	Pain killer
Verbascum thapsus L. (Scrophulariaceae)	mullein	flower	Respiratory tonic
Vernonia anthelmimtica	Kali jiri	seed	Round worms
Vitis sp. (Vitaceae)	grape	leaves	Unknown illness
Zea mays L. (Poaceae)	cornsilk	Silk (style, stigma)	Udder edema
Zingiber officinale Roscoe (Zingiberaceae)	ginger	rhizome	Diarrhea, scours

PROFENDER® Topical Solution (emodepside/praziquantel)

"The public's exposure to zoonotic parasites is of a magnitude not generally recognized by some in the veterinary and medical communities," "The general public, particularly families with young children, need to be aware of the risk and take the appropriate steps to limit their exposure." "Profender provides stress-free treatment for cats and easy-to-use administration for owners, ultimately improving owner compliance and their pet's health."

A topical application of Profender is absorbed through the skin and enters the circulation, allowing both active ingredients, emodepside and praziquantel, to exert their effects directly on target parasites in the gastrointestinal tract. This new formulation is the first topical dewormer for cats with efficacy against most common intestinal parasites — ascarids, hookworms, and tapeworms. Profender is available in three convenient dose sizes — Small (.35ml for 2.2 lbs to 5.5 lbs) Medium (.70ml for > 5.5 lbs to 11 lbs), and Large (1.12ml for >11 lbs to 17.6 lbs).

Leading parasitologists (CAPC) recommend year-round anthelmintics for cats. 2 Strategic deworming is a planned parasite control program that involves targeted deworming of pets to treat and control clinical disease and limit environmental contamination.

In addition to strategic deworming, Profender is also a gap deworming tool. Gap deworming is the practice of deworming to fill the gaps in intestinal parasite treatment and control left by monthly heartworm preventatives/intestinal parasite combination products. Heartworm preventatives are administered at treatment intervals based on the lifecycle of heartworms, not intestinal parasites, and most do not kill immature and/or migrating stages. Heartworm preventatives don't prevent pets from acquiring new infections between doses and they have a varied parasitic spectrum. This creates a situation where a pet may shed potentially zoonotic eggs into the environment, as often as monthly, even if they are on a fully compliant heartworm regimen. When gaps and infection occur, Profender makes deworming easier for the cat. In addition to affecting a cat's health, intestinal parasites pose a risk to owners and their families.

Zoonotic diseases can be transmitted via intestinal parasites, and children, pregnant women, and immunocompromised people are especially vulnerable. Backyards, sandboxes, public parks, and beaches accessible to dogs, cats, and wildlife often are contaminated with parasite eggs from an infected animal's feces.

Cat owners can limit their risk of exposure by practicing good personal hygiene and having children wash their hands after playing with pets and playing in potentially infected environments.

OIE launches WAHID, unique global animal health database

The World Animal Health Information Database (WAHID) interface is now available on the OIE web Site and operational. This new extensive database is a milestone in OIE efforts to improve the transparency, efficiency and speed with which animal health information is disseminated throughout the world.

Complementary to the on-line notification made by OIE Member Countries through the World Animal Health Information System (WAHIS) launched in April 2006, WAHID offers all available data on animal diseases, including zoonoses, per country, region, month and year. Among others, the database also compiles country animal population, exceptional epidemiological events maps, global animal diseases distribution maps or comparative disease status between two countries. The latter application can help define health hazards linked to the trade of live animals and animal products between countries.

"WAHID is designed to provide high quality animal diseases information to all stakeholders including veterinary services, international organisations, trading partners, academics, the media and the larger public. All can access and monitor with us the evolution of animal diseases in one or several countries or regions of the world," Dr Karim Ben Jebara, Head of the OIE Animal Health Information Department explained.

The new web interface will replace Handistatus II that compiles data from 1996 to 2004. Handistatus II will disappear when all this data is transferred into the more user-friendly WAHID.

WAHIS and WAHID are the unique system worldwide in the field of animal health information. WAHID can be found on the OIE website home page or on the following link: www.oie.int/wahid.

HOMEOPATHIC FIRST-AID FOR ANIMALS

Homeopathy (homoeopathy / homœopathy) is a system of medicine that bases its therapeutics on the principle of 'let likes be cured by likes' - 'similia similibus curentur'. The medicines used may be derived from animal, vegetable or mineral sources and, in latter times, remedies have also been derived from man-made substances. The initial requirement for treatment is knowledge of what effect a particular remedy or substance will have on a healthy body (i.e. what signs and symptoms it can provoke in a healthy body). The signs and symptoms presented by a sick animal or person are then compared to this 'symptom picture' of the various medicines, choosing that medicine which is the closest 'match'.

There is no risk of: a) toxic side-effects, b) medicine residues in farm animal products, c) 'doping' or residues in sporting animals, d) stimulation of antibiotic resistance. Laboratory animal research is not required for its development.

The strategy of a homeopathic consultation is to find the correct stimulus for the body's inherent healing potential (i.e. the correct homeopathic remedy) and, as an essential adjunct to this, to remove or to minimise any factors and influences that could obstruct or impede that healing process. For this reason, attention to the patient's diet is an essential part of the procedure, with a conscious attempt to feed each species as naturally and as healthily as possible, in line with its evolved needs.

Information concerning the effect of substances on the healthy body comes primarily from three sources:

- Provings in which healthy human volunteers take the remedy under investigation and record the effects. Modern proving protocols employ 'blinding' techniques to avoid bias and the placebo effect.
- Toxicology reports where appropriate.
- Clinical Experience

Although many of the remedies have, as their source, substances which, in material doses, are toxic, the process of homeopathic preparation removes the toxic properties, leaving only a healing potential.

The process of homeopathic preparation involves three distinct stages:

1. Solution

The substance is put into solution, using a water/alcohol solvent. This solution is known as a 'mother tincture'.

Insoluble substances first undergo a process of trituration, which entails the thorough mixing and grinding together of the material with fixed amounts of lactose, for three successive stages. Following this a tincture as above is prepared.

2. Dilution

The various potencies used are determined by the degree of dilution employed. Two dilution scales are used. One is based on a 1/10 scale and results in the 'decimal' range, designated by the symbols 'x' or 'd'. The other employs a 1/100 scale and this produces the 'centesimal' or 'c' or 'CH' potencies. There is a third method (LM potencies) but this is more complex.

3. Succussion

This process takes place between each dilution and involves a vigorous agitation of the solution. It is this which is vital for the creation of a homeopathic remedy, as opposed to mere dilution.

HOMEOPATHIC FIRST-AID MEDICINES

- **Aconitum** - This remedy treats shock, both mental and physical and will also assist in the treatment of acute febrile conditions, such as viral or bacterial diseases.
- **Apis** - Urticarial swellings, oedema and fluid in joints will often respond to this remedy, apart from its benefits for insect bites and stings. It may also help urine retention, if this is physiological.
- **Arnica** - Arnica is homeopathy's great injury remedy. Its use will minimise bruising and speed healing. It also has 'antiseptic' properties.
- **Belladonna** - High fevers with head, ear, throat or eye pain are especially helped by this remedy. Very painful abscesses may also respond.
- **Bryonia** - Arthritis, rheumatism, pneumonia, peritonitis or mastitis, when the animal refuses to move, are the main areas of use of Bryonia.
- **Calendula** - Used as a lotion, this remedy speeds healing of cuts, grazes or open wounds, in addition to helping the animal to fight septic infection of such injuries.
- **Cantharis** - This medicine helps most cases of cystitis.
- **Carbo veg.** - This is nicknamed the 'homeopathic corpse reviver', on account of its ability to help patients that are in a state of collapse.
- **Caulophyllum** - The birth process, at all stages, is helped by Caulophyllum.
- **Chamomilla** - Teething in young dogs and trouble from teething in any species will benefit from use of this remedy.
- **Colocynthis** - Colic in horses would be the most common first-aid use of Colocynthis.
- **Euphrasia** - Named 'eyebright', this remedy helps many eye conditions, including conjunctivitis from cold winds. It also helps in cases of sneezing and nasal allergy.
- **Hamamelis** - Bleeding from wounds and orifices would indicate Hamamelis, in many cases.

- **Hepar sulph**. - This is nick-named the 'homeopathic antibiotic', so effective is it in helping patients to fight septic, purulent infections.
- **Hypericum** - Use this remedy whenever there is a painful graze or damage to tissues rich in nerve endings (e.g. teats, toes and tail).
- **Ledum** - Use this whenever puncture wounds occur, from whatever injury. There are reputed anti-tetanus properties, in addition to its ability to help such wounds heal correctly, from the depths outwards.
- **Nux vomica** - If an animal has stolen too much rich food or has had access to poisons, Nux vomica should help recovery from the resultant intoxication.
- **Rhus tox**. - This suits most cases of rheumatism and arthritis, that are worse for first movement but 'limber up'.
- **Ruta** - Ligaments, tendons and other fibrous tissues constitute the main areas of benefit of this remedy.
- **Silica** - Helps the body to drive out foreign bodies, e.g. grass seeds. The power of this remedy, way beyond its simple chemical capability, is evidence of the power of crystals.
- **Symphytum** - Symphytum treats bone injuries of any type, speeding healing.
- **Urtica** - This remedy treats nettle rash (urticaria) and helps the flow of milk from the mammary gland.

WILDLIFE and HOMEOPATHIC MEDICINES

1. **Aconitum napellus** (Acon) – Extremely useful for INTENSE FEAR. Severe shock, especially shock from fright or accident. Symptoms are intense, painful, and acute (occur quickly). Hemorrhages are bright red. May be very restless or timid. Senses are acute. Remote affects of fright or terror. Acute inflammation and infection. Acon is often the first remedy given to an adult or older juvenile wild animal brought into rehabilitation since they are in shock and terrified from being captured and handled by a predator (human). In cases where fear is a primary reason for selecting Acon, it is often only given one time at a 30c, 200c or 1m potency. If initially selected due to animal's severe fear, it may be followed a short time later (15 to 30 minutes) by another remedy for another condition, such as Arn.

2. **Arnica montana** (Arn) – Often selected as the first remedy for TRAUMATIC INJURY, such as bruises, head trauma, sprains, fractures. Extremely useful in treating injuries, falls, blows, contusions and shock from injury. Patient does not want to be touched. Cannot get comfortable. Sore, lame, bruised feeling with tendency for bruises to hemorrhage. Some vertigo (dizziness) after head trauma. Overuse of muscles. Tends to be cool. A very common homeopathic medicine used with wildlife since so many wild animals arrive in rehabilitation as a result of trauma (falls, accidents). Considered when a trauma, however remote, may have caused the problem.
3. **Arsenicum album** (Ars) – Useful for sudden weakness, restlessness and anxiety. Prostration seems out of proportion from the illness. CADAVEROUS ODORS, such as from diarrhea. Intense thirst; drinks little and often, which distresses the stomach and may be vomited immediately. Loss of appetite, with thirst. Twitching, trembling extremities. A wide variety of conditions can result in these symptoms, including exposure to some toxins and viruses; infections; eating rotten food, especially fruit or meat; or emotions. .
4. **Calendula** (Cal) – Supports healing of open, torn, cut, lacerated, ragged or suppurating wounds. NOT USED WITH DEEP PUNCTURES. Hemorrhage after lacerations or scalp wounds. Promotes healthy granulations. Can be used topically (dissolved in water) or orally. Continue to follow standard wound management protocols.
5. **Carbo vegetabilis** (Carb-v) - General WEAKNESS, easily tired. EXHAUSTING DISEASE (e.g., respiratory distress, diarrhea, dehydration). ICY COLD and does not want heat. Some digestive problems.
6. **Cinchona officialis** (China) – Used to treat debility from FLUID LOSS; PROFUSE, EXHAUSTING DISCHARGES, including diarrhea, hemorrhage, loss of vital fluids. Variety of gastro-intenstinal and stool problems. Oversensitive to noise. Used conjunction with the administration of isotonic fluids.
7. **Gunpowder** (Gunp) - Blood poisoning or septic suppurations after wounds. Wounds that are expected to become infected or septic (sometimes used prophylatically). Continue to follow standard wound management protocols. External use of Calendula may be complementary in some cases.
8. **Hepar sulphuris** (Hep) – Small wounds fester and become infected. OVERSENSITIVE to all impressions, cold, pain, noise, odors. Easily irritated. Chilly. The higher potencies may abort suppuration (30c), the lower may promote it (less than 30c). There are other homeopathic medicines used for different types of infections.

9. **Hypericum** (Hyper) – The great remedy for INJURIES TO THE NERVES, especially fingers, toes, nails, tail, coccyx. Punctured or lacerated wounds. Useful for excessive painfulness or crushing wounds. Concussions to the spine or brain. Spasms after injury. Effects of shock.
10. **Ignatia** (Ign) – Conditions arriving from profound emotion, such as GRIEF or fright. Takes deep breath for relief (sighs, yawns). Hungry but loses appetite. Some neurological symptoms. Especially considered when an animal with close connections to mate, family, flock, or herd is separated from them, such as geese, corvids, raptors, fawns or juvenile rabbits. Often only a single dose of an Ign 30c or 200c has been needed in such cases.
11. **Ledum** (Led) – PUNCTURE wounds, including bites, stings, injections, and other intentional wounds. Puncture wound feels cold. Supports puncture healing from 'inside out'. Bruises are swollen, puffy, and purple. Avoids placing weight on painful foot.
12. **Lycopodium** (Lyc) – Affects NUTRITION; WEAKNESS OF DIGESTION. Some diarrhea; bloat after eating. Easy satiety (becomes full after eating a small amount). Many gastrointestinal and urinary symptoms, including lienteric stool. Malnutrition. Symptoms may move from right to left. Awakens angry.
13. **Nux vomica** (Nux-v) – DIGESTIVE DISTURBANCES, especially after eating improper diet or overeating. Angry, irritable, impatient. Cannot bear noises, odors, light, etc. Possible vertigo. Easily chilled.
14. **Natrum sulphuricum** (Nat-s) – Head symptoms AFTER INJURY TO THE HEAD (follows Arnica well). Mental dullness. Vertigo. Head tips to the side. Many head symptoms. Some spinal injuries. Some gastrointestinal symptoms.
15. **Phosphorus** (Phos) – SUDDENNESS of symptoms. Hemorrhage of bright red blood. WOUNDS BLEED MUCH EVEN IF SMALL. SUDDEN RESPIRATORY DIFFICULTY. Many respiratory symptoms. Indifferent. Great weakness after stool, debilitating diarrhea.
16. **Podophyllum** (Podo) – Profuse, offensive, gushing, INVOLUNTARY and PAINLESS LIQUID STOOL. PROLAPSED RECTUM during or after stool. It is still necessary to follow other protocols to reduce diarrhea and dehydration, such as treating for parasites.
17. **Ruta graveleons** (Ruta) - BONE BRUISE. Sprains (Ruta would be given after Arnica). Restlessness. Injured tendons and joints. Weakness in limbs from bruising.

18. **Symphytum** (Symph) – Injuries to BONE, PERIOSTEUM, and CARTILAGE including FRACTURES. Used after Arnica for bone injuries. Eye injury and pain after blow or blunt trauma; TRAUMATIC INJURIES OF THE EYE. Follow standard fracture management protocols, such as stabilizing the fracture and restricting patient's movements. Symph should NOT be administered until after the fracture is set.

Chapter 2
Anti-Infective / Antiparasitic Agents

ANTIBIOTICS

- AMIKACIN
- AMOXICILLIN
- AMOXICILLIN + SULBACTAM COMBINATION
- AMOXICILLIN + CLOXACILLIN
- AMOXYCILLIN + CLAUVULANATE
- AMPICILLIN
- AMPICILLIN + CLOXACILLIN
- APRAMYCIN
- BACITRACIN
- BENZATHINE PENICILLIN & other penicillin
- CEPHALOSPORIN
  - CEFADROXIL
  - CEFOPERAZONE
  - CEFOTAXIME
  - CEFTIOFUR
  - CEFTRIAXONE
  - CEPHALEXIN
  - CEPHALORIDINE
- CHLORAMPHENICOL
- CIPROFLOXACIN
- CIPROFLOXACIN combination
- CLOXACILLIN
- DANOFLOXACIN

- DOXYCYCLINE
- DOXYCYCLINE + NEOMYCIN
- ENROFLOXACIN
- ERYTHROMYCIN
- ERYTHROMYCIN + SULPHADIAZINE + TRIMETHOPRIM
- FLUMEQUINE
- FORTIFIED PROCAINE PENICILLIN
- FURALTADONE
- FURAZOLIDONE
- FURAZOLIDONE+METRONIDAZOLE
- FURAZOLIDONE+NITROFURAZONE
- GENTAMICIN
- JOSAMYCIN & combination
- KANAMYCIN
- LEVOFLOXACIN
- LINCOSAMIDES
  - CLINDAMYCIN
  - LINCOMYCIN & combination
- METRONIDAZOLE COMBINATION
- NALIDIXIC ACID
- NITROFURAZONE
- NORFLOXACIN
- NORFLOXACIN+METRONIDAZOLE
- NORFLOXACIN+TINIDAZOLE
- OFLOXACIN & combination
- PEFLOXACIN
- POLYMIXIN B
- ROXITHROMYCIN
- STREPTOMYCIN
- STREPTOMYCIN COMBINATION
- SULPHONAMIDE+TRIMETHOPRIM

- SULPHONAMIDES: SULPHADIMIDINE, SULPHACHLORPYRIDAZINE, SULPHAGUANIDINE, SULPHA METHOXY PYRIDAZINE, SULPHAQUINOXALINE
- TETRACYCLINE, TETRACYCLINE COMBINATION
  - OXYTETRACYCLINE
  - CHLORTETRACYCLINE
- TIAMULIN
- TOBRAMYCIN
- TYLOSIN
- VIRGINIAMYCIN

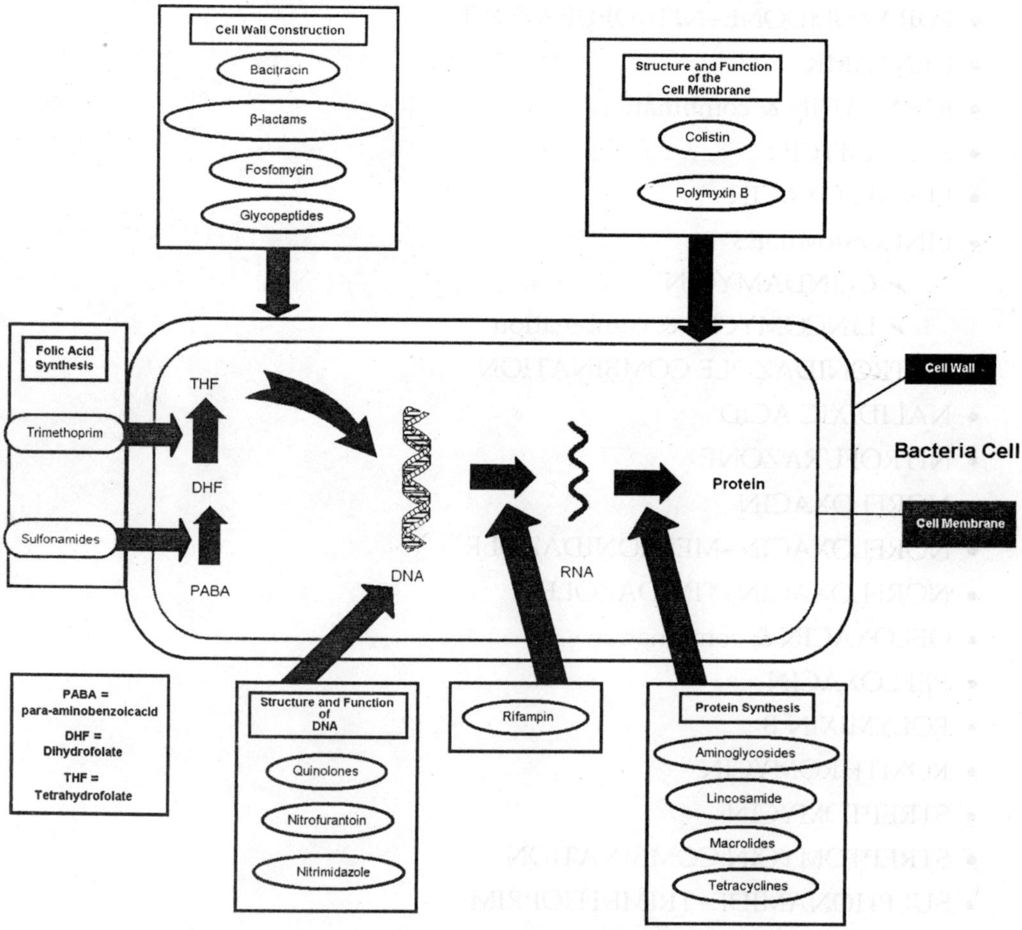

DIAGRAM : MECHANISM OF ACTION OF DIFFERENT ANTIBIOTICS

AMIKACIN

a semisynthetic derivative of kanamycin. Amikacin, like other aminoglycoside antibiotics, is a bactericidal agent that exerts its action at the level of the bacterial ribosome. Amikacin has been shown to be effective against many aminoglycoside-resistant strains due to its ability to resist degradation by aminoglycoside inactivating enzymes known to affect gentamicin, tobramycin and kanamycin. It is active against most of the gram negative and some gram positive bacteria. Antimicrobial spectrum includes Pseudomonas, Proteus E coli, Klebsiella, Staphylococcus, Serratiae. It is not active against anaerobes.

Indications: Gram negative bacillary infections specially septicaemias, respiratory tract and uterine infections, peritonitis, burns and postoperative infections, due to E coli, pseudomonas, proteus, Klebsiella. Also in intra-abdominal infections, meningitis, bone and joint infections. Also against Serratia and Staphylococcus.

DOSAGE:

- Horse: 5 – 7.5 mg/kg q 12 hr, IM, IV or SC, BID; 2-3 gm intrauterine.
- Dog : 10 mg/kg BID; IM, SC

CONTRAINDICATION: contraindicated in dogs with seriously impaired renal function.

Product	Company	Presentation	Composition
AMIKAVET inj	Novitech	2 ml, 10 ml vial	Each ml contains 250 mg Amikacin
AMBIOTIC	Neon labs	2 ml vial	Each ml contains 250 mg Amikacin
MIKACIN inj	Aristo	2 ml vial	Each ml contains 250 mg Amikacin

AMOXICILLIN

(amino penicillin), semisynthetic penicillin with extended spectrum of activity including many gram negative bacteria besides gram positive bacteria. It is well absorbed orally, food does not interfere with absorption, mostly excreted unchanged in urine. Not sensitive to mycobacteria and viruses. Actinomyces are susceptible. Pseudomonas and beta lactamase producing organisms not susceptible.

Indications: Upper respiratory tract, urinary tract infections, meningitis, skin and soft tissue infections, selected cases of enteric fever. First line drug in most ENT infections like otitis media and sinusitis. Bronchiectasis with cystic fibrosis. Respiratory Tract Infection (RTI), Mastitis, Urinary Tract Infection (UTI), Wound, GIT infection, Haemorrhagic Septicemia, Metritis, Salmonellosis, Fowl typhoid, E. coli infection, Chronic Respiratory Disease, Necrotic enteritis.

DOSAGE

Dog/cat: 10-20 mg BID IM, IV, Oral;

Cattle/Horse/Pig: 10 mg/Kg Bwt BID IM,IV, Oral;

Poultry: 40 mg/kg BW in water/day.

Product	Company	Presentation	Composition
Amoxirum tab	Virbac	**2 x 10 tab pack**	Each tab contains amoxicillin 1.5 gm
Amoxirum forte inj.	**Virbac**	**300 mg vial, 3000 mg vial**	Each 300 mg vial contains amoxicillin 500 mg; Each 3000 mg vial contains amoxicillin 3000 mg
Amoxysol powder	Pfizer	500 gm pack	Amoxycillin : 50 % w/w
AmoxStron powder	Neospark	50 gm pack	Amoxycillin : 50% w/w
Hipen inj	Cadila Health care	250 mg vial	Amoxycillin: 250 mg
Delamin tab	HAL	125 mg tab	Amoxycillin: 125 mg
Mox syrup	Rexel	Syrup 30ml	Amoxycillin: 125 mg/ ml
Mox syrup	Rexel	Syrup 60ml	Amoxycillin: 125 mg/ 5 ml
Mox syrup	Rexel	Syrup 60ml	Amoxycillin: 250 mg/5 ml
Venmox Vet	Venky's Ltd	100 g and 500 g	Amoxycillin Trihydrate equivalent to Amoxycillin 10% w/w
Novamox Powder	Cipla	100gm, 250gm	Amoxicillin 20% w/w
Novamox 75%	Cipla	25gm,200g m, 500 gm sachet	Amoxycillin 150gm/200gm powder
Vetmox Palatable Suspension	Cipla	Bottle of 60ml	Amoxycillin 50mg / ml (as Trihydrate)
Amoxycip LA	Cipla	100ml vial	Amoxycillin Trihydrate 15 % w/v long acting
Novamox 20%	Cipla	100g, 200gm, 1kg container	Amoxycillin Veterinary Oral Powder BP Vet 20% w/w

AMOXICILLIN + SULBACTAM COMBINATION: Sulbactam Na blocks Beta lactamase enzyme, rendering the organism more susceptible to **Amoxicillin's** rapid bactericidal action at concentration readily attainable in the body.

Indicated in respiratory tract infection, mastitis, urinary tract infection, wound infection, calf scours, osteomyelitis, septicemia, otitis; Birds- Necrotic enteritis,

Infectious coryza, Colisepticemia, Fowl cholera, Fowl typhoid, Wing rot, Salmonellosis, CRD.

DOSAGE

Large animal: 3 g daily IV or IM. In serious condition, frequency may be increased at 12 hr interval.

Small animal: 300 mg daily IV or IM.

In case of contagious and environmental mastitis, infuse 300 mg Amoxyrum forte/teat after dilution in 5 ml sterile water.

Safe during lactation and pregnancy.

Product	Company	Presentation	Composition
ACROMIN FORTE inj	Novitech	4.5 gm vial	**4.5 gm vial** contains Amoxicillin 3g + sulbactam sodium 1.5 g.
Amoxirum forte Inj	Virbac	300 mg, 3 g vial	**300 mg vial** contains Amoxycillin 200 mg + Sulbactam sodium 100 mg. **3 gm vial** contains Amoxycillin 2g + sulbactam sodium 1 g.
Amoxirum forte tablet	Virbac	2 tab x 10 blister box	Each tab contains Amoxycillin 1500 mg
PETROMO X Inj	Novartis	3 g vial	**3 gm vial** contains Amoxicillin 2g + sulbactam sodium 1 g.

AMOXICILLIN+CLOXACILLIN: Cloxacillin is a highly penicillinase and acid resistant penicillin, usually given in combination with Amoxycillin or ampicillin for various staphylococcal infections. It is rapidly but incompletely absorbed from GIT, absorption is better on an empty stomach. Highly effective against staphylococcus and streptococcus species.

Indicated in mixed bacterial infection including RTI, UTI, Genital tract infection, GIT infection, Skin and soft tissue infection, septicemia, BQ, HS, Calf scour.

DOSAGE

All animals : 4 -10 mg/kg Bwt IV, IM. Poultry: 1 gm / 2 - 4 ltr water

Product	Company	Presentation	Composition
ACROMIN inj	Novitech	**3** gm vial	Each 3 gm vial contains Amoxicillin Na 1.5 gm + Cloxacillin Na 1.5 gm
Amclox	Novartis	2 gm vial	Each 2 gm vial contains Amoxicillin Na 1gm+Cloxacillin Na 1gm
AmoClox 2500 Injection	Neospark	2.5gm vial, 3 gm vial	Amoxicillin Na 1.25gm+Cloxacillin Na 1.25 gm / 2.5 g vial Each 3 gm vial contains Amoxicillin Na 1.5 gm + Cloxacillin Na 1.5 gm
Centamox	Century	2 gm vial	Each 2 gm vial contains Amoxicillin Na 1gm+Cloxacillin Na 1gm

Chemclox	Vetcare	2 gm & 3 gm vial	Each 2 gm vial contains Amoxicillin Na 1gm + Cloxacillin Na 1gm Each 3 gm vial contains Amoxicillin Na 1.5 gm + Cloxacillin Na 1.5 gm
Crilmox	Cattle remedies	2 gm vial	Each 2 gm vial contains Amoxicillin Na 1gm + Cloxacillin Na 1gm
Hipenox	Sarabhai zydus	1g, 2 gm vial	Each 1 gm vial contains (Amoxicillin Na 500 mg +Cloxacillin Na 500 mg) Each 2 gm vial contains (Amoxicillin Na 1gm+Cloxacillin Na 1gm)
Inimox	Indian immunological	2 gm, 4 gm vial	2 gm vial contains (Amoxicillin Na 1gm+Cloxacillin Na 1gm) 4 gm vial contains (Amoxicillin Na 2gm+Cloxacillin Na 2gm)
Intamox	Neovet	500mg, 2 gm, 2.5gm, 4 gm vial	(Amoxicillin Na 250mg +Cloxacillin Na 250 mg)/500 mg vial (Amoxicillin Na 1gm+Cloxacillin Na 1gm)/2g vial (Amoxicillin Na 1.25gm+Cloxacillin Na 1.25 gm)/2.5 g vial Amoxicillin Na 2 gm+Cloxacilin Na 2 gm)/ 4 g vial
Klomivet inj	Lyka	2 gm vial	Amoxicillin Na 1gm+Cloxacillin Na 1gm
Megamycin inj	Pfizer	2 gm vial	Amoxicillin Na 1gm+Cloxacillin Na 1gm
Megamycin Forte	Pfizer	3.0 gm vial	Amoxicillin Na 1.5 gm + Cloxacillin Na 1.5 gm
MLA Bolus	French remedies	2 bolus pack	Amoxicillin Na 1gm + Cloxacillin Na 1gm + Lactic acid bacillus 120 million spores
Moxel	Alembic	500mg, 2 gm vial	(Amoxicillin Na 250mg +Cloxacillin Na 250 mg) (Amoxicillin Na 1gm+Cloxacillin Na 1gm)
Synchron	Cadila pharma	2 gm vial	Amoxicillin Na 1gm+Cloxacillin Na 1gm
Novaclox-2000	Cipla	2gm vial with WFI 20ml	Amoxycillin 1gm+Cloxacillin 1gm Inj
Panamoxin bolus	Panacia pharma	2 boli strip	Amoxicillin Na 1gm + Cloxacillin Na 1gm

AMOXICILLIN + CLAUVULANATE

Beta-lactamase resistant; Clavulanic acid is a b-lactamase inhibitor. Clavulanic acid inhibits Beta lactamase and makes organisms susceptible to Amoxicillin e.g. S. aureus, coagulase negative staphylococcus, E coli, Proteus, Klebsiella, Shigella, Yersinia enterocolitica, H influenza. M fortuitum M. bovis, M. kansii, Pseudomonas, Serratia, and Citrobacter remain resistant. It is generally combined with Amoxicillin to extend its action.

Indications: Skin and soft tissue infections, intraabdominal and gynaecological sepsis, urinary, biliary and respiratory tract infections. Selected cases of gonorrhoea, sinusitis, various catarrhal infections. RTI, Otitis, skin inf., mixed infection, UTI, Wound, GIT infection, H.S., Metritis, Salmonellosis, E. coli inf.

DOSAGE:

Dog/cat: 12.5-25 mg/kg bwt BID Oral

Product	Company	Presentation	Composition
Augmentin	Smith Kline Beecham	30 ml syrup	Amoxycillin (200 mg) + Clauvulanic Acid (28.75 mg)/ 5 ml
Augmentin	Smith Kline Beecham	1.2 gm vial	Amoxicillin (1000 mg) + Clauvulanic Acid (200 mg)/ vial
Clavet Tablets	Cipla	Pack of 250's	Amoxicillin 40mg + Clavulanic acid 10mg
Clavet Tablets	Cipla	Pack of 100's	Amoxicillin 400mg + Clavulanic acid 100mg
Clavet Tablets	Cipla	Pack of 100's	Amoxicillin 200mg + Clavulanic acid 50mg
Clavet Palatable Drops	Cipla	30 ml bottle,15 ml bottle	Clavulanic acid 12.5mg[as Clavulanate Potassium] + Amoxicillin 50 mg [as Amoxicillin trihydrate]
Clavet Injection	Cipla	10ml	Clavulanic acid 35mg[as Clavulanate Potassium]+Amoxicillin 140mg[as Amoxicillin trihydrate]

AMPICILLIN (amino penicillin)- It is a semisynthetic penicillin with extended spectrum of activity including many gram positive bacteria and most gram negative bacteria excluding Brucella, Klebsiella, Serratia, Burkholdia, Mycobacterium, Mycoplasma. It is well absorbed orally, food interferes with absorption, primarily excreted in kidney with t½ of 1 hour.

Indications : Urinary tract infections, lower respiratory tract infections including bronchitis, sinusitis, otitis media, meningitis gonorrhoea, bacillary dysentery, paratyphoid infections, cholecystitis, sub-acute bacterial endocarditis, septicemias and mixed infections. RTI, Mastitis, UTI, Wound, GIT infection, H.S., Metritis,

Salmonellosis, fowl typhoid, E. coli inf., CRD.

Dosage

- Dog/cat: 11 - 22 mg BID IM,IV, Oral q 12 hr;
- Horse: 11 - 22 mg BID IM, IV q 8 hr
- Cattle/Pig: 10 mg/kg bwt QID IM,IV, Oral
- Poultry : 30g (10 %) / 6000 chicks

Product	Company	Presentation	Composition
Ampicillin inj	Cadila	1g, 2 g, 2.5g	Ampicillin Na 1g/vial, 2g/vial, 3g/vial
Bacipen inj	Alembic Limited	2.5 g. 2g	Each vial contains: Ampicillin sodium BP (Vet) Equivalent to 2g &2.5g anhydrous Ampicillin.
Caticillin inj Vet	Cattle remedies	2.5 gm vial	Ampicillin sodium BP (Vet) Equivalent to 2.5g anhydrous Ampicillin
Roscillin oral powder	Ranbaxy	30 gm pack	Ampicillin 10%w/w
Vetampin inj	Wockhardt	2 gm vial	Ampicillin sodium BP (Vet) 2 gm
Ampisyn 20%	Cipla	100gm, 1/2 kg,1kg container	Ampicillin Oral powder 20% w/w

AMPICILLIN + CLOXACILLIN

Makes the combination penicillinase resistant. Active against all penicillinase producing Staphylococcus, Streptococci, Gonococci, Neisseria and Hemophyllus, Not active against resistant gram negative and methicillin resistant Staphylococci. Metritis, mastitis, septicemia, mixed infections, PUO.

DOSAGE

All animals : 4 -10 mg/kg Bwt IV, IM. Poultry: 1 gm / 2 - 4 ltr water

Product	Company	Presentation	Composition
AC-VET inj	Neovet	2 gm vial	Ampicillin Na and Cloxacillin Na (1gm + 1 gm) / 2 gm vial
AC-VET FORTE inj	Neovet	3 gm vial	Ampicillin Na (1.5gm) and Cloxacillin Na (1.5 gm) / 3 gm vial
AC-VET MAX inj	Neovet	4 gm vial	Ampicillin Na and Cloxacillin Na (2gm + 2 gm) / 4 gm vial
Betalactin	Vet care	2 gm vial	Ampicillin Na and Cloxacillin Na (1gm + 1 gm) / 2 gm vial
Biolox Injection	Jeps Pharma	2 gm vial	Ampicillin Sodium I.P. equivalent to Anhydrous Ampicillin 1 gm. Cloxacillin Sodium I.P. equivalent to Cloxacillin 1 gm

Catlox inj	Cattle remedies	2 gm vial	Ampicillin Na and Cloxacillin Na (1gm + 1 gm) / 2 gm vial
Megapen inj	Aristo	500mg, 1gm, 2 gm, 2.5gm vial	Ampicillin Na and Cloxacillin Na (250mg + 250mg) / 500 mg vial Ampicillin Na and Cloxacillin Na (1gm + 1 gm) / 2 gm vial Ampicillin Na and Cloxacillin Na (1.5gm + 1.5 gm) / 2 gm vial
Vetclox Forte inj	Sarabhai Zydus	2 gm vial	Ampicillin Na and Cloxacillin Na (1gm + 1 gm) / 2 gm vial
Vetclox Plus	Sarabhai Zydus	10 ml tube (One tube/quarter)	Each tube has Ampicillin Na: 75 mg Cloxacillin Na: 200 mg

APRAMYCIN

it is used to control gram-negative infections including E. coli, salmonellae, Proteus, Mycoplasma. Poor oral absorption. It is ***toxic in cats***.
Dosage: All species (except feline) : 20 mg/kg BID, IM.

Apracin powder	Cipla	50 gm container	Apramycin Sulphate equivalent to 50gm Apramycin activity

BACITRACIN

Mixed bacterial Infections; performance promoter; improves litter quality; reduces ammonia level, improves health status and increases carcass yield.

DOSAGE

Poultry: 150 – 200 g / ton feed; Cattle, Buffalo, Pig : 5 -10 g/animal orally

Product	Company	Presentation	Composition
Albac 15% powder	Ranbaxy	25 kg pack	Zinc bacitracin 15% w/w
Bacitracin powder	Micro	1 kg, 5 kg, 25 kg pack	Zinc bacitracin 10% w/w
BMD powder	Ranbaxy	1 kg, 5 kg, 25 kg pack	Bacitracin methylene disalicylate 10% w/w
ALBMD	Alembic Limited	1 kg, 5 kg, 25 kg pack	Granulated Bacitracin Methylene Disalicyalte 100g (42, 00,000 U) per kg.

BACITRACIN +DICLAZURIL combination

Bazuvet Powder	Cipla	5kg, 500gm	Zinc bacitracin 10% + Diclazuril 0.2%

PENICILLIN

Act by inhibiting bacterial peptidoglycan cell wall synthesis. Good efficacy against Streptococci, Meningogocci, Gonococci, Pneumococci, Anthrax, Diptheria, Leptospirosis, clostridium etc. It has a narrow spectrum activity limited primarily to gram positive bacteria specially Streptococci, Pneumococci, C. diphtheriae, B. anthracis, Clostridium tetani, Listeria and Treponema. It is acid labile, destroyed by gastric acid. It is primarily given as I.M. injection, and is mainly excreted unchanged by kidneys. It is available as two types of preparations, namely:

1. Crystalline penicillin (Sodium penicillin G injection).
2. Repository penicillin G – these are insoluble salts, they release penicillin G slowly from the site of injection. Two such preparations are available :

a) Procaine penicillin G injection
b) Benzathine penicillin G injection

Indications : Streptococcal infections like pharyngitis, otitis media, scarlet fever, rheumatic fever, pneumcoccal infections like pneumonia and meningitis, meningococcal meningitis. It is the drug of choice in syphilis, diphtheria, tetanus and gas gangrene, rare infections like anthrax, actinomycosis, trench mouth, rat bite fever, Listeria and pasturella infections.

BENZATHINE PENICILLIN

Indications : mixed bacterial infections. Anthrax, Actinomycosis, Black leg, Tetanus, Mastitis, H.S., Strangles, Erysipelas.

DOSAGE:

Cattle, Horse, sheep, goat, swine : 12000 IU / kg bwt, deep IM; Dog: 40000 IU/kg bwt IM

Product	Company	Presentation	Dose rate	Composition
Longacillin –vet 48 inj	HAL	vial	12000 IU / kg bwt IM	Penicillin: 48 lac IU/vial
Longacillin –vet 24 inj	HAL	vial	12000 IU / kg bwt IM	Penicillin: 24 lac IU/vial
Longacillin –vet 12 inj	HAL	vial	12000 IU / kg bwt IM	Penicillin: 12 lac IU/vial
Longacillin –vet 6 inj	HAL	vial	12000 IU / kg bwt IM	Penicillin: 6 lac IU/vial
Pencom inj	Alembic	6 lac vial	12000 IU / kg bwt IM	Penicillin: 6 lac IU/vial
Pencom inj	Alembic	12 lac vial	12000 IU / kg bwt IM	Penicillin: 12 lac IU/vial
Pencom inj	Alembic	24 lac vial	12000 IU / kg bwt IM	Penicillin: 24 lac IU/vial

CEPHALOSPORINS

CLASSES:

- **FIRST GENERATION**: Active against Gm positive aerobic cocci and few of Gm negative including E. coli, Proteus, Klebsiella, Salmonella, Enterobacter. Ex. Cephalothin, Cephapirin, Cefazolin, Cephalexin, Cepharadine, Cefadroxil
- **SECOND GENERATION**: More active against Gm negative bacteria. Ex.

Cefamandole, Cefoxitin, Cefotiam, Cefachlor, Cefuroxime, Ceforanide, Cefotetan, Cephamycins.

➢ **THIRD GENERATION** : More active against Gm negative bacteria including *Pseudomonas aeruginosa*. Able to penetrate Blood-Brain Barrier. Indicated in bacterial meningitis. Ex. Ceftiofur, ceftriaxone, Cefsulodin, Cefotaxime, Cefoperazone, Moxalactam

DOSAGE:

- ➢ Cephalothin: 20-35 mg/kg IM, IV TID
- ➢ Cephapirin : 30 mg/kg IM, IV QID
- ➢ Cefazolin: 20-25 mg/kg IM, IV TID
- ➢ Ceftriaxone : 15-50 mg/kg BWt IM, IV
- ➢ Cefapirin : 20 – 30 mg/kg BWt IM, IV
- ➢ Cefoxitin : 15 – 30 mg/kg BWt IM, IV
- ➢ Cefotetan : 30 mg/kg Bwt IM, IV
- ➢ Cefotaxine : 10 – 50 mg/kg BWt IM, IV
- ➢ Ceftazidime : 30 – 50 mg/kg IM, IV
- ➢ Cephalexin : 10- 30 mg/kg PO TID
- ➢ Cefadroxil: 22 mg/kg, P.O. BID
- ➢ Ceftiofur: 1.1 mg/kg, IM, SID (specially for Pasteurella infection)

Cephalosporins exhibit synergistic effect with aminoglycosides.

CEFADROXIL

Cephalosporin. It is a first generation cephalosporin and a close congener of cephalexin; has good tissue penetration-exerts more sustained action at the site of infection; can be given 12 hourly despite a t½ of 1 hr. It is active against several gram positive organisms including coagulase - positive, coagulase negative, penicillinase producing strains of Staphylococcus and some gram negative organisms. It is not active against Proteus, Pseudomonas, Enterobacter, Morganella, Serratia, Listeria. It is also not active against Methicillin-resistant staphylococcus.

Indications : Infections due to Staphylococci or streptococci, like pharyngitis, tonsillitis, urinary tract infection, skin and soft tissue infections.

DOSAGE

- ➢ Dog: 10-30mg/kg bwt TID IM

Treatment should be given for 48 hrs. After patient becomes asymptomatic and in case of infections with b-hemolytic streptococcus, treatment should be continued for 10 days. Reduced dose in renal impairment. Special precautions : Specially during abnormal liver function test.

Product	Company	Presentation	Dose rate	Composition
Droxyl tab	Torrent	500 mg tab	10-30mg/kg bwt	Cefadroxil 500mg/tab
Droxyl suspension	Torrent	30 ml bottle	10-30mg/kg bwt	Cefadroxil 250mg/5ml
Lydroxil syrup	Lyka	40 ml bottle	10-30mg/kg bwt	Cefadroxil 125mg/5ml

CEFOPERAZONE			
A third generation cephalosporin, cefoperazone sodium contains a piperazine side chain giving it antipseudomonal activity. It occurs as white, crystalline powder and is freely soluble in water and poorly soluble in alcohol. At room temperature, cefoperazone sodium has a maximum solubility in compatible IV solutions of 475 mg/ml (at concentrations >333 mg/ml vigorous and prolonged shaking may be required).Cefoperazone exerts its bactericidal effect by inhibiting the bacterial cell wall synthesis. **INDICATIONS**: It is one of few cephalosporin antibiotics effective in treating Pseudomonas bacterial infections which are otherwise resistant to these antibiotics. Mastitis. RTI, GIT infiections, Pyrexia of unknown origin. **Incompatible** with some TPN mixtures, doxapram HCl, gentamicin sulfate, hetastarch, labetolol HCl, meperidine HCl, odansetron HCl, perphenazine, promethazine, and sargostim. No teratogenic effects. Hypersensitivity reactions could potentially occur. If administered via the IM route, pain at the injection site. **DOSE:** 20 mg/kg bwt IV, IM			
Product	**Company**	**Presentation**	**Composition**
Mastiwok	Wockhardt	10 ml Intramammary syringe	Each syringe contains cefoperazone Na 250 mg (single dose treatment)
CEFOPERAZONE COMBINATION			
Salzone inj	Marc	3 gm, 4 gm vial	3gm vial contains Cefoperazone (2 gm) + Sulbactam (1 gm); 4 gm vial contains Cefoperazone (3 gm) + Sulbactam (1 gm);

CEFOTAXIME			
(Third generation cephalosporin): **Indication : RTI**, UTI, Skin & soft tissue infection, Tuberculosis. **Dose :** Dog: 25-50mg/kg bwt/day IM/IV			
Product	**Company**	**Presentation**	**Composition**
ORITAXIM (VET)	Cadila	'2 gm. Vial	Cefotaxime Sodium IP equivalent to Cefotaxime 2000 mg.
Vetaxim inj Vet	Cattle Remedies	500 mg, 2 gm	Cefotaxime 500mg/ vial and 2g / vial
Lyforan inj	Lyka	vial	Cefotaxime 250mg/vial
Lyforan inj	Lyka	1 g vial	Cefotaxime 1g/vial
Omnatax inj	Hoechst	vial	Cefotaxime 250mg/vial
Omnatax inj	Hoechst	1 g vial	Cefotaxime 1g/vial

CEFTIOFUR			
Third gen cephalosporin. Moderate activity against gram positive (Staphylococcus, Streptococcus, Actinomyces) and highly effective against gram negative bacteria (Pasteurella, Hemophilus, Fusobacterium, Actinobacillus pleuropneumoniae, Moraxella bovis, Bacteriodes melaninogenicus, Burkholdolia (Earlier known as Pseudomonas). Susceptible to Beta lactamase enzymes. Able to penetrate Blood Brain Barrier. Indicated in bacterial meningitis, bronchopneumonia, bovine respiratory disease, foot rot, metritis, pyometra, urinary tract infection, early chick mortality. **DOSAGE** : 1.1-2.2 mg/kg bwt/day IM (Ruminant, horse, swine, elephant, camel); SC (poultry, dog)			
Product	**Company**	**Presentation**	**Composition**
XCEFT inj	Alembic	500 mg, 1 gm, 4 gm	Ceftiofur Na 500 mg/vial of 500 mg; 1 gram ceftiofur Na / vial of 1 gm; 4 gm ceftiofur Na / vial of 4 gm
Cefattak tablets	Cipla	Pack of 10's (2x5's)	Cefadroxil 1000mg
CeftiCure injection	Cipla	1gm, 2gm & 4 gm vial	Ceftiofur for injection[as Ceftiofur sodium] 1gm, 2gm & 4 gm/ vial

CEFTRIAXONE			
Third generation cephalosporin, highly effective against enterobacteriaceae and gonorrhea. Stable against b-lactamase. Effective against Pseudomonas spp. **Indications** : Enteric fever, shigellosis, gastroenteritis, meningitis, infective endocarditis, pneumonia and other respiratory tract infections, acute bacterial otitis media, pelvic inflammatory disease, bacteremia and sepsis, urinary tract, bone and joint infections, severe skin and soft tissue infections, syphilis. PUO, Mixed infection. **DOSAGE** 10 mg/kg bwt/day IM, SC, IV (all animals)			
Product	**Company**	**Presentation**	**Composition**
Intacef	Neovet	0.5 gm, 2 gm , 3 gm vial	Ceftriaxone 500mg, 2 gm, 3 gm per vial in different presentation
TRICEF inj Vet	Cattle Remedies	2 gm	Ceftriaxone 2 gm/vial
WOCEF	Wockhard t	0.5 gm pack vial	Ceftriaxone 500mg/vial
CEFTOCID inj	Marc	3 gm	Ceftriaxone 3 gm/vial

AXONE (VET) inj.	Cadila	2 gm. Vial	Ceftriaxone Sodium USP equivalent to Ceftriaxone 2000 mg.
TGCEF-VET inj.	Stallen	3 gm vial	Ceftriaxone Na 3 gm / vial
ZICEF inj	ZIP healthcare	3 gm vial	Ceftriaxone 3 gm per vial
CEFTRIAXONE COMBINATION			
C.S.Forte inj	Genesis pharma	3 gm vial	Each vial contains ceftriaxone 3 gm + sulbactam 1 gm
IntacefTazo inj	Intas	562.5 mg, 2250 mg, 3375 mg vial	Each 562.5 mg vial contains ceftriaxone (500 mg) and tazobactam (62.5 mg); Each 2250 mg vial contains ceftriaxone (2000 mg) and tazobactam (250 mg); Each 3375 mg vial contains ceftriaxone (3000 mg) and tazobactam (375 mg)

CEPHALEXIN

orally acting and one of the most commonly used first generation cephalosporin. It is active against Gram-positive organisms like Staphylococcus aureus (including penicillinase - producing strains), Streptococcus pneumoniae (penicillin-susceptible strains), Streptococcus pyogenes and Gram-negative organisms including Escherichia coli, Haemophilus influenzae, Klebsiella pneumoniae, Moraxella (Branhamella) catarrhalis, Proteus mirabilis.

Note — Methicillin-resistant staphylococci and most strains of enterococci is resistant to it cephalexin. It is not active against most strains of Enterobacter spp., Morganella morganii, Proteus vulgaris. Pseudomonas spp. or Acinetobacter and Penicillin-resistant Streptococcus pneumoniae.

Indications : Infections due to Staphylococci or streptococci like pharyngitis, tonsillitis, urinary tract infection, skin and soft tissue infections, prostatitis, metritis, pyometra, cervicitis, otitis media and bone infections.

DOSAGE

- Dog: 10-30mg/kg bwt TID Oral;
- Cattle/Buffalo : 5-10 mg/kg bwt BID Oral.
- Poultry : 20g /day /1500 chicks in water

Interactions : Cephalexin decreases metformin excretion by inhibition of tubular secretion via organic cationic transporter systems.

Product	Company	Presentation	Composition
Ceflax powder 7.5%w/w	Neospark	20g pack	Cephalexin 7.5% w/w

Lixen powder 7.5%w/w	Virbac	20 g pack	Cephalexin 7.5% w/w (dose : 20 gm/3000 chicks orally)
Lixen bolus 1.5 g	Virbac	bolus	Each bolus contains Cephalexin 1.5g (one bolus per 150 kg Bwt)
Lixen IU suspension	Virbac	Bottle of 4 gm (60 ml on reconstitution)	Each 4 gm contains Cephalexin 1.5g
Lixen pet	Virbac	Bottle of 60 ml	Each 5 ml contains Cephalexin 250 mg (5-10 ml lixen pet twice daily)

CEPHALORIDINE

first generation cephalosporin. Mainly effective against Gram positive bacteria. RTI, UTI, Skin and soft tissue infection

DOSAGE:

Dog: 15-30mg/kg bwt/day IM/IV

Product	Company	Presentation	Composition
Ceporan inj	Virbac pharma	1g vial 500mg vial	500mg Cephaloridine / 500 mg vial; 1g Cephaloridine / 1 gm vial

CHLORAMPHENICOL

Bacteriostatic. (Bactericidal against *Hemophilus*). It is a neutral nitrobenzene derivative. Act by inhibiting microbial protein synthesis by binding to 50 S ribosome and impairing peptidyl transferase activity. Mixed infections including mycoplasma, salmonella, rickettsia, anaerobic oraganisms. Widely distributed in CSF and other tissues and excreted via urine and milk.

DOSAGE

Dog: 45-60 mg/kg bwt/day PO, IV, IM; Horse: 50 mg/kg bwt P.O., IM, IV; Bovine: 20-30 mg/kg bwt BID IM

Product	Company	Presentation	Composition
Neochlor inj	Vet care	10 ml vial 30 ml vial	Chloramphenicol 100mg/ml
Neochlor forte powder 20% w/w	Vet care	50gm pack	Chloramphenicol 20%w/w
Chlormycetin susp.	Parke Davis	60 ml bottle	Chloramphenicol 125mg / 4ml
Simercetin inj	Biomedica	10 ml vial	Chloramphenicol 100mg/ml

CIPROFLOXACIN

fluoroquinolone. Bactericidal. Ciprofloxacin is rapidly absorbed orally, but food delays absorption. It is excreted primarily in urine.

Indications : Urinary tract infections, gonorrhoea, chancroid, bacterial gastroenteritis, typhoid, bone, soft tissue, gynaecological and wound infections caused by resistant Staph, respiratory infections, tuberculosis, gram negative septicaemias, meningitis, prophylaxis of infections in neutropenic / cancer and other suspectible patients, conjunctivitis by gram negative bacteria. Surgical prophylaxis, bacterial diarrhoea, prostatitis. RTI, UTI, GIT inf, Skin inf., Bone and joint infection, Mixed infections.

Dosage : oral :

Small animal: 5-15 mg/kg bwt BID PO, IV.

Intravenous. : 100mg slow infusion (gonorrhoea) (single dose) or 100mg 2 times (UTI) or 200-400mg 2-4 times slow infusion (RTI and other infections)

Status in

1. Pregnancy : Use with caution
2. Lactation : Contraindicated
3. Old age : Use with caution. Dose Interval not less than 12 hours.

Interactions : Sucralfate, Rifampicin and Chloramphenicol affect blood level. Antacids reduce absorption. Contraindicated in young animals. C/I with nitrofurans.

Product	Company	Presentation	Composition
CFLOX inj	NEOVET	15 ml vial	each ml contains 40 mg ciprofloxacin lactate
C-FLOX POWER injection	NEOVET	15 ml vial	each ml contains 100 mg ciprofloxacin lactate
Ciprobid tab	Cadila health care	Tab	250 mg/tab
Ciprobid inj	Cadila health care	50 ml, 100 ml vial	2 mg/ml
CIPTAS-L tab	Neovet	Strip of 6 tabs	each tab contains ciprofloxacin 250 mg + Lactobacillus sporogenes 20 m CFU
Strox inj IV	Dabur	100 ml vial	2 mg/ml
V-ciprol	Varsha labs	Powder 100g, 500 g	10% w/w
VETCIP inj	Sushima	10 ml vial	each ml contains 40 mg ciprofloxacin lactate
VETCIP bolus	Sushima	1 x 2 boli	each bolus has Ciprofloxacin 2500 mg + Lactobacillus 20 million CFU + Co chloride 20 mg

Ciplox 10%	Cipla	1/2 litre , 1 litre ,100ml	Ciprofloxacin Oral Suspension 10%
Siproxin 40 Injection	Neospark	30 ml Vial	Each ml contains: Ciprofloxacin Lactate equivalent to Ciprofloxacin I.P. 40 mg

CIPROFLOXACIN combination

Mixed infections, Mycoplasma inf, Coryza, Wing rot, Fowl cholera, Colibacillosis, Salmonellosis. Diarrhea of mixed bacterial and/ or protozoal origin
GI infections caused by gram negative bacteria like E. coli, salmonella, shigella spp., gram positive bacteria, aerobes, anaerobes and protozoa- Eimeria spp. Amoeba and Giardia

Product	Company	Presentation	Dose rate	Composition
AV-Floxin 2000 powder	AHV	500 g	500 g/metric ton feed of poultry	(Ciprofloxacin 20 g + Norfloxacin 20 g) / kg powder
C-FLOX-TZ bolus	NEOVET	strip of 2 boli	1 boli per large animal BID	Each bolus contains Ciprofloxacin 1500 mg + Tinidazole 1800 mg
C-FLOX-TZ tablet	NEOVET	strip of 10 tabs	1 tab per small animal	Each tab contains Ciprofloxacin 250 mg + Tinidazole 300 mg
CIPTAS-TZ oral suspension	Neovet	75 ml, 100 ml bottle	5-10 ml per 25 kg body weight, BID for 3-4 days in sheep, goat, cattle	Each 5 ml contains Ciprofloxacin 125 mg Tinidazole 150 mg
CTZ forte	Genesis pharma	1x4 boli	1 bolus for 300 kg bodyweight per os	Each bolus contains Ciprofloxacin 1500 mg + Tinidazole 1800 mg

Griptol suspension	Neovet	60 ml bottle	5-10 ml per 25 kg body weight, BID for 3-4 days	Each 5 ml contains Ciprofloxacin 125 mg Tinidazole 150 mg
VETCIP-TZ I/U	Sushima	60 ml vial	60 ml I/U	each 5 ml contains Ciprofloxacin 125 mg + Tinidazole 150 mg
VETCIP-TZ bolus	Sushima	strip of 2 boli	1 boli per large animal BID	Each bolus contains Ciprofloxacin 1500 mg + Tinidazole 1800 mg

CLOXACILLIN

(penicillinase resistant penicillin. Cloxacillin is a highly penicillinase and acid resistant penicillin, usually given in combination with Amoxicillin or ampicillin for various staphylococcal infections. It is rapidly but incompletely absorbed from GIT, absorption is better on an empty stomach. Highly effective against staphylococcus and streptococcus species.

Indications: Skin and soft tissue infections, staphylococcal infections, selective cases of lower respiratory tract and post-operative infections and septicemia, endocarditis, tonsillar abscesses. Staphylococcal inf., Skin inf., Spondylitis, Mastitis.

Contraindications : Hypersensitivity to penicillins, hepatic disease and jaundice

Special precautions : Same as Penicillins

Status in

1. Pregnancy : Use with caution.
2. Lactation : Use with caution.

Interactions : Probenecid and sulphonamides increase serum levels.

DOSAGE

Small animal: 4 - 10 mg/kg bwt QID, IM.

Product	**Company**	**Presentation**	**Dose rate**	**Composition**
Bioclox inj	Biochem	Inj 250 mg, 500 mg	10 mg/kg bwt	250 mg/vial 500 mg/vial
Klox syrup	Lyka	40 ml bottle	10 mg/kg bwt	125 mg/5ml
Klox inj	Lyka	Inj 250 mg, 500 mg	10 mg/kg bwt	250 mg/vial 500 mg/vial

DANOFLOXACIN It is quinolone carboxylic acid. Indicated in deep seated respiratory, urinary, intestinal infections and skin. Dose rate: Dog: 10-20 mg/kg bwt PO bid				
Advocip injection	**Cipla**	**50 ml vial**	10-20 mg/kg bwt PO bid	**Danofloxacin 25 mg/ml [as Danofloxacin mesylate]**
Advocip Powder	**Cipla**	**75 gm sachet**	10-20 mg/kg bwt PO bid	**Danofloxacin 12.5 gm[as Danofloxacin mesylate]**

DOXYCYCLINE

(Tetracycline Congener). Bacteriostatic. Doxycycline is the safest tetracycline, specially in patients with renal impairment. The t½ is shortened by simultaneous use of barbiturates and phenytoin.

Indications : First line of drug in nonspecific urethritis, atypical pneumonia, clamydial infections specially Lymphogranuloma venererum cholera, rickettsial infections, granuloma inguinale, brucellosis, Lyme's disease. Second order drug in trachoma, nonspecific cervicitis. Also used in dental and respiratory infections. RTI, H.S., B.Q., Anthrax, UTI, Haemoprotozoan inf, Leptospirosis, Mixed infection, Early chick mortality.

DOSAGE: Small animal: 5 – 10 mg/kg bwt/day PO. Large animal: 1-2 mg/kg bwt/day PO

Product	**Company**	**Presentation**	**Dose rate**	**Composition**
Bidox soluble granules powder	Merind	10 g, 50g, 250 g	10g/40 lit water or as per direction	100 mg/gm powder
Megadox powder	Neospark	100 g, 500 gm	2g/lit water or as per direction	2.5 % w/w
Vendox Vet	Venky's India Ltd	100 g and 500 g	*Prevention* 1st day – 1 g/L of water 2nd day and 3rd day – 0.5 g/L of water *Treatment* 1st day – 2 g/L of water 2nd day onwards – 1 g/L of water for 2 – 4 days	Doxycycline 2.50 g/ 100 gm powder

Doxivet Tablets	**Cipla**	**15 tablets,10tablets**	Large animal: 1-2 mg/kg bwt/day PO	**Doxycycline 100 mg**
Doxivet	**Cipla**	**2.5gm Syringe**	Large animal: 1-2 mg/kg bwt/day PO	**Doxycycline 100 mg/Gm oral paste**
Doxivet Tablets	**Cipla**	**10 tablets**	Large animal: 1-2 mg/kg bwt/day PO	**Doxycycline 20 mg**
Doxycip 20%	**Cipla**	**100gm,1/2 kg container ,1 kg container**	Large animal: 1-2 mg/kg bwt/day PO	**Doxycycline Oral powder 20% w/w**
Doxycip 50%	**Cipla**	**100gm,1/2 kg container, 1 kg container container**	Large animal: 1-2 mg/kg bwt/day PO	**Doxycycline Oral powder 50% w/w**

DOXYCYCLINE + NEOMYCIN

Neomycin has Very good activity against gram (-) ve bacilli and some gram +ve cocci however Pseudomonas and Strep. pyogenes are not sensitive. High ototoxicity and nephrotoxicity. Low oral availability.

Indications : Presurgical GI antibacterial. Rarely for bacterial and fungal diarrhoeas. Neomycin sulfate has been shown to be effective adjunctive therapy in hepatic coma by reduction of the ammonia-forming bacteria in the intestinal tract. The subsequent reduction in blood ammonia has resulted in neurologic improvement. SALMONELLA, FOAL PNEUMONIA, Leptospirosis, RTI, BQ, HS, CRD, Fowl cholera, Inf. Synovitis, Early chick mortality.

DOSAGE

Poultry: 1 gm/5-10 liter water for 5 days oral.

Product	**Company**	**Presentation**	**Dose rate**	**Composition**
Bidox –N	Merind	50 g pack	Poultry: 1 gm/5-10 liter water	(Doxycycline: 100 mg + Neomycin 100mg)/gm powder
Neodox	Vet care	Strip of 6 boli	1 bolus / 80 kg body wt for 5 days in cow/buffaloes Per os.	Each bolus contains Neomycin SO4 (400 mg) +

				Doxycycline (160 mg)
Docmycin WSP	ALEMBIC LTD	50g tamper proof PVC bottle.	1g in 10 litres of drinking water for 3 - 4 days for 200 chicks. Repeat the dose after 4th week.	Each gram contains: Neomycin Sulphate equivalent to 100mg of base Doxycycline HCl : 100mg
Vendox –N	Venky's	50 g powder pack	Poultry: 1 gm/5-10 liter water	(Doxycycline: 100 mg + Neomycin 100mg)/gm powder

DOXYCYCLLINE + COLISTIN COMBINATION: Indicated in growth promotion for poultry and fishery.

LAYBROMIX powder	Virbac	1 kg, 5 kg bag	500 gm-1 kg per ton feed in broilers	Each kg contains Colistin sulfate 1000 mg; Doxycycline 10,000 mg

ENROFLOXACIN

Fluoroquinolone. Bactericidal. It has antibacterial activity against a broad spectrum of Gram negative and Gram positive bacteria It inhibits bacterial enzyme DNA gyrase and reduces supercoiling with disruption of spatial arrangement of DNA. It is rapidly absorbed from the digestive tract, penetrating into all measured body tissues and fluids.

Indicated in Mycoplasmosis, Coli septicemia, Mastitis, Metritis, Salmonella, Leptospirosis, GIT inf., RTI, BQ, HS, CRD, Fowl cholera, Inf. Synovitis, Early chick mortality.

DOSAGE

Large animal: 2.5-5 mg/kg BW oral, IM, IV.

Contraindicated in dogs and cats known to be hypersensitive to quinolones.

Product	Company	Presentation	Composition
Enrocare	Vet care	20 ml vial	Enrofloxacin : 100 mg/ml
Enrocin oral soln	Ranbaxy	100 ml, 500 ml, 1000 ml pack	Enrofloxacin : 100 mg/ml
Enrodac-10	Sarabhai Zydus	Injection 15 ml vial	Enrofloxacin : 100 mg/ml
ENROFLOX	Agrovetma	flask x 100	enrofloxacin 200 mg, excipients in a long

20 LA inj	rket	mL (1 mL / 40 kg of b.w.)	acting vehicle q.s.ad. 1 mL
ENROTREAT 10 % W/V Injection	Cadila Vet	50 ml.,15 ml.	Each ml. contains : Enrofloxacin – 100 mg. Benzyl Alcohol B.P. – 2% w/v (as preservative). Water for Injection I.P. – q.s.
ENROTREAT 10% ORAL SOLUTION	Cadila	'500 ml.,5000 ml.	Each ml. contains : Enrofloxacin – 100 mg. Aqueous Base – q.s.
ENROX injection	ALEMBIC LTD	Vial of 15ml & 100 ml	Each ml contains: Enrofloxacin: 100mg
ENROX oral liquid	ALEMBIC LTD	Bottle of 100ml pack, Jar of 1litre and 5litre	Each ml contains: Enrofloxacin: 100mg
Floxidin inj	Intervet	15 ml, 50 ml vial	Each ml (Floxidin 10% inj) contains 100 mg enrofloxacin.
Floxidin oral soln 5%w/v, 10 %w/v	Intervet	100ml, 250 ml	Enrofloxacin:5% w/v Enrofloxacin:10 % w/v
FORTIUS inj	Virbac	30 ml vial	Each ml contains 100 mg enrofloxacin (single shot treatment)
FLOCURE inj	Stallen	20 ml vial, 100 ml vial	Each ml contains 100 mg enrofloxacin
QUININTAS inj	Neovet	15 ml, 50 ml, 100 ml	Each ml contains: Enrofloxacin: 100mg
ROFLOX inj	Novartis	15 ml vial	Enrofloxacin: 100 mg/ml
Enrovet 10% inj	Cipla	50ml Vial100 ml Vial	Enrofloxacin 10% Inj
Enrovet 10% oral solution	Cipla	100ml bottle,500 ml can,1000 ml can	Enrofloxacin 10% oral solution 30ml bottle
Enrovet 2.5% oral solution	Cipla	100 ml bottle, 500ml can	Enrofloxacin 2.5%
Enrovet 5% inj	Cipla	50 ml Vial, 100ml Vial	Enrofloxacin 5% w/v
Quinrocin Injection	Neospark	Vials of 15 ml, 50 ml and 100 ml	Each ml contains Enrofloxacin : 100 mg

ERYTHROMYCIN			
Macrolide. Bacteriostatic. Antimicrobial spectrum is narrow, includes mostly gram positive and few gram negative organisms, Campylobacter and Mycoplasma are highly sensitive. Erythromycin base is acid labile. It is given as enteric coated tablets, it is widely distributed in the body, crosses serous membranes and placenta but not blood-brain barrier. Indications : Alternative to penicillin in streptococcal pharyngitis, tonsillitis, mastoiditis and most respiratory infections and syphilis. Drug of choice for atypical pneumonia caused by Mycoplasma and for chancroid. Second line of drug for Campylobacter enteritis, chlamydia trachomatis, penicillin resistant staphylococcal infections. Mixed infection, RTI, Dysentery, BQ, Actinomycosis, Swine erysipelas, CRD, Ornithosis, Infectious synovitis, Inf. Coryza. A growth promoter, ensures higher weight gain. Improves the feed conversion ratio. It also works as antistress agent. DOSAGE Large animal: 2.2-4.4 mg/kg BW oral; Dog: 10-40 mg/kg BW oral. Poultry : 50 mg/ltr water			
Product	**Company**	**Presentation**	**Composition**
Althrocin soluble powder	Alembic	100 gm pack	Erythromycin 50mg/g powder
Althrocin liquid	Alembic	60 ml bottle	Erythromycin: 25mg/ 5 ml; 250 mg/5 ml
ALTHROCIN-FS	Alembic	100 gm pack	Each gram contains: Erythromycin Thiocyanate B.P.(Vet) equivalent to 20 mg Erythromycin base.
Erycip 11% Powder	Cipla	200gm sachet, 1kg container	Erythromycin 22gm Soluble Powder
Erycip 35% Powder	Cipla	1Kg container	Erythromycin Thiocyanate soluble powder
Erycip 5% Powder	Cipla	1/2 kg container	Erythromycin Thiocyanate soluble powder (50mg Erythromycin B
COMBINATION			
ERYSRIM powder	Themis	100 gm pack (@1 gm/20 kg Bwt TID (large animal) Orally.	Erythromycin 15 g + Sulphadiazine 15 g + Trimethoprim 3 g /100 gm

Neostrep Plus Powder	Cipla	12 gm sachet	Erthromycin thiocynate 3500mg + Oxytetracycline HCl 500mg + Streptomycin sulphate 3500mg + Neomycin sulpahte 1000mg + Colistin sulphate 25000000 IU + Vitamin A-500000 IU + Vitamin D3 200000 IU + Vitamin E 200mg + Vitamin B1 200mg + D-Ca pantothenate 1000mg+ Vitamin K 200mg + Vitamin B6 200mg + Vitamin B2 400mg + VitaminB12 1mg + Vitamin PP 2000mg + Vitamin C 200mg + Inositol 100mg
Teryvit powder	Cipla	100 gm container	Erythromycin (as Estolate) 3,000,000 IU+ Tetracycline (as hydrochloride) 3,000,000 IU+ Thiamine hydrochloride (Vitamin B1)40mg+ Riboflavin base (Vitamin B2) 60mg+ Pyridoxine hydrochloride (Vitamin B6) 60mg +Nicotinamide (Vitamin PP)500mg+Calcium pantothenate 220 mg /100 gm

FLUMEQUINE

(prototype quinolone) Bactericidal. CRD, Colibacillosis, Salmonellosis, Coryza.

DOSAGE

Large animal : 6 gm/100 kg Bwt oral.; Poultry : 0.5 – 1 gm/liter water

Product	Company	Presentation	Dose rate	Composition
Fluquin powder 10 % w/w	Cadila	25 gm, 100 gm	Poultry : 0.5 – 1 gm/liter water	10 % w/w
Zydaquin powder	Sarabhai zydus	100 gm	Poultry : 0.5 – 1 gm/liter water	10 % w/w

FORTIFIED PROCAINE PENICILLIN

Mixed infection, RTI, Dysentery, BQ, Actinomycosis, Swine erysipelas, Strangles, Tetanus, HS, Foot rot.

DOSAGE

Large animal: 4,000-10,000 IU /kg BWt IM; Dog: 10,000 – 20,000 IU /kg BW, IM

Product	Company	Presentation	Dose rate	Composition
Fortified Procaine	Alembic	20 lac vial	4,000-10,000 IU /kg BW	(Procaine Penicillin G: 15 lac + Penicillin G

Penicillin inj 20 lac				Sodium 5 lac)/vial
Fortified Procaine Penicillin inj 40 lac	Alembic	40 lac vial	4,000-10,000 IU /kg BW	(Procaine Penicillin G: 30 lac + Penicillin G Sodium 10 lac)/vial
Fortified Procaine Penicillin inj 20 lac	Sarabhai zydus	20 lac vial	4,000-10,000 IU /kg BW	(Procaine Penicillin G: 15 lac + Penicillin G Sodium 5 lac)/vial
Fortified Procaine Penicillin inj 40 lac	Sarabhai zydus	40 lac vial	4,000-10,000 IU /kg BW	(Procaine Penicillin G: 30 lac + Penicillin G Sodium 10 lac)/vial
G-Pen Injection	Cipla	4 vials of 20ml & 4 ampoules of WFI 10ml	4,000-10,000 IU /kg BW IM	Penicillin G sodium-5,000,000IU
OTHER PENICILLINS				
Kaypen	HAL	Tab strip of 10's	10 mg/kg BW TID in dog	125mg/tab; 250 mg/tab
PAM inj	Sarabhai zydus	10 ml Vial	Large animals: 8000 IU/kg bwt, IM Dog: 3 – 6 lac IU total dose, IM	Procaine penicillin G: 3 lac IU / ml
Benpen Injection	Cipla	4 vials of 20 ml & 4FFS ampoules of WFI 10ml	4,000-10,000 IU /kg BW	Penicillin G Benzathine esteyl-3,600,000 IU per vial
PENICILLINS in combinations				
Bistrepen-V inj	Alembic	2.5 g vial	Large animal 1-2 vial daily I/M	(Procaine penicillin-V 15 lac. + Benzyl Penicillin 5 lac + streptomycin sulphate 2.5 g) / vial

Dicrysticin-S inj	Sarabhai Zydus	Vial 2.5 g	Large animal 2 ml/ 50 kg BW I/M	(Procaine penicillin G 15 lac. + Penicillin G 5 lac + streptomycin sulphate2.5 g) / vial
Munomycin forte inj	Virbac	2.5 g vial	Large animal 1-2 vial daily I/M	(Procaine penicillin-V 15 lac. + Benzyl Penicillin 5 lac + streptomycin sulphate 2.5 g) / vial
Gass cutter	Piya	Tab	4 tab / calf orally	Each tab contains Streptomycin SO4 250 mg + Neomycin SO4 100 mg + Vitamin A 25000 IU
Stre Pen Powder	Cipla	100 gm	100 gm per cattle PO daily	Each gram contains Streptomycin as sulphate –133 mg + Procaine penicillin G – 45mg + Pantothenic acid –5,850mcg +Nicotinamide – 16,600mcg +Folic acid – 410mcg+ Vitamin A –6,600IU +Vitamin B2 – 1,690mcg+ Vitamin B6 –2,500mcg + Vitamin B12 – 2.5mcg + Vitamin D3 –1,660 IU+ Vitamin E – 2,500mcg + Vitamin K3 (as Menadione sodium bisulphate) 2,500 mcg.

FURALTADONE

Nitrofuran. Bactericidal. Mixed infection, RTI, Dysentery, Coccidiosis, colisepticemia, CRD, Salmonellosis.

Dosage : Large animal : 20-25 mg /kg BW oral. Poultry : 0.5-1.0 gm / liter water for 5 days

Product	Company	Presentation	Dose rate	Composition
Furasol powder	Pfizer	30 g, 450 gm pack	Poultry : 0.5-1.0 gm / liter water	FURALTADONE:20 % w/w

20 % w/w				
Microsol powder	Micro	50 g, 500 gm pack	Poultry : 0.5-1.0 gm / liter water	FURALTADONE:20 % w/w

FURAZOLIDONE: (Nitrofuran). Bactericidal. **Indications** : Usually used with metronidazole for diarrhoea due to Giardiasis, bacillary dysentery and food poisoning. Mixed infection, RTI, Dysentery, Coccidiosis, colisepticemia, CRD, Salmonellosis. Intrauterine infection.

DOSAGE:

Large animal : 10 mg /kg BW/day oral. Dog: 4 mg /kg BW/day oral; Poultry : 0.5-1.0 gm / liter water for 5 days

Product	**Company**	**Presentation**	**Composition**
Neftin 200	Pfizer	1 kg, 5 kg	Each kg of Premix contains Furazolidone ...... 200 g
Profidone 200 powder	Sarabhai zydus	1 kg, 5 kg	Each kg of Premix contains Furazolidone ...... 200 g
V-FUR 200	Venky's India	1 kg	Each kg of Premix contains Furazolidone ...... 200 g
KOX – CARE	Vesper Pharmaceuticals	Powder	Each kg of Premix contains Furazolidone ...... 200 g
PESUREA	Indian Immunologicals	Bolus	Each bolus contains Furazolidone ...... 500 mg
UTEX	Novartis India	Bolus	Each bolus contains Furazolidone ...... 500 mg

FURAZOLIDONE+NITROFURAZONE: Caecal and intestinal Coccidiosis.

Product	**Company**	**Presentation**	**Dose rate**	**Composition**
Avicox powder	Micro labs	5 kg, 25 kg	500 kg / ton feed upto 14th week of age or as per advise	Furazolidone 3.6% w/w + Nitrofurazone 25 % w/w
Bifuran	Pfizer	5 kg pack	500 kg / ton feed upto 8th week of age or as per advise	Furazolidone 3.6% w/w + Nitrofurazone 25 % w/w

FURAZOLIDONE+METRONIDAZOLE: diarrhea, bovine Coccidiosis, protozoal GIT inf., UTI.				
Product	**Company**	**Presentation**	**Dose rate**	**Composition**
CULEX bolus	Univet	8x4 boli	1 bolus / 50 kg bwt bid	Each bolus contains Furazolidone 200 mg + Metronidazole 1g
Dependal-M	Smith Kline Beecham	Tab 10's	1 tab TID orally	Each tab contains Furazolidone 100 mg + Metronidazole 300 mg
Diamet	Novartis	Strip of 4 boli	1 bolus / 50 kg bwt bid	Each bolus contains Furazolidone 200 mg + Metronidazole 1g
Diofur-M bolus	Cattle Remedies	12x4 bolus packing	1 bolus / 50 kg bwt bid	Each bolus contains Furazolidone 200 mg + Metronidazole 1g
Fazole	Vet care	Strip of 4 boli	1 boli/50 kg bwt Per os. Intrauterine: 2-4 boli in cow, 1-2 boli in sheep/goat	Metronidazole (1 gm) + Furazolidone (0.2 gm) per bolus
Metrofural Bolus	Alembic	Blister of 4 boli and Box of 10 blisters	Large animals: 4-6 boli/day for 3-5 day, Small animal : 1-2 boli/day for 3-5 days,	Each bolus contains: Metronidazole:1,000mg Furazolidone : 500 mg Loperamide HCl : 7.5 mg
MARCOGYL bolus	Marc India Ltd	Blister of 4 boli and Box of 10 blisters	Large animals: 2-4 boli/day for 3-5 day, Small animal : 1-2 boli/day for 3-5 days,	Each bolus contains: Quinolone :1,000mg Furazolidone : 500 mg Kaolin : 2 gm
MARCOGYL LM	Marc India Ltd	Blister of 4 boli and Box of 10 blisters	Large animals: 4-6 boli/day for 3-5 day, Small animal : 1-2 boli/day for 3-5 days,	Each bolus contains: Metronidazole:1,000mg Furazolidone : 500 mg Loperamide HCl : 7.5 mg

PESULIN MFL BOLUS	Zydus Cadila	4 Boli pack	Large animals: 4-6 boli/day for 3-5 day, Small animal : 1-2 boli/day for 3-5 days,	Each bolus contains: Metronidazole:1,000mg Furazolidone : 500 mg Loperamide HCl : 7.5 mg

GENTAMICIN: (aminoglycoside). Bactericidal. It is more potent, has a broader spectrum of action , effective against Psuedomonas aeruginosa and most strains of Proteus, E. coli, Klebsiella, Enterobacter, Serratia. Staphylococeus and Listeria monocytogenes. It is ineffective against M. tuberculosis.

Indications : Preventing and treating respiratory infections in critically ill patients; burns, urinary tract infection, pneumonia, lung abscesses, osteomyelitis, middle ear infection, septicaemia etc, meningitis caused by gram negative bacilli. Bacterial neonatal sepsis peritonitis, skin and soft tissue infections. Bone and joint infections, cystic fibrosis, biliary tract infection, brucellosis, Cat Scratch disease, gastroenteritis, Listeriosis and gynaecological infection, endometriosis, UTI, Mastitis-metritis-agalactia syndrome, RTI, GIT inf., CRD, Colibacillosis.

DOSAGE

Large animal : 4.4 mg/kg Bwt IM,IV.; Dog: 4.4 mg/kg Bwt IM,IV.; Poultry : 3-5 mg/kg Bwt IM,IV. Ointment preparation has 0.1 %. Ophthalmic ointment has 0.3% concentration. Contraindicated in pregnancy.

Product	**Company**	**Presentation**	**Dose rate**	**Composition**
Aminocin Injection	Neospark	Vials of 30 ml and 100 ml	2-5 mg of Gentamicin / kg body weight by either Intramuscular or Intravenous or Subcutaneous route.	Each ml contains Gentamicin Sulphate I.P. equivalent to 40 mg of Gentamicin base
Catlogenta inj Vet	Cattle remedies	10ml, 30 ml vial	4 mg/kg Bwt BID, IM	Gentamicin : 40mg/ml
Gentamicin	Alembic	30 ml vial	4 mg/kg Bwt BID, IM	Gentamicin : 40mg/ml
Gentamicin	Cadila pharma	30 ml, 90 ml vial	4 mg/kg Bwt BID, IM	Gentamicin : 40mg/ml
Gentamicin	Vet care	30ml, 100 ml vial	4 mg/kg Bwt BID, IM	Gentamicine sulphate : 40 mg /ml
Gentamicin Inj.	Laborate Pharmace	40 ml vial 30 ml vial	4 mg/kg b.wt. BID, IM	Each 2 ml contains Gentamicin sulphate I.P.

	utical Ltd.			80 mg
Ranbamycin	Ranbaxy	30 ml, 90 ml vial	4 mg/kg Bwt BID, IM	Gentamicin : 40mg/ml
Cipmycin 10%	Cipla	10 ml, 50 ml & 100 ml vial	4 mg/kg Bwt BID, IM	Gentamycin 10% Injection
Cipmycin 5%	Cipla	10ml,50ml &100ml vial	4 mg/kg Bwt BID, IM	Gentamycin 5% Injection
GENTAMICIN EARDROP :Acute and chronic otitis externa or otitis media perpetuated by bacteria and/or fungi Yeast infection like malassezia pachydermatitis				
Pomisol	Neovet Neovet Pharmaceutical	15 ml and 30 ml bottles	Ear should be thoroughly cleaned and dried before use of medication. administer liberally 8-10 drops in each affected ear twice daily. massage in well.	Gentamicin: 0.3% w/v Clotrimazole: 1.0 % w/v Betamethasone dipropionate: 0.025% w/v Lignocaine hydrochloride: 2.0 w/v
GENTAMYCIN COMBINATION				
Gentadox powder	Cipla	100 gm sachet, 500 gm, 1kg container	10 mg/kg bodyweight PO or mixed in feed	Gentamycin 10% & Doxycycline 10% Powder

JOSAMYCIN & Combination

it is a macrolide with 16 membered ring. Active against most gram positive aerobic and anaerobic bacteria.

DOSAGE: Large animal : 8-15 mg/kg Bwt bid, IM,IV, oral.

Drug interaction: Should not be used with chloramphenicol and licosamides.

Product	Company	Presentation	Composition
Duobact powder	Cipla	100gm sachet	Josamycin 180,000IU + Trimethoprim 100gm/1000mg

KANAMYCIN

(aminoglycoside). Bactericidal. It is a semisynthetic derivative of kanamycin. It is active against most of the gram negative and some gram positive bacterias. Antimicrobial spectrum includes Pseudomonas, Proteus E coli, K lebsiella, Staphyloccoccus, Serratiae. It is not active against anaerobes.

Indications : Gram negative bacillary infections specially septicaemias, respiratory tract infections, peritonitis, burns and postoperative infections, due to E coli, pseudomonas, proteus, klebsiella. Also in UTI intraabdominal infections, meningitis, bone and joint infections. Also against Serratia and Staphylococcus. Only used in multi drug resistant tuberculosis. UTI, Mastitis-metritis-agalactia syndrome, RTI, GIT inf., Colibacillosis.

Dosage : Large animal : 12-15 mg/kg Bwt IM,IV, SC, SID or BID.

Dog: 5 mg/kg Bwt IM,IV. Prolonged administration may result cochlear and vestibular damage.

Product	Company	Presentation	Dose rate	Composition
Kancin	Alembic	500 mg, 1 gm vial	5-10 mg/kg Bwt	Kanamycin : 500 mg/vial, 1 gm/vial
Kanamycin	Biochem	500 mg, 1 gm vial	5-10 mg/kg Bwt	Kanamycin : 500 mg/vial, 1 gm/vial

LEVOFLOXACIN

Levofloxacin is a synthetic chemotherapeutic agent used to treat severe and life threatening bacterial infections. Levofloxacin is commonly referred to as a fluoroquinolone (or quinolone) drug and is a member of the fluoroquinolone class of antibacterials. It functions by inhibiting DNA gyrase, a type II topoisomerase, and topoisomerase iv, which is an enzyme necessary to separate replicated DNA, thereby inhibiting cell division.

Indication: metritis, retention of placenta, pyometra

Adverse Reactions: spontaneous tendon ruptures and irreversible peripheral neuropathy. Such reactions may manifest long after therapy had been completed and in severe cases may result in life long disabilities. Hepatoxicity has also been reported.

Product	Company	Presentation	Composition
LENOVO I.U.	Intas	30 ml, 60 ml bottle	Product contains levofloxacin & alpha tocopherol

LINCOSAMIDES

derivatives of amino acid and a sulfur containing octose. Highly active against gram positive cocci and anaerobic pathogens. Clindamycin is more active analog of lincomycin.

Drug interaction: They should not be combined with bactericidal agent and macrolides.

CLINDAMYCIN

Dose: cattle (10 mg/kg, IM, bid), pigs (10 mg/kg, IM, bid), Dogs (20 mg/kg, PO, sid)

Clinvet Liquid	Cipla	20 ml Bottle	Dogs, cats (20 mg/kg, PO)	Clindamycin 25 mg/ml

LINCOMYCIN

Bactericidal. It is a lincosamide, has similar antibacterial and toxic properties, but is less potent and produces a higher incidence of diarrhoea and collitis as compared to clindamycin, deaths have occured. Thus, it has been largely replaced by clindamycin. It is absorbed orally and excreted mainly in bile with plasma t½ of 5 hours. Used in pharyngitis, chronic bronchitis, osteomyelitis, endocarditis, sinusitis, UTI, Mastitis, metritis, RTI, Skin Inf, GIT inf., Colibacillosis, Mixed infections.

DOSAGE:

Large animal : 10 mg/kg Bwt bid, IM,IV, oral; Dog: 15-25 mg/kg Bwt BID, IM,IV.
Pig: 11 mg/kgBW BID IM.

Product	Company	Presentation	Dose rate	Composition
Alincomycin premix powder	Vetnex	1 kg pack	Dog: 15-25 mg/kg Bwt BID, IM,IV	Lincomycin 0.88% w/w
Alincomycin vet inj	Vetnex	5 ml vial	Dog: 15-25 mg/kg Bwt BID, IM,IV	Lincomycin 300mg/ml
Lynx syrup	Wallace	60 ml bottle	Dog: 15-25 mg/kg Bwt BID,	Lincomycin 125mg/ml
Lynx inj	Wallace	1ml, 2ml ampoule	Dog: 15-25 mg/kg Bwt BID, IM,IV	Lincomycin 300 mg/ml
LINCOMYCIN + SPECTINOMYCIN COMBINATION				
Linco-spectin inj	Unichem	20 ml vial	Dog: 15-25 mg/kg Bwt BID, IM,IV	Each ml contains Lincomycin HCl 50 mg + Spectinomycin SO4 : 100mg
Linco-SP 100 Soluble Powder	Cipla	1 Kg	cattle: 10 mg/kg Bwt bid, oral	Lincomycin 33.3gm + Spectinomycin 66.7gm
Linco-SP 44 Premix	Cipla	1 Kg	1 kg powder per ton feed	Lincomycin HCl 22 gm + Spectinomycin sulphate 22gm

METRONIDAZOLE combination:

Metronidazole (C6H9N3O3): a nitroimidazole anti-infective medication used mainly in the treatment of infections caused by susceptible organisms, particularly anaerobic bacteria and protozoa. Indicated in diarrhea, dysentery, uterine infection of mixed origin. Metronidazole is a prodrug. It is converted in anaerobic organisms by the redox enzyme pyruvate-ferredoxin oxidoreductase. The nitro group of metronidazole is chemically reduced by ferredoxin (or a ferredoxin-linked metabolic process) and the products are responsible for disrupting the DNA helical structure,

thus inhibiting nucleic acid synthesis. Metronidazole is selectively taken up by anaerobic bacteria and sensitive protozoal organisms because of the ability of these organisms to reduce metronidazole to its active form intracellularly.			
MARCOGYL LM	Marc India Ltd	Blister of 4 boli and Box of 10 blisters	Each bolus contains: Metronidazole:1,000mg Furazolidone : 500 mg Loperamide HCl : 7.5 mg
Centrogyl-LM	Genesis pharma	1x2 boli strip	Each bolus contains metronidazole 100mg + furazolidone 500 mg + loperamide 7.5 mg
FAZOLE bolus	Vetcare	4 boli pack	Each bolus contains: Metronidazole:1,000mg Furazolidone : 200 mg
METROFUR PLUS	Torque Pharma	10 Tab	Metronidazole 200mg, Loperamide HCL 1.5mg
METROGYL COMPD	J.B. Chemicals	15 Tab	Metronidazole 400mg, Diloxanide Furoate 500mg
METROGYL DG GEL	Lekar Pharma	10g, 20g, 30g Gel	Metronidazole 1%, Chlorhexidine 0.25%)
METROGYL P	Lekar Pharma	15g Oint, 125g, 100ml Sol.	Povidone iodine 5%, Metronidazole 1%)
METROGYL V GEL	Lekar Pharma	10g Gel	Metronidazole 10mg per g
METROGYL-F	J.B. Chemicals	10 Tab	Metronidazole 400mg, Furazolidone 100mg
METROGYL-F	J.B. Chemicals	30ml, 60ml Sus	Metronidazole 200mg, Furazolidone 40mg/5ml
METRONOR	P.C.I.	30ml Syrup	Metronidazole 100mg, Norfloxacin 100mg
METRONORM	Modern Pharma	30ml Susp	Norfloxacin 100mg, Metronidazole 100mg/5ml
DEPENDAL-M	GSK	10 Tab	Furazolidone 100mg, Metronidazole (as benzoate 300mg
DEPENDAL-M	GSK	60ml Sus	Furazolidone 25mg, Metronidazole 75mg, per 5ml
Spiragyl tablets	Cipla	Pack of 10's Container 500 tabs.	Metronidazole 125mg + Spiramycin 750,000IU

NALIDIXIC ACID
(Quinolone) Bactericidal. UTI, enteritis. It is a synthetic quinolone antimicrobial

agent which is mainly excreted in urine and is effective against usual urinary pathogens. It is active against gram negative bacteria, specially coliforms : E.coli, proteus, Klebsiella, Enterobacter, Shigella but not Pseudomonas. Is absorbed orally, highly plasma protein bound and partly metabolized in liver and excreted in urine.
Indications : Urinary tract infections (given after sensitivity testing as resistance is high).

DOSAGE

Dog : 50 mg/kg Bwt bid, oral;

Product	Company	Presentation	Dose rate	Composition
Gramoneg tab	Ranbaxy	Strip of 4 tab	50 mg/kg Bwt	Nalidixic acid 500 mg/tab
Gramoneg susp.	Ranbaxy	30 ml	50 mg/kg Bwt	Nalidixic acid 300 mg/5 ml

NEOMYCIN

(Aminoglycoside): Bactericidal. Bacterial enteritis, GIT infection.
Large animal: 2.5-5.0 mg/kg bwt BID IM, IV; 10mg/kgBW orally; Dog : 20mg/kgBW orally.

Product	Company	Presentation	Dose rate	Composition
Neocare forte powder	Vet care	50 g, 250 g	50 mg/kg BW oral	Neomycin : 25 % w/w
Neocare powder	Vet care	250 g	250 mg/1250 layers oral	Neomycin : 12.5 g/250g
Neobact 30%	Cipla	100gm, 250gm, 500gm container	10 mg/kg BW orally	Neomycin Sulfate Oral powder 30%
Unimycin injection	Vet care	30 ml vial	2.5 – 5.0 mg / kg b wt. IM,IV, SC (cattle/horse /sheep/swine)	Neomycin SO4 : 140 mg per ml
Unimycin bolus	Vet care	Strip of 4 boli	1 bolus / 45 kg body wt for 5 days in cow/buffaloes Per os.	Neomycin SO4 : 350 mg per bolus
NEOMYCIN in COMBINATION				
Vendox-N	Venky's India Ltd	100 g powder	*Prevention of early chick mortality* 1 g per 10 ml	Neomycin Sulphate B.P. 100 mg Doxycycline

			water for 3 to 4 days. Repeat after 4th week *or as per direction*	Hydrochloride (equivalent to Doxycycline)100 mg
C-Dox Forte Powder	Jeps Pharma	50 gm. Bottle 100 gm. Bottle	*Prevention of early chick mortality* 1 g per 10 ml water for 3 to 4 days.	Neomycin Sulphate 10% w/w, Equivilant to Neomycin 10% w/w. Doxycycline Hcl 10% w/w.
Neodox bolus	Vetcare	strip of 6 boli	*1 bolus/80 kg bwt PO per day*	Neomycin Sulphate B.P. 400 mg Doxycycline Hydrochloride (equivalent to Doxycycline)160 mg
Neoplus Powder	Cipla	Pack of 6 sachets x12 gm	1 sachet per day per large animal	Neomycin -2.4gm + Sulphaguanidine –24 gm + Kaolin –24 gm +Pectin –2.4 gm

NITROFURAZONE

Nitrofurazone is bactericidal for most pathogens that commonly cause surface skin infections, including Staphylococcus aureus, Streptococcus, Escherichia coli, Clostridium perfringens, Enterobacter aerogenes, and Proteus organisms. Indicated in skin problems, intrauterine and repeat breeding problems.

Product	**Company**	**Presentation**	**Dose rate**	**Composition**
Furazone	vetsfarma	120 ml suspension	For Infertility and Repeat Breeders : Instil 30 ml Furazone solution in the uterus 4 to 48 hrs. pre and post insemination. For Genital Infections : Instil 30 - 90 ml of Furazone	Solution for Intra-uterine Infections Nitrofurazone I.P. 0.2%w/v

			solution in the infected part.	

NORFLOXACIN

Fluoroquinolone. Bactericidal. It has similar spectrum of activity as nalidixic acid. Active against many gram +ve and negativesps. including Penicillinase producing, methicillinase resistant and Pseudomonas.

Indications : Primarily used in urinary and genital tract infections, bacterial diarrhoeas and acute gonococcal infections. UTI, Genital tract infection. Mixed G+ve and –ve etiology.

DOSAGE

Dog : 22mg/kgBW BID orally.

Product	Company	Presentation	Dose rate	Composition
Norflox distab	Cipla	Strip of 10's	22mg/kgBW	100mg/tab; 200 mg/tab; 400 mg/tab
Uroflox	Torrent	Strip of 10's	22mg/kgBW	400 mg/tab
NORFLOXACIN+METRONIDAZOLE: Mycoplasma, Infectious coryza, Salmonellosis, Pasteurellosis, Diarrhea of mixed etiology				
Triflox –M powder	Trichem	250 gm, 500 gm	500 gm / ton of feed	Each 500 g pack contains Norfloxacin 250g + Metronidazole 250g
NORFLOXACIN+TINIDAZOLE: Diarrhea of mixed etiology				
NT-ZOLE bolus	Cattle Remedies	5x4 bolus pack	1 bolus/50 kg BW orally per day	Each bolus contains norfloxacin + tinidazole

OFLOXACIN

mixed bacterial infection. It is the most potent fluroquinolone. Ofloxacin is relatively lipid soluble; oral bioavailability is high. Food does not interfere with its absorption. It is excreted largely unchanged in urine. Activity against many gram +ve and negative resistant strains, chlamydia, anaerobes, mycoplasma and legionella.

Indications : Chronic bronchitis and other respiratory or ENT infections, genito-urinary and gastro-intestinal diseases. May be used in gonorrhoea and nongonococcal urethritis, tuberculosis and leprosy as an alternative multidrug therapy.

Dosage

Cattle: 1800 mg/300 KG bw P.O.

OLONE	Rodec	2 boli pack	2 boli per large animal	Each bolus contains 900 mg Ofloxacin
ZIOF bolus	ZIP healthcare	1 gm x 2 bolus	2 bolus for adult cow	Each bolus contains 1000 mg ofloxacin

OFLOXACIN COMBINATION Indicated in mixed intrauterine infections				
OFTIN – TZ oral suspension	Kwality pharnace utical	60 ml suspension	Intrauterine 30 – 60 ml daily in	Each 5 ml contains ofloxacin 50 mg+tinidazole 150 mg
CURACIN-OZ	VETSFAR MA	60 ml suspension	Intrauterine In Repeat breeding : Instil 30 ml Curacin oz bd. In Infected uterus : Instil 30 - 60 ml Curacin oz per Infected horn daily	Each 5 ml contains ofloxacin 50 mg+ ornidazole 125 mg

PEFLOXACIN

Fluoroquinolone. Bactericidal. It is the methyl derivative of norfloxacin. It is more lipid soluble and has longer t½. Dose of pefloxacin needs to be reduced in liver disease but not in renal insufficiency. Active against many gram +ve and negativeand resistant microbes. Not against anaerobes.

Indications : Primarily used in urinary and genital tract infections, bacterial diarrhoeas. Also used in selected cases of gonorrhea and typhoid, RTIs, bone and joint infection, pactereimeia septicemia

DOSAGE

Large animal: 5-10 mg/kg BW/day, IV, oral; Dog : 10-40mg/kgBW BID, oral, IV.

Product	**Company**	**Presentation**	**Composition**
Pelox injection	Wochardt	100 ml vial	400mg/ml
Pelwin tab	Wochardt	Strip of 4's	400mg/tab
Pelwin infusion	Wochardt	100 ml vial	400mg/ml
Pelwin-DS powder	Wochardt	500 g pack	100 mg/gm

POLYMIXIN B

Bactericidal. Ocular infection, systemic Gram negative infection. It is a polypeptide with average molecular weight of 30,000 which exerts oncotic pressure similar to albumin and is not antigenic. It is not metabolised in the body, is excreted slowly by kidney and expanstion of plasma volume lasts for 12 hours.

Indications : Treatment of burns, hypovolemic and endotoxic shock, severe trauma and extensive tissue damage. Contraindications : Severe anaemia, cardiac failure, pulmonary edema, renal insufficiency. Known hypersensitivity to the constituents of the preparation.

Adverse drug reactions : Hypersensitivity reactions are rare like flushing, rigor, urticaria, wheals, wheezing and hypotension.
Status in
1. Pregnancy : Use only if clearly indicated.
2. Lactation : Use only if clearly indicated.
3. Old age : Use only if clearly indicated.
DOSAGE
Dog : 2.2 mg (10,000 IU)/kg BWt/day IM. Nephrotoxic in prolong use. Do not use with neuromuscular agents

Product	Company	Presentation	Dose rate	Composition
Aerosporin inj	Burrough's Wellcome	5 lac unit vial	2.2 mg (10,000 IU)/kg BWt	Polymixin 5 lac unit / vial

ROXITHROMYCIN (Macrolide): Bacteriostatic. RTI, UTI, skin and genital infection. It is a semi-synthetic long acting acid stable macrolide. It is more potent against Branh. catarrhalis, Gard. vaginalis and legionella. It has good enteral absorption and tissue penetration, an average plasma t½ of 12 hours. Bactericidal spectrum includes Staph., Strep., Corynebacterium, listeria, Gardeneralla, Legionella, Mycoplasma, Chlamydia.
Indications : Respiratory, ENT, skin and soft tissue and genital tract infections, UTI, cirrhosis.
DOSAGE: Dog : 2.5 mg/kg BWt BID Oral.

Product	Company	Presentation	Composition
Biorox tab	Biochem	Strip of 10's tab	150 mg Roxithromycin/tab
Roxisara disp. Tab.	Sarabhai	Strip of 6's tab	50 mg Roxithromycin / tab; 150 mg Roxithromycin / tab

STREPTOMYCIN: (Aminoglycoside). Bactericidal for Gm negative bacteria. Pasteurellosis, Salmonellosis, Brucellosis, Poll evil, Pink eye, Leptospira, Tuberculosis. During pregnancy, affects 8th cranial nerve of foetus. Prolong use results neurotoxicity, damaging vestibular and auditory mechanism.
DOSE RATE : All animals: 11 mg/kg BW IM q 12 hr (25 mg/kg in canine leptospirosis). Cow : 0.5 g/quarter. Poultry : 44 – 99 mg/kg

Product	Company	Presentation	Composition	
Ambistryn – S Inj	Sarabhai	1 g , 0.75 g vial	Streptomycin 1 g /vial, 0.75 g/vial	
STREPTOMYCIN COMBINATION				
Bistrepen-V inj	Alembic	2.5 g vial	Large animal 1-2 vial daily I/M	(Procaine penicillin-V 15 lac. + Benzyl Penicillin 5 lac + streptomycin sulphate 2.5 g) / vial

Dicrysticin-S inj	Sarabhai Zydus	Vial 2.5 g	Large animal 2 ml/ 50 kg BW I/M	(Procaine penicillin G 15 lac. + Penicillin G 5 lac + streptomycin sulphate2.5 g) / vial
Munomycin forte inj	Virbac	2.5 g vial	Large animal 1-2 vial daily I/M	(Procaine penicillin-V 15 lac. + Benzyl Penicillin 5 lac + streptomycin sulphate 2.5 g) / vial
Gass cutter	Piya	Tab	4 tab / calf orally	Each tab contains Streptomycin SO4 250 mg + Neomycin SO4 100 mg + Vitamin A 25000 IU
Stre Pen Powder	Cipla	100 gm	100 gm per cattle PO daily	Each gram contains Streptomycin as sulphate –133 mg + Procaine penicillin G –45mg + Pantothenic acid –5,850mcg +Nicotinamide –16,600mcg +Folic acid –410mcg+ Vitamin A –6,600IU +Vitamin B2 –1,690mcg+ Vitamin B6 –2,500mcg + Vitamin B12 –2.5mcg + Vitamin D3 –1,660 IU+ Vitamin E –2,500mcg + Vitamin K3 (as Menadione sodium bisulphate) 2,500 mcg.

SULPHONAMIDES

Bacteriostatic and antiprotozoan. Act as competitive inhibitors of bacterial dihydropteroate synthase and thus blocks the synthesis of folic acid from paraaminobenzoic acid and dihydropteroic acid. Acidification of urine tends to make them insoluble and thus predisposes to Crystalluria. Sodium bicarbonate renders the urine alkaline and thus hastens their renal excretion. Urea increases their solubility. Hematuria, obstruction of renal tubules are seen after prolonged therapy; peripheral neuritis, jaundice, anemia, cyanosis(dogs), decreased weight gain & egg prodn., thin rough shelled eggs are also observed.

Indicated in Actinobacillosis, Actinomycosis, colibacillosis, ehrlichiosis, hemorrhagic septicemia, infectious keratitis, polyarthritis, mastitis, nocardiosis, pneumonia, salmonellosis, strangles, coccidiosis, toxoplasmosis. Silver sulfadiazine is effective against nearly all bacteria and fungi.

CLASSES:

- **Standard Use Sulfonamide:** sulfathiazole, sulfamethazine (sulfadimidine), sulfamerazine, sulfadiazine, sulfapyridine.
- **Highly soluble Sulfonamide for Urinary Tract Infection:** sulfisoxazole (sulfafurazole), sulfisomidine.
- **Poorly soluble Sulfonamide for Intestinal infection:** sulfaguanidine, sulfasalazine (used for ulcerative colitis in dogs),
- **Potentiated sulfonamide:** Trimethoprim / sulfadiazine, trimethoprim / sulfamethoxazole, trimethoprim / sulfadoxine, ormetoprim / sulfamethoxine.
- **Sulfonamide use Topically**: sulfacetamide, sulfathiazole, mafenidine, silver sulfadiazine

SULPHADIMIDINE (sulfamethazine, sulphamezathine): a sulphapyrimidine.
DOSE: All animals: 110 mg/Kg BW PO, IV, SC for 4 days

Product	Company	Presentation	Composition
Diadin	Pfizer	Bolus 5 g	Sulphadimidine 5 g / bolus
Entradin Injection	Neospark	100 ml vial	Each ml contains:Sulphadimidine Sodium I.P. : 333 mg
Sulfamin bolus	Indian Immunological	Bolus 5 g	Sulphadimidine 5 g / bolus
Sulfamin inj	Indian Immunological	100 ml, 450 ml vial	Sulphadimidine 333 mg / ml
Sulpha bolus	Sarabhai zydus	Bolus 5 g	Sulphadimidine 5 g / bolus
ALDINE	Alembic Limited	Strip of 4 bolus	Each bolus contains: Sulphadimidine I.P.: 5g
PABADINE bolus	NEOVET	strip of 4 bolus	Sulphadimidine 5 g / bolus
Sulphadimidine	Novartis	100 ml ampoule	Sulphadimidine 333 mg / ml
Sulphadimidine sodium inj	Prima vet care	100 ml, 450 ml vial	Sulphadimidine 333 mg / ml
Sulfacip Inj	Cipla	Bottle of 100ml	Sulphadimidine sodium inj 33.33%
SULPHACHLORPYRIDAZINE			
ESB3	Novartis	100 gm pouch	Sulphachlorpyridazine 30%
SULPHAGUANIDINE			
Sulfagut bolus	KAPL	Bolus	Sulphaguanidine 5 g / bolus

SULPHA METHOXY PYRIDAZINE Dose : 1 ml / 10 kg bwt IM, IV, SC			
Aldazin long acting	Vetnex	Inj 30 ml vial	Sulpha Methoxy Pyridazine 250mg/ml
SULPHAQUINOXALINE			
Coxiquin Forte	Vet care	30 gm pack	Sulphaquinoxaline
SULPHONAMIDE+TRIMETHOPRIM Trimethoprim is a diaminopyrimidine related to the antimalarial drug pyrimethamine which selectively inhibits bacterial dihydrofolate reductase (DHFRase). Human folate metabolism is not interfered at antibacterial concentartions of trimethoprim. Individually both sulfonamide and trimethoprim are bacteriostatic, but the combination becomes cidal against many organisms.			
Bactrisol dispersible powder	Vetnex	100 g, 500 g, 1 kg Given @ 1 g/ltr water	Each gm has Sulphadiazine : 100 mg Trimethoprim : 20 mg
BESTOPRIM	Univet	Bolus Blister of 4 boli 4 boli daily (Large animal)	Each bolus has Sulphamethoxazole : 2 gm Trimethoprim : 400 mg
Biotrim inj	Indian Immunolog ical	30 ml vial	Each ml has Sulpha diazine 400 mg + Trimethoprin 80 mg
COSUMIX PLUS	Novartis	250 gm pouch	Sulphachlorpyridazine 10% + Trimethoprim 2%
Cosumix plus powder	Novartis	10 g, 100 g, 250g	Each 5 g contains Sulphachlorpyridazine 500 mg + Trimethoprim 100 mg
Genprim bolus	Genesis pharma	1x2 boli	Each bolus contains sulphamethoxazole 2gm + trimethoprim 400 mg
MARCOPRIM bolus	Marc	Bolus Blister of 4 boli	Each bolus has Sulphamethoxazole : 2 gm Trimethoprim : 400 mg
Oriprim	Sarabhai Zydus	Injection 30 ml vial	Each 5 ml has Sulphamethoxazole : 400 mg Trimethoprim : 80 mg
Oriprim	Sarabhai Zydus	Bolus Blister of 4 boli	Each bolus has Sulphamethoxazole : 2 gm Trimethoprim : 400 mg
Oriprim U	Sarabhai Zydus	Bolus strip of 4 boli	Each bolus has Sulphamethoxazole : 0.5 gm

		2- 4 boli IU after parturition daily (Large animal)	Trimethoprim : 0.1 g
RAPSOPRIM DS bolus	Raps Health Care	4 boli pack 4 boli daily (Large animal)	Each bolus has Sulphamethoxazole : 2 gm Trimethoprim : 400 mg
Sulpha	Sarabhai Zydus	Strip of 2 boli 1-2 bolus/50 kg Bwt or as per direction	Each bolus has Sulphadimidine: 5g
Sulprim 24	Vet care	30 ml vial 1 ml / 16 kg bwt IM or slow IV.	Each ml has Sulphadiazine : 200 mg Trimethoprim : 40 mg
Sulprim DS	Vet care	30 ml vial 1 ml / 32 kg bwt IM only	Each ml has Sulphadiazine : 400 mg Trimethoprim : 80 mg
Sulcoprim boli	Concept	Bolus Blister of 4 boli 4 boli daily (Large animal)	Each bolus has Sulphadiazine : 2 gm Trimethoprim : 400 mg
TREPIN I/V INJ.	Cadila	30 ML vial	Each 5 ml. contains : Trimethoprim B.P. (Vet) - 80 mg. Sulphamethoxazole I.P. - 400 mg. Aqueous Base - q.s.
V-cozine	Varsha lab	100 g, 750 g pack 1 g/4 kg BWt (calf) or as per direction	Sulphadiazine 10% w/w + Trimethoprim 2%w/w
Woktrin tab	Wochardt	Tablets	Each tab contains Sulphadiazine 1gm + Trimethoprim 200mg
Cobact powder	Cipla	100 gm sachet, 1kg container	Sulfamethazine 200 mg + Trimethoprim 40mg/g
Cotrim Powder	Cipla	1 Kg	Sulphamethoxypyridazine 69% + Trimethoprim 21%
Equix Granules	Cipla	100gm	Trimethoprim 6.67% w/w + Sulfadiazine 33.33%w/w
Equix Oral Paste	Cipla	Syringe of 37.5 gm	Trimethoprim 67 mg+ Sulfadiazine 333 mg/Gmof oral paste
Sparktrim I/M Injection	Neospark	Vial of 30 ml	Each ml Contains Sulphadiazine I.P. : 400 mg

			Trimethoprim I.P. : 80 mg
ZIPRIM - DS bolus	ZIP healthcare	4 boli strip	Each bolus contains sulphamethoxazole 2 gm + trimethoprim 400 mg
SULPHONAMIDE COMBINATION			
Ciplacin Tablet	Cipla	20 tablets	Each tablet contains : Sulphadiazine BP vet 1.58g, Sulphamerazine BP vet 1.58g, Sulphapyridine BP 1.59g, Streptomycin sulphate BP vet 0.313g
Diasulf Suspension	Cipla	225ml	Each ML contains:Sulphadimidine 21.3mg + Sulphaquanidine 21 Sulphadimidine 21.3mg + Sulphaguanidine 21.3mg + Sulphadiazine 28.4mg + Streptomycin sulfate 7.6mg+Neomycin sulpfate 1.8mg+Hyoscine hydrobromide 0.02mg+Sodium chloride 11.33mg+Calcium gluconate 2.2mg+Magnesium sulphate0.6mg+Potassium sulphate-3.6mg+Kaolin 103.3mg+Pectin 7.1mg+Glycine 20.9mg
Tripar Powder	Cipla	100gm sachet	Sulfadimidine Sodium 180 gm + Pyrimethamine HCl 15 gm + Furaltadone HCl 50 gm + Tetracycline HCl 10 gm + Vitamin A palmitate 10,000,000 IU + Vitamin K3 5 gm
Sulfacox Powder	Cipla	100gm,500gm sachet, 1kg container	Sulphadimerazine-860gm,Diaveridine -105gm

TETRACYCLINES			
Bacteriostatic. There are three naturally occurring tetracycline namely Oxytetracycline (OTC), chlortetracycline (CTC), demthylchlortetracycline (DCTC). Semisynthetic derivatives include tetracycline (TTC), rolitetracycline, methacycline, minocycline, doxycycline, lymecycline. Based on elimination time, these drugs may be classified into short acting (TTC, OTC, CTC), intermediate acting (DCTC, methacycline) and long acting (doxycycline, minocycline). Clinical use of tetracycline has declined to a large extent because of availability of more selective and less toxic antimicrobial agents. Indications : Initial treatment of mixed infections, Lymphogranuloma venereum, granuloma inguinale, atypical pneumonia, cholera, brucellosis, plague, relapsing fever. May be used in selected cases of tetanus, anthrax, syphillis, chancroid, tularemia. Occasionally in UTI and pneumonia. **DOSAGE:** TETRACYCLINE – All animals : 4.4 – 11 mg/kg IM; Dog- 7 mg/kg IM, IV BID; 20 mg/kg PO TID; Oxytetracycline - Dogs --- 7 mg/kg IM, IV BID; 20 mg/kg PO TID; Cattle, Sheep, pigs : 5 -10 mg/kg IM, IV SID; Horse : 5 mg/kg IV SID. Doxycycline --- Dogs --- 5 -10 mg/kg PO SID; 5 mg/kg IV SID.			
Product	**Company**	**Presentation**	**Composition**
Neocyclin	Neovet	500 mg Bolus	Tetracycline : 500mg/bolus
Resteclin	Sarabhai	250 mg tab	Tetracycline : 250mg/tab
Steclin	Sarabhai	500 mg Bolus	Tetracycline : 500mg/bolus
Tetracycline HCl	Intervet	100g, 1 kg jar	Tetracycline : 50mg/gm powder
Steclin bolus	Sarabhai Zydus	Bolus Strip of 4 boli	Each bolus has Tetracycline HCl: 500 mg
Terramycin egg formula powder	Pfizer	125 g pack	500 mg/g powder
Tetracycline bolus	Alembic Limited	Strip of 4 boli and Box of 15 strips.	Each bolus contains: Tetracycline HCl I.P.: 500 mg
V-cycline powder	Varsha labs	100 g pack	Tetracycline 30% w/w
Wolicycline inj	Wochardt	30 ml vial	Tetracycline 50mg/ml
Wolicycline-DS inj.	Wochardt	30 ml vial	Tetracycline 100mg/ml

TETRACYCLINE COMBINATION			
Codrinal powder	Intervet	20g, 100g pack	Each gm contains TSM ethyl urethane 0.55 g +Tetracycline HCl 0.05g [Dose : 4g / ltr water orally/day (poultry)]
Tetra Plus Powder	Cipla	100gm,250gm,500gm sachet, 1kg container	Tetracycline Hcl-125gm + Vitamin A palmitate –15,000,000IU + Vitamin D3 –3,000,000IU +Vitamin E –15,000IU +Vitamin K3-1gm+Vitamin B1- 1gm +Vitamin B2 –2.5gm+Vitamin B6 –1gm +Vitamin B12 –6mg +Vitamin C-25m +Vitamin PP –17.5gm +Ca Pantothenate –7.5gm+Folic acid –50mg+ Lysine Hcl-25gm + DL-Methionine –25gm ,

CHLORTETRACYCLINE

Bacteriostatic. Mixed infections including Salmonella, rickettsia. Synovitis, Blue comb. Contraindicated in pups and pregnant animals. It is not given by IM, imtramammary, being irritant. It is useful in enteric and ocular infection.

DOSAGE

Small animal: 25-50 mg/kg bwt/day PO; Large animal: 10-20 mg/kg bwt BID oral

Product	Company	Presentation	Composition
Chlortetracycline powder	Novartis	25 kg	Chlortetracycline 15 %
CTC 15 %	Osco	25 kg	Chlortetracycline 15 %

OXYTETRACYCLINE

Tetracycline congener, Bacteriostatic.

Indications: RTI, H.S., CCBP, B.Q., Mastitis, Strangles, UTI, Genital tract infection; Abscess, diarrhoea, foot rot, metritis, enteritis, bacterial pneumonia, calf scour and secondary bacterial complications associated with viral disease Mixed G+ve and –ve etiology.

DOSAGE

Large animal: 5-10 mg/kg BW/day IM,IV, oral; Dog : 10-20mg/kgBW BID IM, IV. Avoid in pups and pregnant animals

Product	Company	Presentation	Composition
Alcyclin-O inj	Alembic Limited	Injection 30 ml, 100 ml	Each ml contains Oxytetracyline Dihydrate: 50mg
INTAMYCIN-LA inj	Neovet	30 ml, 50 ml inj	Each ml contains Oxytetracycline Dihydrate 200 mg

Oxaclin LA inj.	Intervet	30 ml , 50 ml bottle	Each ml contains Oxytetracycline Dihydrate 200 mg
Oxytetracycline hydrochloride injection	Ranbaxy	30 ml , 50 ml, 100 ml vial	Each vial contains oxytetracycline HCl: 50 mg
Oxytetracycline Injection	Alembic ltd	Vial of 30ml, 50ml and 100ml.	Each ml contains Oxytetracycline Hydrochloride injection I.P. : 50mg
Oxytetracyline inj	Sarabhai Zydus	30 ml, 50 ml, 100 ml vial	Each ml has Oxytetracyline HCl: 50 mg
Oxytetracyline LA inj	Sarabhai Zydus	Injection 30 ml vial	Each ml has Oxytetracyline HCl: 200 mg [20 mg/kg bwt q 72 hrs. IM only]
OXYTETRACYCLINE Tab	Pfizer	Tablets	Each tab contains Oxytetracyline HCl: 500 mg
OTC Vet 10% Inj	Cipla	100 ml vial , 50 ml vial	Oxytetracycline 10% Inj
OTC-Vet LA 20% Inj	Cipla	10ml,50ml, 100ml, 250ml vial	Oxytetracycline 20% long acting Injection
OTC 20% powder	Cipla	100gm Sachet, 1kg container	Oxytetracycline 20% powder
OTC Spray	Cipla	200ml,300m l,500ml	Oxytetracycline 2g + Gentian violet – 0.7g
OTC Vet LA 30%	Cipla	100 ml	Oxytetracycline 30% long acting Injection
OTC-Vet LA 30% Inj	Cipla	10ml,50ml,100ml, 250ml vial	Oxytetracycline 30% long acting Injection
OTC-Vet 5% Inj	Cipla	50ml vial , 100ml vial	Oxytetracycline 5% Inj
OTC-Vet Tablets	Cipla	8 tablets, 500tabs. in a container	Oxytetracycline Hcl 500mg
UltrOx Injection	Neospark	Vials of 30 ml and 100 ml	Oxytetracycline Injection I.P. (Vet) - 50 mg/ml

UltrOx–DS Injection	Neospark	Vials of 30 ml and 100 ml	Oxytetracycline Injection I.P. (Vet) - 100 mg/ml
UltrOx / LA Injection	Neospark	Vials of 30 ml and 100 ml	Oxytetracycline Injection I.P. (Vet) - 200 mg/ml
OXYTETRACYCLINE WITH VITAMINS			
Oxyplus Powder	Cipla	100gm sachet, 500gm, 1kg	Oxytetracycline Hcl –60mg + Vitamin A –2.250 IU + Vitamin D3 – 450 IU +Vitamin B2 –2.9mg +Vitamin B12 –2.2mcg +Vitamin K3 –0.8mg + Vitamin E –1mg + Nicotinamide –13.5mg + Calcium pantothenate – 4.65mg
OTC Plus Powder	Cipla	180gm sachet	Oxytetracycline Hcl-55.56mg + Neomycin(as Neomycin sulphate)-38.89mg+Vitamin A – 1111.11 IU +Vitamin D3 –222.22 IU +Vitamin B12 –4.44mcg + Nicotinamide 8.89 mg + Ca-d-Pantothenate –3.33mg + Vitamin K3 –0.44mg + Vitamin E –0.33 IU + Vitamin B2 – 1.78mg

TIAMULIN

Bacteriostatic. Active against gram positive bacteria, mycoplasma, anaerobes including Treponema hyodysenteriae. Indicated in swine dysentery and mycoplasmal arthritis. Pneumonia, CRD, Coryza, RTI. Large animal: 6-8 mg/kg BW. Avoid in last month of pregnancy and in breeding boars. Do not use with anticoccidials like monensin, salinomycin.

DOSAGE: Large animal/dog : 8.8 mg/kg IM; Pig: 15 mg/kg IM for mycoplasmal pneumonia.

Product	Company	Presentation	Dose rate	Composition
Mycomulin 45% sol. granules	Concept	30 gm pack	1g / 20 ltr water orally or as advised by doctor	Tiamulin : 45%w/w
Tiamutin 10% inj	Novartis	15ml, 100 ml vial	Pig: 15 mg/kg IM	Tiamulin 100 mg /ml
Tiamutin 45% sol granules	Novartis	100 g, pack	5g / 20ltr water/ 1000 birds/day or as per direction	Tiamulin 45 % w/w

Mycomulin 10% Feed Premix	Cipla	1 Kg	500 gm - 1 kg per ton feed	Tiamulin Hydrogen Fumarate 10%
Mycomulin 25% Feed Premix	Cipla	1 Kg	500 gm - 1 kg per ton feed	Tiamulin Hydrogen Fumarate 25%

TOBRAMYCIN

aminoglycoside. Bactericidal. Septicemia, UTI. Actions and uses are similar to gentamicin but superior against Pseudomonas. **Contraindicated** in pregnancy. Do not use with other aminoglycoside.

DOSAGE: Dog: 1mg/kg BW TID SC, IM, IV

Product	Company	Presentation	Dose rate	Composition
Tobacin inj	Aristo	2ml vial (20mg/ 60mg / 80mg) / vial	1mg/kg BW	Tobramycin : 20mg/vial; 60mg/vial; 80mg/vial
Tobraneg inj	Ranbaxy	Ampoule	1mg/kg BW	Tobramycin: 10mg / 20mg / 40mg / 60mg / 80mg / ampoule

TYLOSIN

Macrolide. Bacteriostatic. More active at higher pH. Active against most aerobic and anaerobic gram positive bacteria, mycoplasma, rikettsiae. Indicated in pneumonia, Otitis, Metritis, Dysentery, Arthritis, coryza, CRD, Coccidiosis.

DOSAGE: Cattle: 10-20mg/kgBW oral, IM, BID; Dog: 20-40 mg/kg BW oral; Pig: 10 mg/kg IM, SID; Poultry: 250 - 290 gm/1000 layers in drinking water.

Product	Company	Presentation	Dose rate	Composition
Solutyl	Venky's	30 g, 100 g, 500 g, and 5 kg pack sizes	176 mg per kg body weight of birds for 3 days. However, treatment may be continued upto 5 days depending upon severity of infection.	Tylosin Tartrate I.P. 62.5 % w/w

Tylomix	Venky's	500 g, 1000 gm	For Breeders: Mix 500 g Tylomix ™ Premix per metric ton of complete feed from 20th week upto depletion of flock or as per advice of doctor	Each kg of premix contains Active ingredient Tylosin as Tylosin Phosphate ...... 100 g
TROX soluble powder	Virbac	60g, 120g	Mix 500 g Tylomix ™ Premix per metric ton of complete feed from 20th week upto depletion of flock	Tylosin tartrate 50%w/w
Tylocip 15 % LA	Cipla	100ml Vial	Cattle: 10-20mg/kgBW, IM	Tylosin 15 % w/v Long Acting injection
Tylocip 20 % inj	Cipla	100 ml vial	Cattle: 10-20mg/kgBW, IM	Tylosin 20 % inj.
Tylocip powder	Cipla	100gm, 1kg container	Cattle: 10-20mg/kgBW oral,	Tylosin 20% soluble powder
Tylocip 50 % powder	Cipla	100 gm container	Cattle: 10-20mg/kgBW oral	Tylosin 50 % soluble powder
Tylocip 10 % inj	Cipla	50 ml vial	Cattle: 10-20mg/kgBW, IM	Tylosin 10 % inj.
Tylocip 5 % inj	Cipla	50 ml vial	Cattle: 10-20mg/kgBW, IM	Tylosin 5 % inj.
TYLOSIN+ FOSFOMYCIN COMBINATION				
Tylofos	Cipla	100g, 1kg, 5kg, 20kg, 40kg	Mix 500 g powder per metric ton of complete feed	Fosfomycin 20% +Tylosin 5%

VIRGINIAMYCIN

an antibiotic of the streptogramin class that has been used in animal feeds to prevent disease and improve growth. Used to prevent necrotic enteritis in chickens and to treat laminitis in horses.

Dosage (Per 1000kg of feed.)

Broilers : 20g from day 1 to marketing.

Layer Chicks/ Growers 20g upto point of lay & 10g. 10g from point of lay till end.

Breeders : 20g to 40g from point-of-lay to end-of-lay.

Indications/Uses Performance enhancers in Layers Broilers Breeders Reduces cost in Feed Mills.			
Stafac 500	Pfizer	Plastic bucket of 5kg	Each kg contains Virginiamycin.....500g

MISCELLANEOUS ANTIBIOTIC PREPARATION (Topical appln.)			
OTC Spray	Cipla	200ml, 300ml, 500ml	Oxytetracycline HCL 5gm + Gentian violet 0.7gm
DC Spray	Cipla	200 m	Dichlorophen 7.5% w/w
Sulfatop ointment	Cipla	100mg	Sulphadiazine 400mg/ gm ointment
Dustit Powder	Cipla	40gm dusting powder	Coumaphos-3gm, Propoxur-2gm, Sulphanilamide-5gm
Oxolin Powder	Cipla	100gm sachet	Oxolinic acid 20% w/w

ANTIFUNGAL PRODUCTS

- AMPHOTERRICIN B
- CLOTRIMAZOLE
- GRISEOFULVIN
- KETOCONAZOLE
- MICONAZOLE
- NYSTATIN
- HERBAL ANTIFUNGAL PREPARATIONS

ANTIFUNGAL PRODUCTS
AMPHOTERRICIN B

Mechanism of action : The polyenes have high affinity for ergosterol present in fungal cell membranes, cell permeability is markedly-increased leading to cell lysis. Amphotericin - B (AMB) is active against a wide range of yeasts and fungi-Candida albicans, Histoplasma capsulatum, Cryptococcus neoformans, Blastomyces dermatitidis, Coccidioides Torulopsis, Rhodotorula, Aspergillus, Sporothrix etc. It is obtained from Streptomyces nodosus. It is not absorbed; can be given orally for intestinal candidiasis. It is administered i.v. as a suspension made with the help of deoxycholate (DOC), it gets widely distributed in the body, but penetration in CSF is poor. The terminal elimination t½ is 15 days. About 60% of AMB is metabolized in the liver. Excretion occurs both in urine and bile

Indications : Life threatening fungal infections such as aspergillosis, cryptococcosis, blastomycosis, systemic candidiasis, coccidioido-mycosis, histoplasmosis, zygomycosis including mucormycosis. Amphotericin B may be useful in the treatment of mucocutaneous leishmaniasis. It is used orally in candidial oesophagitis.

Dosage :

- Systemic mycoses: Dog: 0.25-0.5 mg/kg BW IV q 48 hrs
- Histoplasmosis: Dog: 1.8 mg/kg BW IV x 7 days

(Drug should be diluted in dextrose solution for IV application. NaCl soln. should not be used as a diluent)

Contraindications : Renal impairment.

Amphotericin B overdoses can result in cardio-respiratory arrest

Adverse drug reactions : Acute reaction with I.V. infusion including chills, fever and generalised pain, nausea and vomiting. Thromboflebitis of the injected vein can occur. Nephrotoxicity occurs with prolonged use with azotemia, reduced g.f.r., acidosis, hypokalemia and anaemia.

Status in

1. Pregnancy : Use only when benefits outweigh risks.
2. Lactation : Use only when benefits outweigh risks.
3. Old age : May be used.

Interactions : Flucytosine : Supra additive action with AMB; Rifampin, minocycline: Potentiate AMB; Aminoglycosides, vancomycin, cyclosporine and other nephrotoxic drugs : Enhance risk of renal impairment.

FUNGIZONE I.V.	Sarabhai	vial	50 mg/vial

CLOTRIMAZOLE

The polyenes have high affinity for ergosterol present in fungal cell membranes, cell permeability is markedly-increased leading to cell lysis. Indicated in dermatophycoses. Used for topical application.

CANESTEN cream	Bayer	15g Cream	10mg/g
CANESTEN solution	Bayer	15ml Sol.	1% w/v
IMIDIL	Lyka	30 gm powder, 15 gm cream, 15 ml soln.	1% w/w powder, cream; 1 % w/v soln.

GRISEOFULVIN

Mechanism of action : It is active against most dermatophytes including Epidermophyton, Trichophyton, Microsporum etc, but not against Candida and other fungi causing deep mycosis. Griseofulvin interferes with mitosis, multinucleated and stunted fungal hyphae result from its action. Absorption is improved by taking it along with fat. Griseofulvin gets deposited in keratin forming cells of skin, hair and nails; it is specially concentrated and retained in tinea infected cells. Because it is fungistatic and not cidal, the newly formed keratin is not invaded by the fungus.

Indications : Dermatophyte disease of skin, hair and nails.

Dosage

Cattle: 7.5 mg – 10 mg/kgBW/Day for 30 days orally.

Dog: 20 mg/kgBW/Day for 30 days orally.

Contraindications : Known hypersensitivity. Teratogenic if used during pregnancy.

Interactions : Warfarin, oral contraceptives: Griseofulvin decreases efficacy of these drugs; Phenobarbitone : Decreases efficacy of griseofulivn.

GRISOVIN-F.P.	Glaxo pharma	10's tablets	250 mg griseofulvin/tablet; 500 mg griseofulvin/tablet

KETOCONAZOLE

Oral absorption of ketoconazole is facilitated by gastric acidity, in the blood it is largely bound to albumin and RBCs. Hepatic metabolism is extensive; metabolites are excreted in urine and faeces. Elimination of ketoconazole is dose dependent :t½ varies from 1½ to 6 hours. Penetration in CSF is poor : not effective in fungal meningitis.

Indications : Systemic candidiasis, chronic mucocutaneous candidiasis, oral thrush, candiduria, blastomycosis, coccidioidomycosis, histoplasmosis, chromomycosis, and paracoccidioidomycosis, severe recalcitrant cutaneous dermatophyte infections who have not responded to topical therapy or oral griseofulvin.

Dosage

- Dogs/cats : 10 mg/KgBW orally

Contraindications : Known hypersensitivity.

Special precautions : Hepatic impairment.

Adverse drug reactions : Nausea and vomiting; loss of appetite, headache paresthesia, rashes and hair loss. Found to decrease androgen production from testes and to displace testosterone from protein binding sites. Gynaecomastia, loss of hair and libido and oligozoospermia in men and menstrual irregularities occur in some women. Mild and asymptomatic elevation transaminases occurs in 5% patients. Thrombocytopenia.

Status in

1. Pregnancy : Use with caution
2. Lactation : Use with caution
3. Old age : Use with caution.

Interactions : Antacids, H2 blockers, PPIs : Decrease oral absorption of ketoconazle; Rifampicin, isoniazid, phenytoin, phenobarbitone : Increase metabolism of ketoconazole; Warfarin, sulfonylureas, phenytoin, cyclosporine, diazepam, nifedipine, indinavir : Ketoconazole raises the blood levels of these drugs.

FUNGICIDE 200	Torrent	10's tabs	200 mg/tab
NIZRAL	J&J	10's tabs	200 mg/tab

MICONAZOLE:

It is an imidazole antifungal with similar action to clotrimazole.

Indications : Ringworm. Candidial infections of vulva, penis and oral cavity, tinea cruris and tinea pedis.

Dosage : Apply 2-3 times a day to the affected area for 2-3 weeks.

Contraindications : Hypersensitivity.

Special precautions : For external use only.

Adverse drug reactions : Local : Burning, irritation and redness, contact dermititis.

Systemic : I.V administration : cardiac arythemias, phloebitis, pruritis, anaphylactic reactions and cardiac arrest.

Status in

1. Pregnancy : Use with caution.
2. Lactation : Use with caution.

Interactions : I.V. administration potentiate hypoglycenic drugs and anticoagulants. Increased cardiotoxicity with cisapride, astemizole, terfenadine.

MICOGEL cream	Cipla	15 g tube	2 % w/w miconazole
ZOLE	Rexcel	15 gm oint, 15 ml lotion, 15 gm powder	oint has 2% w/w, Lotion has 2 % w/v; powder has 2 % w/w miconazole.

NYSTATIN

Mechanism of action : Obtained for S. *noursei,* it is similar to AMB in antifungal action and other properties. It has higher systemic toxicity, it is used only locally. It is not absorbed orally; can be used for monilial diarrhoea.

Indications : Primarily used for vaginal ,cutaneous, corneal , conjunctival and intestinal candidiasis, Coccidiomycosis, Blastomycosis.

Dosage

- Dogs: 22,000 units/Kg BW/day orally

Contraindications : Known hypersensitivity.

Status in

1. Pregnancy : Use with caution.
2. Lactation : May be used.
3. Old age : May be used.

MYCOSTATIN	Sarabhai Zydus	tablet	each tab contains 5 lac units.

HERBAL ANTIFUNGAL PREPARATIONS

CHARMAID	Dabur	caps	herbal
TEEBURB	Natural Remedies	caps	herbal

ANTIPROTOZOAL DRUGS

ANTICOCCIDIALS

- AMPROLIUM/ AMPROLIUM COMBINATION
- CLOPIDOL
- DINITOLMIDE/ combination
- LASALOCID
- MADURAMYCIN
- MONENSIN
- METRONIDAZOLE:/ combination
- ROBENIDINE
- SALINOMYCIN
- SODIUM SULPHA DIMETHYL PYRIMIDINE
- SULPHADIMIDINE
- TINIDAZOLE/ combination

ANTIHAEMOPROTOZOAN

- BUPARVAQUONE
- DIMINAZINE ACETURATE
- ISOMETAMIDIUM
- LITHIUM ANTIMONY THIOMALATE
- OXYTETRACYCLINE
- QUINAPYRAMINE CHLORIDE AND QUINAPYRAMINE SULFATE
- SURAMIN

ANTIPROTOZOAL DRUGS
ANTICOCCIDIALS:
For prevention and treatment of coccidiosis caused by Eimeria spp. in ruminants, birds and Isospora spp. in pig and dogs.

- **BENZENEACETONITRILES:** example: clazuril, Diclazuril
- **IONOPHORES:** example: Lasalocid, Maduramycin, Monensin, Narasin, Salinomycin.
- **QUINOLONES:** example: Decoquinate, Methylbenzoate.

<table>
<tr><td colspan="4">

• **SULFONAMIDES:** Coccidiostat. Act as competitive antagonist of GABA. Effective for treatment at schizont stage.

- **Sulfachloropyrazine**: chicken: 0.03% in water.
- **Sulfadimethoxine**: Broilers: 125 ppm in feed. Dog: 55 ppm P.O.x 21 days.
- **Sulphadimidine**: Intestinal and caecal coccidiosis. Dose: 200mg/kg BW oral
- **sulfamethoxine-amprolium**: chicken: 125+75 ppm in feed.
- **sulfamethoxine- diaveridine**: Rabbit: 100-125 ppm in feed x 3 days.
- **sulfamethoxaine-ormetoprim**: poultry: 125+75 ppm in feed.
- **sulfaquinoxaline**: poultry: 125 ppm in feed.
- **sulfaquinoxaline-pyrimethamine**: chicken: 0.005 % + 00015 % in water.

AMPROLIUM:
Coccidiostat. Thiamine antagonist. Inhibits thiamine uptake by coccidia. Acts on first gen schizont preventing differentiation of merozoites. **Indicated in** cecal and intestinal coccidiosis.
Dose rate: cattle: 10 mg/kg BW oral. Chicken: 125-250 ppm in water. Avoid in layer birds. May cause thiamine deficiency in host resulting nervous symptoms.
AMPROLIUM-Ethopabate: Poultry: 125+40 ppm in feed
APRINOCID: coccidicidal/static. Poultry: 60 ppm in feed
CLOPIDOL: coccidiostatic. For preventive. Poultry: 125-250 ppm in feed
DINITOLMIDE: coccidicidal/static. Poultry: 125 ppm in feed
FURAZOLIDONE: antiprotozoal. Chicken: 55-110ppm in feed
HALOFUGINONE hydrobromide: coccidicidal/static. Chicken: 3 ppm in feed.
IODOQUINOL: coccidicidal, amebicidal. Cattle: 5 gm/227 Kg/day PO
NICARBAZIN: coccidicidal/static. Broilers: 125 ppm in water.
NITROFURAZONE: Coccidiostatic. chicken: 82 ppm in water for 5 days
ROBENIDINE: guanidine coccidiostat.
TOLTRAZURIL: coccidicidal/static. Broilers: 25ppm in water.
SALINOLMYCIN : coccidiostat. 6.0 %w/w 1 kg/ton feed of poultry

</td></tr>
<tr><td colspan="4">AMPROLIUM</td></tr>
<tr><td>Amprolium powder 20% w/w</td><td>Neospark</td><td>30 gm, 150 gm</td><td>Amprolium HCl 200 mg/gram (poultry: 30-60 gm / 25 ltr water)</td></tr>
<tr><td>AMPROLIUM SOLUBLE powder 20 %w/w</td><td>Virbac</td><td>150 gm sachet and 1 kg bag</td><td>20% w/w (30-60 gm / 25 ltr water)</td></tr>
<tr><td>Vetpro 20%</td><td>Cipla</td><td>100gm sachet, 500gm, 1kg container</td><td>Amprolium 20% soluble powder</td></tr>
<tr><td>Vetpro E powder</td><td>Cipla</td><td>100gm sachet, 500gm, 1kg container</td><td>Amprolium 25% +Ethopabate 1.6% Powder</td></tr>
</table>

Vetpro 60%	Cipla	100gm sachet, 500gm, 1kg container	Amprolium 60% soluble powder
Vetpro Plus Powder	Cipla	100gm sachet	Amprolium Hcl-200mg,Sulfaquinoxaline base-200mg,Vit K3 –2mg
AMPROLIUM COMBINATION			
Amprolium and Ethopabate premix	Wockhardt	5 kg powder	Each kg pwder contains Amprolium HCl 250 gm and Ethopabate 16g
COXIMAR powder	Virbac	30 gm pouch (poultry: 30g / 50 ltr water)	Amprolium HCl 16.67% w/w + sulfaquinoxaline 16.67% w/w
COXIQUIN FORTE	Vetcare	30 gm pouch (poultry: 30g / 50 ltr water)	Amprolium HCl 16.67% w/w + sulfaquinoxaline 16.67% w/w
CLOPIDOL			
COXIDOL	Venky's	1 kg, 10 kg, 25 kg	25 % w/w
COXYMIX	Agvet	1 kg, 10 kg, 25 kg	25 % w/w
Clopicip 25% powder	Cipla	10kg, 25kg	Clopidol 25%
DINITOLMIDE			
COXYBAN	Agvet	10 kg, 25 kg	25 % w/w (poultry @ 500gm/ton feed)
DOT powder	Wockhardt	5 kg	25 % w/w (poultry @ 500gm/ton feed)
VELDOT powder	Venky's	1 kg, 5 kg	25 % w/w (poultry @ 500gm/ton feed)
DINITOLMIDE combination			
ETHCOXI powder	Concept	100 gm, 1 kg	Dinitolmide 25% w/w + Ethopabate 1.6 % w/w
UNISTAT powder	Unichem	5 kg, 25 kg	Dinitolmide 25% w/w + Ethopabate 1.6 % w/w
LASALOCID			
AVATEC powder	Piramal	600 gm	15 % w/w (poultry @ 600gm/ton feed)
MADURAMYCIN			
ionophore coccidiostat. Disturbs osmotic balance and cellular reaction in parasite in sporozoite and merozoite stage of coccidia. Indicated in prophylaxis of coccidiosis.			

Dose rate: 1 % powder 500 gm/tonne of poultry feed.			
COCCIWIN	Sarabhai zydus	1 kg, 20 kg	1 % w/w
MONACOX powder	Vetnex	20 kg	1 % w/w
Ramycox 1% Granules	Cipla	1 kg & 5 kg	Maduramycin 1% [Granular]
MONENSIN			
ionophore coccidiostat. Disturbs osmotic balance and cellular reaction in parasite in sporozoite and merozoite stage of coccidia. Indicated in prophylaxis of coccidiosis. **Dose** rate: 1 % powder 1000 gm/tonne of poultry feed.			
COBAN-100	Ventry's	1 kg, 5 kg	100 gm / kg powder
METRONIDAZOLE			
action attributed by DNA damage. Indicated in intestinal amebiasis, trichomoniasis, giardiasis, gingivitis, Balantidium, Bovine trichomoniasis. **Dose**: Dogs: 20-50mg/kgBW oral; 20 mg/kgBW IV ; Cattle: 20 mg/kgBW IV			
FLAGYL	Rhone poulenc	10 Tab, 30ml, 60ml Susp	200mg; 400mg; 200mg/5ml,
FLAGYL-I.V.	Rhone poulenc	100ml I.V. pack	500mg/5ml
METROGYL	J.B. Chemicals	10 Tab, 30ml, 60ml Susp, 20g Gel;	200mg; 400mg; 200mg/5ml, Gel 1%;
METROGYL	J.B. Chemicals	100ml I.V. pack	500mg/5ml
METROGYL	Unique	10 Tab, 30ml, 60ml Susp, 20g Gel;	200mg; 400mg; 200mg/5ml, Gel 1%;
METROGYL	Unique	100ml I.V. pack	500mg/5ml
METRONIDAZOLE combination			
indicated in diarrhea, dysentery, uterine infection of mixed origin.			
MARCOGYL LM	Marc India Ltd	Blister of 4 boli and Box of 10 blisters	Each bolus contains: Metronidazole:1,000mg Furazolidone : 500 mg Loperamide HCl : 7.5 mg
FAZOLE bolus	Vetcare	4 boli pack	Each bolus contains: Metronidazole:1,000mg Furazolidone : 200 mg
METROFUR PLUS	Torque Pharma	10 Tab	Metronidazole 200mg, Loperamide HCL 1.5mg
METROGYL	J.B. Chemicals	15 Tab	Metronidazole 400mg,

COMPD			Diloxanide Furoate 500mg
METROGYL DG GEL	Lekar Pharma	10g, 20g, 30g Gel	Metronidazole 1%, Chlorhexidine 0.25%)
METROGYL P	Lekar Pharma	15g Oint, 125g, 100ml Sol.	Povidone iodine 5%, Metronidazole 1%)
METROGYL V GEL	Lekar Pharma	10g Gel	Metronidazole 10mg per g
METROGYL-F	J.B. Chemicals	10 Tab	Metronidazole 400mg, Furazolidone 100mg
METROGYL-F	J.B. Chemicals	30ml, 60ml Sus	Metronidazole 200mg, Furazolidone 40mg/5ml
METROHEX	Dr. Reddy's Lab	10g	Metronidazole 1%, Chlorhexidine Gluconate 0.25% w/v
METRONOR	P.C.I.	30ml Syrup	Metronidazole 100mg, Norfloxacin 100mg
METRONORM	Modern Pharma	30ml Susp	Norfloxacin 100mg, Metronidazole 100mg/5ml
DEPENDAL-M	GSK	10 Tab	Furazolidone 100mg, Metronidazole (as benzoate 300mg
DEPENDAL-M	GSK	60ml Sus	Furazolidone 25mg, Metronidazole 75mg, per 5ml
Spiragyl tablets	Cipla	Pack of 10's Container 500 tabs.	Metronidazole 125mg + Spiramycin 750,000IU
ROBENIDINE: guanidine coccidiostat. Inhibits oxydative phosphorylation in mature first generation schizont stage. Indicated for prophylaxis of coccidiosis. Avoid use in layers. **Dose**: 500gm (6.6%) / tonne feed.			
ROBINEX	Stallen	20 kg	6.6% w/w
SALINOMYCIN: Dose : 60 ppm in broiler feed.			
COXISTAC	PFIZER	5 kg pack	6 % w/w
SACOX 120 powder	Intervet	25 kg	12 % (poultry: 250-500 gm/ton feed)
COXIAL	Alembic	Kraft paper bag of 10kg	Salinomycin Sodium 12% microgranulated W/W (Broilers - Mix 500g into 1 tonne of broiler feed or as per direction)
Coxstop	Cipla	250gms, 25kgs.	Salinomycin 12% powder

SODIUM SULPHA DIMETHYL PYRIMIDINE: sulphonamide anticoccidial. For details, refer to antibiotic section.			
SULPHADIMIDINE: sulphonamide anticoccidial. Dose: 200 mg/kgBW orally. For details, refer to antibiotic section.			
TINIDAZOLE: action attributed by DNA damage. Indicated in intestinal amebiasis, trichomoniasis, giardiasis, gingivitis, Balantidium, Bovine trichomoniasis. **Dose**: Dogs: 30-50mg/kgBW oral. Avoid during pregnancy.			
FASIGYN	Pfizer	4 Tab	500mg
FASIGYN	Pfizer	2 Tab	1000mg
TINIBA	Cadila	10x10's tab	300mg, 500mg,1000mg
TINIBA INFUSION	Zydus Cadila	400ml Inf.	800mg
TINIDAZOLE combination			
TINIBA-N	Zydus Cadila	10 Tab	Norfloxacin 400mg, Tinidazole 600mg
TINIBA DF	Zydus Cadila	10 Tab	Tinidazole 150mg, Diloxanide furoate 250mg
ZIL	Sarabhai zydus	10 Tab	300mg, 600mg
TOLTRAZURIL Dose : 25 ppm in water (Broiler)			
Cipcox 2.5 %	Cipla	100ml, 500ml, 1ltr, 20 ltrs.	Toltrazuril 2.5 % Liquid
Cipcox 5 %	Cipla	100ml, 500ml, 1ltr, 20 ltrs.	Toltrazuril.5 % Suspension

ANTIHAEMOPROTOZOAL PRODUCTS **BUPARVAQUONE** antitheilerial. Avoid intravenous/subcut administration. **Dose:** cattle/bufflao: 2.5mg/kg IM.			
BUTALEX	Sarabhai zydus	20 ml pack	50mg/ml
Buprocip	Cipla	40 ml Inj	Buparvaquone 50mg/ml inj
DIMETRIDAZOLE Antihaemoprotozoal compound			
Helmett Soluble powder	Cipla	500gm	40% w/w
DIMINAZINE ACETURATE Babesicidal, Trypanocidal, Bactericidal action. Dose: 0.8-1.6g/100kgBW IM (Max dose is 9 gm total). C/I in camels.			

BERENIL RTU	Intervet	20 ml vial	70mg/ml
BERENIL granules	Intervet	5 gm, 22.5 gm vial granular form	0.444 gm/gm powder
ProZant Vet Injection	Neospark	Presentation: 20 ml Vial	Each ml contains: Diminazene Aceturate : 70 mg Phenazone B.P : 375 mg Water for Injection I.P. : QS
Dimaze inj	Wochardt	30 ml vial	Each ml contains: Diminazene Aceturate : 70 mg
Nilbery inj.	Intas	30 ml, 90 ml vial	Each ml contains: Diminazene Aceturate : 70 mg
PROZOMIN inj	Virbac	vial 30 ml	Each ml contains Diaminazine Diaceturate 70 mg, Phenazone 375 mg
Target inj.	Marc	20ml, 30 ml, 90 ml vail	Each ml contains Diaminazine Diaceturate 70 mg, Phenazone 375 mg
Trycip plus granules	Cipla	2.36 gm sachet, 23.6 gm sachet	Diminazene diaceturate 1.05gm +Vitamin B12 1mg /2.36 gm
Trycip granules	Cipla	2.36 gm sachet, 23.6 gm sachet	Diminazene diaceturate 1.05gm/2.36 gm granules sachet
Trycip Forte Granules	Cipla	23.6gm sachets	Diminazene Diaceturate 10.5gm + Vitamin B12 0mg + Antipyrine 13.1gm
Trycip Inj.	Cipla	30 ml, 50ml vial	Diminazene diaceturate 70 mg / ml & Phenazone BP 375 mg / ml
Trytil granules	Lyka	22.5 gm vial granular form	0.444 gm Diminazene diaceturate /gm powder

IMIDOCARB

Indicated in Babesiosis and anaplasmosis.

Dose (SC, IM): Horse: 2.4 mg/kg; Cattle: 1.5 mg/kg; Dog: 6 mg/kg. For prophylaxis: Cattle: 3 mg/kg SC, IM

Babex Injection	Cipla	100ml	Imidocarb dipropionate 12%

ISOMETAMIDIUM

antitrypanosoma drug. A phenathridine aromatic amidine compound. Inhibits kinetoplastic topoisomerase type II.

Dosage: Therapeutic:125 mg/adult animal deep I/M; Prophylactic: 250 mg/adult animal deep I/M.

Trypadium Injection	Cipla	Box 0f 10 sachet each of 125mg	Isometamidium chloride 125 mg [Powder for Injection]
Surral inj.	Alembic	vial	Isometamidium chloride 250 mg per vial with DW
LITHIUM ANTIMONY THIOMALATE Indicated for nasal granuloma @ 15-20 ml IM q week x 3 dose; Papillomatosis @ 15-20 ml IM on alternate days; filariasis/leishmaniasis @ 1-2.5 ml on alternate day.			
Lithimony	Indian Immunologicals	50 ml vial	6 % w/v
OXYTETRACYCLINE anaplasmosis, theileriosis, ehrlichiosis. Dose: 10-20 mg/kg BW IV (Product details in antibiotic section)			
QUINAPYRAMINE CHLORIDE AND QUINAPYRAMINE SULFATE A 2:1 minxture (10g+6.6g) prosalt is used. Inhibits growth and cell division of haemoprotozoans. Indicated in surra, trypanosomiasis. Dose: All animals: 5 mg/kg BW S/C (10 % soln in cattle and 5 % soln. in horses).			
ANTRYCIDE PROSALT	GLAXO	vial 2.5 gm	Quinapyramine sulphate 1.5 gm+ Q. chloride 1 gm in each vial (@ 2.5ml / 100 kg BW S/C after adding 15 ml water for inj.)
TEVANSI	VETNEX	vial 2.5 gm	Quinapyramine sulphate 1.5 gm+ Q. chloride 1 gm in each vial (@ 2.5ml / 100 kg BW S/C after adding 15 ml water for inj.)
TRIQUIN-S	Wockhardt	vial 2.5 gm	Quinapyramine sulphate 2 gm/vial (@ 2.5ml / 100 kg BW S/C after adding 15 ml water for inj.)
Vetquin	Cipla	2.5gm vial	Quinapyramine Sulphate 1.5gm + 1gm Quinapyramine Chloride In
Quinocip Injection	Cipla	15ml	Quinapyramine sulphate-3.0gm
SURAMIN Indicated for Rx of Trypanosoma infection. **Dose**: 7-10 mg/kgBW IM as 10 % soln. Dog: 30-50 mg/KgBw IM.			
GILPOL	G. Loucatos	vial	1 gm/vial
NAGANOL	Bayer	vial	5 gm/vial
PHENYLARSINE COMPOUND Indicated in haemoprotozoal infection.			

Ciplarsan	Cipla	100 mg	Bis(aminoethylthio) – 4 - melaminophenylarsine dihydrochloride 100 mg [Sterile freeze dried powder for injection]

ANTIPARASITIC PRODUCTS

Endoparasiticides

- ALBENDAZOLE
- FENBENDAZOLE COMBINATION
- FENBENDZOLE
- LEVAMISOLE
- MEBENDAZOLE
- MILBEMYCIN OXIME
- MORANTEL CITRATE
- OXYCLOZANIDE
- OXYCLOZANIDE COMBINATION
- PIPERAZINE
- PRAZIQUANTEL
- PYRANTEL PAMOATE
- RAFOXANIDE
- TRICLABENDAZOLE
- TRICLABENDAZOLE COMBINATION
- TETRAMISOLE

ECTOPARASITICIDES

- AMITRAZ
- CARBAMATES
- COUMAPHOS
- CYPERMETHRIN
- DELTAMETHRIN
- DIAZINON

- DICHLORVAS
- FIPRONIL
- FLUMETHRIN AND COMBINATION
- GAMMA BEZENE HEXACHLORIDE
- GAMMA BEZENE HEXACHLORIDE AND COMBINATION
- IMIDACLOPRID
- LUFENURON
- FENVALERATE
- ORGANOPHOSPHORUS COMPOUND
- POLYHERBAL ECTOPARASITIC / MULTIPURPOSE FORMULATIONS

Ectendoparasiticides

- DORAMECTIN
- IVERMECTIN
- CLOSANTEL

ENDOPARASITIC PRODUCTS

ALBENDAZOLE

Benzimidazole anthelmintic.

Mechnaism of action: Causes inhibition of microtubules polymerisation by binding to b tubulin, also may cause decrease in glucose transport and uncoupling of oxidative phosphorylation, in the nematodes. Absorption of albendazole after oral administration is moderate but inconsistent. Albendazole sulfoxide is widely distributed in the body, enters brain and is excreted in urine with a t½ of 8.5hours. Thus, albendazole is able to exert antihelmintic activity in tissues as well. It is vermicidal, ovicidal, larvicidal in action. It is indicated in Nematode, cestode and trematode infestation.

Dose rate: **Ruminants**, horses, pig: 5-10 mg/kg body weight once orally; **Dog** and cat: 25-50mg/kgBW for 3 days. Contraindicated in first trimester of pregnancy.

Indications : Ascariasis, hookworms, enteroviasis, tapeworm and strongyloidosis, trichinosis. Drug of choice of cystic hydatid disease and neurocysticercosis. Given with diethylcarbamazine for lymphatic filariasis.

Contraindications : Known hypersensitivity.

Special precautions : Hepatic impairment.

Status in

1. Pregnancy : Use with caution
2. Lactation : Use with caution.

Interactions : Fats increase absorption.

Product	Company	Presentation	Composition
ALBACRIL 150	Cattle Remedies	10 x 10 tabs	Albendazole 150 mg / tab
ALBACRIL 1500	Cattle Remedies	6 x 2 tabs	Albendazole 1500 mg / tab
ALBACRIL 3000	Cattle Remedies	3 x 2 boli	Albendazole 3000 mg / bolus
ALBACRIL suspension	Cattle Remedies	30 ml, 60 ml	Albendazole 25 mg / ml
ALBOMAR micronised bolus	Virbac	2 boli /blister	Albendazole 1500 mg / bolus
ALBOMAR micronised suspension	Virbac	30, 60, 90, 500 ml glass bottles	Albendazole 2.5% w/v
ALBOMAR micronised tablet	Virbac	10 tab /blister	Albendazole 150 mg / tab
ALBOMAR powder	Virbac	300 gm container	Albendazole 5% w/w
Almicide Tablet / Bolus	Jeps Pharma	25x2's Blister/Strip 5x10's Blister/Strip	Albendazole 150mg., 250 mg. 600 mg., 1500 mg., 2500 mg., 3000 mg.
Almicide Suspension	Jeps Pharma	90 ml. pet bottle, 1 Liter Bottle	Albendazole 2.5% W/V, 5% W/V., 10% W/V.
Benvet 10% susp	Cipla	200ml,1 litre can	Albendazole 10% Suspension
Benvet 1000	Cipla	50 Boli	Albendazole 1000 mg Bolus
Benvet 1500	Cipla	50 Boluses	Albendazole 1500 mg Bolus
Benvet 2.5% susp	Cipla	25ml, 200ml,500ml,1 ltr can	Albendazole 2.5% Suspension
Benvet 250	Cipla	50 Boli	Albendazole 250mg Bolus
Benvet 30%	Cipla	1 kg Container	Albendazole 30% Powder
Benvet 500	Cipla	50 Boli	Albendazole 500 mg Bolus
Benvet 600	Cipla	50 Boli	Albendazole 600 mg Bolus
Benvet Blue Suspension	Cipla	250, 500, 1000ml	Albendazole 25mg + Copper Sulfate 1000mcg + Sodium Selenite 500mcg
Benvet GR 2.5% susp	Cipla	1 ltr can	Albendazole 2.5% Suspension

Benvet GR - 2500	Cipla	40 Boli	Albendazole 2500 mg Bolus
Benvet GR-300	Cipla	50 Boli	Albendazole 300 mg Bolus
Benvet GR-600	Cipla	50 Boli	Albendazole 600 mg Bolus
Benvet Plus Suspension	Cipla	1 ltr	Albendazole 25mg + Copper sulfate 1000mcg + Sodium selenite 500 mcg
CIDAL A susp	Zoic	30 ml	Albendazole 200 mg / 5 ml
MINTHAL BOLUS 200mg	ALEMBIC LTD	Strip of 6boli and box of 5strips.	Each 200mg. Bolus contains: Albendazole I.P.: 200mg
MINTHAL BOLUS 600mg	ALEMBIC LTD	MINTHAL 600mg bolus – Strip of 4boli and box of 5strips.	Each 600 mg. Bolus contains: Albendazole I.P.: 600mg
MINTHAL SUSPENSION	ALEMBIC LTD	Jar of 1 litre.	Each ml contains: Albendazole I.P.: 25mg
<u>ZOMAR 3000MG BOLUS</u>	Cadila	4 Boli,1 Bolus	Each uncoated bolus contains : Albendazole USP. - 3000 mg.
<u>ZOMAR SUSPENSION</u>	Cadila	30 ml., 1 LTR.	Each 5 ml. contains : Albendazole USP - 125 mg. Flavoured syrupy base - q.s. Colour - Carmoisine, Ponceau 4R
ALBENDAZOLE & Combination			
ERAZAN FORTE	Marc	2 boli pack	Each bolus contains Albendazole 500 mg + Oxyclozanide 1000 mg
BITHIONOL SULFOXIDE preparation			
Bisto Tablets	Cipla	Container of 100 sachets each of 1 bolus	Bithionol sulfoxide 2gm

DIETHYL CARBAMAZINE

piperazine derivative.

Mechanism of action : Diethylcarbamazine has a highly selective effect on microfilariae (MF) of suseptible filarial species. Disrupts microtubules and inhibits microtubule polymerization in filarial larvae. The most important action of DEC appears to be alteration of MF membranes so that they are readily phagocytosed by tissue fixed monocytes, but not by circulating phagocytes. DEC is absorbed after oral ingestion, distributed all over the body, metabolized in liver and excreted in

urine. Excretion is faster in acidic urine. Plasma t½ of usual clinical doses is 4-12 hours. **Indicated** for prophylactic threapy against canine heart worm infection or Dirofilariasis. **DOSAGE :** Dogs: 6.6 mg/kg/day for 3-4 weeks,oral. **Contraindications** : Known hypersensitity. **Special precautions** : Renal impairment, hypertension. Antihistaminics and corticosteroids may be required during initiation of therapy to avoid toxic reactions of dying microfilariae and adult worms. Patients with poor health. Adverse drug reactions : Nausea, loss of appetite, weakness, a febrile reaction with rash, pruritus, enlargement of lymph nodes and fall in BP may occur at initiation of therapy. Status in 1. Pregnancy : Contraindicated 2. Lactation : Use with caution. 3. Old age : Use with caution. 4. Neonates : Use with caution.			
BANOCIDE	Burrough Wellcome	Tab, syrup 60ml, 100 ml	50 mg / tab, 100 mg/tab; syrup: 50mg/5 ml, 120 mg/5 ml
HETRAZAN	Cyanamid	Tabs, Syrup 114 ml.	50 mg / tab, 100 mg/tab; syrup: 120 mg/5 ml
FENBENDZOLE Benzimidazole compound. Inhibits polymerization of tubulin in the parasite and blocks the glucose uptake. Interferes activity of enzyme fumarate reductase and blocks energy production in parasite, resulting death.Action is vermicidal, larvicidal, ovicidal with wide margin of safety and non embryotoxic. **Indicated** for nematodal, cestodal and trematodal infections. **DOSAGE :** Cattle, Buffalo, Horse, pig, sheep: 5-7.5 mg/kg BW Oral; Dog: 50 mg/KgBW oral. 5 mg/kg bwt			
CURAMINTH	Sarabhai zydus	Bolus(1.5gm) Tablet (150 mg)	Fenbendazole:1.5 gm/bolus; 150 mg/tablet
FENTAS 1.5 gm	Neovet Intas	strip of 4 bolus	each bolus contains 1.5 gm fenbendazole
FENTAS 3 gm	Neovet Intas	strip of 1 bolus	each bolus contains 3 gm fenbendazole
FENTAS powder	Neovet Intas	6 gm sachet, 60 gm, 120 gm container	Each gram powder contains fenbendazole 250 mg.
Fenzole Bolus / Tablet	Jeps Pharma	5x 10's Blister/Strip 25x2's Blister/Strip	Fenbendazole 1.5 gm., 2.0 gm., 150 mg.
PANACUR	Intervet	150mg tablet; 1.5	each 150 mg tab contains

<table>
<tr><td>bolus/tablet</td><td></td><td>gm bolus (@1.5 gm/300 kg bwt)</td><td>fenbendazole 150 mg; each 1.5 gm bolus contains fenbendazole 1.5 gm</td></tr>
<tr><td>PANACUR Bolus/Tablet</td><td>Intervet</td><td>6 gm sachet, 60 gm, 120 gm container</td><td>Each gram powder contains fenbendazole 250 mg.</td></tr>
<tr><td>RANGFEBEN DA Granules</td><td>Cipla</td><td>Pk. of 50sachets of 12gm each</td><td>Fenbendazole 20%</td></tr>
<tr><td colspan="4">FENBENDAZOLE COMBINATION</td></tr>
<tr><td>FENTAS PLUS</td><td>Neovet</td><td>strip of 6 bolus</td><td>each bolus contains Praziquantel 50 mg + Fenbendazole 150 mg</td></tr>
<tr><td>Eazypet Meltab</td><td>Neovet</td><td>Strip of 2 tablets, box of 10 strips
Dose rate : 1 tablet for 10 kg BW orally</td><td>Each uncoated tablet contains
Praziquantel : 50 mg
Pyrantel Pamoate: 144 mg
Fenbendazole : 150 mg</td></tr>
<tr><td>PRAZITAL PLUS</td><td>Indian Immunologi cal</td><td>strip of 2 tabs one tab/10 kgBW oral</td><td>Each uncoated tablet contains
Praziquantel : 50 mg
Pyrantel Pamoate: 144 mg
Fenbendazole : 150 mg</td></tr>
<tr><td colspan="4">LEVAMISOLE: Mechanism of action : It stimulates the ganglia in worms, causes tonic paralysis which results in expulsion of live worms. Also affects fumarate reductase and energy metabolism. Indications : Ascariasis, Canine hookworm infections. Immunopotentiator.
DOSAGE
Treatment: 7.5 mg/kgBW oral, s/c single dose.
Immunostimulant: 2.5 mg/kgBW oral, s/c single dose.
Contraindications : Known hypersensitivity, preexisting blood disorders.
Status in
1. Pregnancy : Use with caution
2. Lactation : Contraindicated.
Interactions : Disulphiram reaction with alcohol.</td></tr>
<tr><td>ALMIZOL POWDER</td><td><u>Alembic Limited</u></td><td>100 g PACK</td><td>Each gm contains : Levamisole HCL : 300 mg
Dissolve 5 g in 200 ml water (100 g in 4 Litres) One ml of the solution to be given orally / kg.b.wt. or as per direction</td></tr>
<tr><td>Ventrimisole</td><td>VENTRI BIOLOGIC ALS</td><td>100 g and 500 g</td><td>Levamisole Hydrochloride B.P. ...... 30% w/w
Deworming: 50 g per 50 L – for 500 layers or 1000 chicks after starving</td></tr>
</table>

			for 4 hours *Immunostimulant:* 15 g per 1000 birds
LEVAMISOLE HCl 30%	Novartis	HDPE Bottle 1 kg	*Deworming:* 50 g per 50 L – for 500 layers or 1000 chicks after starving for 4 hours *Immunostimulant:* 15 g per 1000 birds Levamisole HCl 30%
Levacip 1000	Cipla	50 Boli	Levamisole 1 gm Bolus
Levacip Powder	Cipla	1/2kg1kg container	Levamisole 10% Powder
Levacip 400 bolus	Cipla	50 Boli Carton	Levamisole 400mg Bolus
Levacip 600 bolus	Cipla	50 Boli Carton	Levamisole 600mg Bolus
LEVAMISOLE COMBINATION			
ENDEX 8.75% suspension	Novartis	HDPE bottle 60 ml, 250 ml	Triclabendazole 5% + Levamisole 3.75 %
ENDEX 19.5 % suspension	Novartis	HDPE bottle 30ml, 60 ml, 250 ml	Triclabendazole 12 % + Levamisole 7.5 %
Levoxy	Cattle Remedies	5x4 bolus 90ml, 1 litre suspension (4 boli / large animal once Orally; 90 ml / cattle / once orally)	Levamisole HCl 1.5 %w/v + Oxyclozanide 3 % w/v
Anthelmect Injection	Cipla	50ml	Closantel [as HCL] 50mg/ml+ Levamisole [as HCL] 100mg/ml
Levoxy Bolus	Cipla	10 x 5 boli	Levamisole HCL 1.125gm + Oxyclozanide 1.4gm
Levoxy Bolus	Cipla	10 x 5 boli	Levamisole HCL 1.125gm + Oxyclozanide 1.4gm
Levoxy Suspension	Cipla	1 litre can	Levamisole Hydrochloride 3% w/v + Oxyclozanide 6% w/v Suspen

MEBENDAZOLE:

Mechanism of action : Similar to albendazole. It has produced nearly 100% cure rate / reduction in egg count in round worm, hook worm (both species), and Trichuris infestations, but is much less active on Strongyloides. The immobilizing and lethal action of mebendazole on worms is rather slow : takes 2-3 days to develop. Absorption of mebendazole from intestines is minimal; 75-90% of an oral dose is passed in the feces. The fraction absorbed is excreted mainly as inactive metabolites in urine/faeces. Destroyes cytoplasmic microtubules in worm's intestinal cells.

Indications :Nematode +/ Cestode infestation. Round worm, hook worm, Trichuris, Hydatid disease.

DOSAGE

Dose: Cattle, Buffalo, Horse, pig, sheep: 10-15 mg/kg BW Oral; Dog/cat: 22 mg/KgBW x 3 days, oral. **Contraindications** : Known hypersensitivity.

Special precautions : Hepatic impairment, monitor blood count.

Status in

1. Pregnancy : Use with caution.
2. Lactation : Use with caution.
3. Old age : May be used.
4. Children : May be given.

Interactions : Fats increase absorption.

MEBEX	Cipla	strip of 6 tabs. Suspension 30 ml; powder 5 gm pouch	Each tab has 100 mg; Suspension has 100mg/5 ml; Powder has 200mg/5gm.
WORMIN bolus/powder	Cadila	strip of 6 tabs. Suspension 30 ml; powder 5 gm pouch	Each tab has 100 mg; Suspension has 100mg/5 ml; Powder has 200mg/5gm.
ZODEX	Concept	Powder 500 gm pouch; pack of 4 boli.	Each tab has 1000 mg; Powder has 500mg/5gm.
MEBENDAZOLE + PRAZIQUANTEL COMBINATION			
Combex Tablets	Cipla	10 tabs,25 tabs	Mebendazole 200mg +Praziquantel 50mg

MILBEMYCIN OXIME: blocks neurotransmission in parasite resulting flaccid paralysis. **Indicated** in canine heart worm disease, ancylostomiasis.

DOSAGE: Dogs: 0.5mg/KgBW oral.

INTERCEPTOR	Novartis	Tab	Each tab contains 2.3 mg, 5.75 mg, 11.5mg, 23 mg.

MORANTEL :

it is a depolarising neuromuscular blocker in nematodes and produces spastic paralysis of worms by cholinomimetic action. Indicated in nematodal infestation.

DOSAGE: Large animal: 10 mg/kgBW oral; Dog: 7.5 mg/kgBW oral; Pig: 15 mg/kgBW oral.			
BANMINTH	Pfizer	Tablet 10x10's	each tab contains 118.8 mg
BANMINTH FORTE	Pfizer	Bolus 5x4's	Each bolus contains 594mg
BANMINTH Oral solution 3 % w/v	Pfizer	solution 500 ml	solution contains 3 % w/v
BANMINTH powder	Pfizer	powder pack 20gm, 100gm	powder contains 9 % w/w
Exworm Tablets	Cipla	Box of 100 boli	Morantel tartarte 150mg
Exworm Tablets	Cipla	Box of 100 boli	Morantel tartarte 750mg
NICLOSAMIDE administered orally has a reputation for excellence against tapeworms and amphistomes. **DOSAGE** Cattle : 1 gm/ 5 kg body weight orally Sheep & goat : 1 gm / 2.5 kg body weight orally Dogs : 1 gm / 2.5 kg body weight orally or as direceted by the Veterinarian.			
Niclex 25 powder	Alved	**PACKAGE** NICLOSAMIDE powder : 100 gms	Niclosamide B.P.(Vet) 25 % w/v
NITROXYNIL: it is substituted phenol compound. Active against liverfluke. **Dose** rate: 10 mg/kg PO			
Nitroxinil 25% w/v	Cipla	250ml,50ml	Nitroxinil 25% w/v
Nitronix Injection	Cipla	250ml,50ml	Nitroxinil 25% w/v
OXIBENDAZOLE +NICLOSAMIDE COMBINATION			
Anthelmex Bolus	Cipla	30 boluses	Oxibendazole 350mg +Niclosamide 3650 mg
OXYCLOZANIDE Oxyclozanide kills the flukes by uncoupling of oxidative phosphorylation in the fluke. Oxyclozanide causes a rapid (0.5 hr.) spastic paralysis of the fluke. Oxyvlozanide quickly reaches its peak concentration in the blood after treatment and its excretion is equally rapid. Therefore Oxyclozanide is effective against the fluke resistance to other Salysalinides e.g. Rafoxanide and Closantel. **Indications** : For the treatment and control of Fascioliasis and Amphistomiasis in cattle, buffaloes,			

sheep and goats. Moneizia tapeworm infestation and in ducks against Notocotylus fluke. Oxyclozanide is only choice of drug for Amphistomiasis. It is the only flukicide with short preslaughter withdrawl period and zero milk discard time.
DOSAGE : ruminants and duck : 10-15 mg/kg P.O.
Oxyclozanide is safe for pregnant, debilated and milking animals.

PRODUCT	COMPANY	PRESENTATION	COMPOSITION/DOSAGE
NEOZIDE bolus	Intas	strip of 4 bolus	each bolus contains 1 gm oxyclozanide 4 bolus per animal once
Clozan Tablet / Bolus	Jeps Pharma	5 x 10's Blister/Strip 25x2's Blister/Strip	Oxyclozanide 200 mg., 1 gm.
NEOZIDE suspension	Neovet	90 ml and 1 ltr bottle	Oxyclozanide 3.4% w/v. (90 ml per cattle PO)
Ocloz Bolus	Cipla	30 Boli	Oxyclozanide (Vet)-1.0gm
TOLZAN – F suspension	Intervet	90ml bottle, 1 litre plastic can	Each ml contains Oxyclozanide 34 mg. (10-15 mg/kg body wt. orally in ruminants)
ALZANIDE	Alembic Limited	1 litre. Bottle	Each ml contains : Oxyclozanide : 3.4 % w/v Cattle & Calves: 10 – 20 mg per kg.b.wt.
Hexanide	Sarabhai zydus	Bolus (1 gm) Suspension (90 ml)	Oxyclozanide: 1 gm/bolus; 3.4% w/v suspension (15 ml/50 kg b wt; 1 bolus/100 kg bwt)
ZANIL suspension	Virbac	100 ml bottle, 1 litre jar	Each 5 ml contains Oxyclozanide IP (Vet) 170 mg.
OXYCLOZANIDE COMBINATION : In ruminants, nematode infestation and fascioliasis.			
TOLZAN PLUS suspension	Intervet	1 litre plastic can (0.33 ml/ kg bwt or 10 ml/30kg b.wt. or 100 ml/300 kg b.wt.)	Each ml suspension contains Tetramisole HCl 30 mg + Oxyclozanide 30 mg
Levoxy	Cattle Remedies	5x4 bolus 90ml, 1 litre suspension (4 boli / large animal once Orally; 90 ml /	Levamisole HCl 1.5 %w/v + Oxyclozanide 3 % w/v

<table>
<tr><td></td><td></td><td>cattle / once orally)</td><td></td></tr>
<tr><td>NEOZIDE PLUS suspension</td><td>Neovet</td><td>90 ml, 500 ml, 1 ltr bottle</td><td>Levamisole HCl 3 % w/v + Oxyclozanide 6 % w/v</td></tr>
<tr><td>Nilzan suspension</td><td>Virbac</td><td>100 ml bottle, 500 ml bottle, 1 litre jar</td><td>Each ml suspension contains Tetramisole HCl 150 mg + Oxyclozanide 150 mg</td></tr>
<tr><td>Flukfree bolus, suspension</td><td>Panacia</td><td>1 bolus per animal
100 ml per animal</td><td>Levamisole HCl + Oxyclozanide</td></tr>
<tr><td>Curazan forte suspension</td><td>Curevet</td><td>100 ml per 300 kg bwt.</td><td>Oxyclozanide + fenbendazole</td></tr>
<tr><td colspan="4">PIPERAZINE: Mechanism of action : Piperazine causes hyperpolarization of ascaris muscle by a GABA agonistic action opening CI- channels that cause relaxation and depress responsiveness to contractile action of ACh. Flaccid paralysis occurs and worms are expelled alive. A considerable fraction of the oral dose of piperazine is absorbed. It is partly metabolized in liver and excreted in urine.
Indications : Second line drug against ascariasis.
DOSAGE
Cattle, Horse, Pig, Dog, Cat: 200-300 mg/Kg BW oral. Poultry: 300-400 mg/Kg BW oral. Repeat once every month Contraindications : Renal insufficiency.
Adverse drug reactions : Nausea, vomiting, abdominal pain, urticaria.
Status in
1. Pregnancy : May be used.
2. Lactation : May be used.</td></tr>
<tr><td>Piperazine Hexahydrate</td><td>Ventri Biologicals</td><td>450 ml and 4.5 Ltr</td><td>Piperazine Hexahydrate ...... 56.3% w/v
4 to 6 weeks: 25 mL per 100 birds in drinking water
6 weeks and above: 40 mL per 100 birds drinking water</td></tr>
<tr><td>Knock 45 liq 45 %</td><td>Sarabhai Zydus</td><td>100ml, 500 ml, 5 ltr.</td><td>45 % w/v piperazine hydrate</td></tr>
<tr><td>Piperazine liquid</td><td>Virbac</td><td>30 ml and 500 ml</td><td>45g piperazine hydrate /100ml</td></tr>
<tr><td>Piperol</td><td>Indian Immunological</td><td>500 ml, 5 ltr jar</td><td>45%w/v piperazine hydrate</td></tr>
<tr><td colspan="4">PRAZIQUANTEL:
Belnogs to group Isoquinolones. Mechanism of action : It is rapidly taken up by</td></tr>
</table>

susceptible worms and appears to act by causing leakage of intracellular calcium from the membranes ® contracture and paralysis. The tape worms lose grip of the intestinal mucosa and are expelled. At relatively higher concentrations, it causes vacuolization of the tegument and release of the contents of tape worms and flukes followed by their destruction by the host. Praziquantel is rapidly absorbed from intestines and undergoes high first pass metabolism in liver which limits its systemic bioavailability. It crosses blood-brain barrier and attains therapeutic concentrations in the brain and CSF. Maximal blood levels are achieved 30-60 minutes after administration. The plasma t½ is short, metabolites are excreted mainly in urine. Avoid in neonates below one month of age.

Indications : Cestode infestation, Schistosomiasis. (kills Both adult and larvae stage)

DOSAGE : Dogs/cat: 5-10mg/kg BW, Oral.

DRONCIT	Bayer	Tab	each tab contains 50mg
PARATAK	Sarabhai Zydus	Tab	each tab contains 50 mg.
PRAZIQUANTEL COMBINATION			
FENTAS PLUS	INTAS	strip of 6 bolus	each bolus contains Praziquantel 50 mg + Fenbendazole 150 mg
Eazypet Meltab	Intas Pharmaceutical	Strip of 2 tablets, box of 10 strips Dose rate : 1 tablet for 10 kg BW orally	Each uncoated tablet contains Praziquantel : 50 mg Pyrantel Pamoate: 144 mg Fenbendazole : 150 mg
PRAZITAL PLUS	Indian Immunological	strip of 2 tabs one tab/10 kgBW oral	Each uncoated tablet contains Praziquantel : 50 mg Pyrantel Pamoate: 144 mg Fenbendazole : 150 mg
WORMNIL Oral Paste	Cipla	32.4 gm Syringe	Abamectin 3.7 mg / Praziquantel 46.2 mg per gm Oral Paste
Prazivet plus XL Tablets	Cipla	10 tabs	Praziquantel 175mg + Pyrantel embonate 504mg + Febantel 525mg
Prazivet Tablets	Cipla	10 Tab	Praziquantel 20 mg + Pyrantel Pamoate 230 mg Tablets
Prazivet plus Tablets	Cipla	20 Tabs	Praziquantel 50 mg +Pyrantel Pamoate 144 mg +Febantel 150mg Tabs
Prazix tablets	Cipla	100 tabs	Praziquantel 50mg + Pyrantel embonate 140mg + Oxantel embonate 545mg

PYRANTEL PAMOATE: Tetrahydropyrimidines.

Mechanism of action : Pyrantel causes activation of nicotinic cholinergic receptors in the worms resulting in persistent depolarization, slowly developing contracture and spastic paralysis. Worms are then expelled. Only 10-15% of an oral dose of pyrantel pamoate is absorbed , this is partly metabolized and excreted in urine.

Indications : Nematode, Ancylostona infestations.

DOSAGE: Horse: 6.6 mg/Kg BW PO; Dog: 5 mg/Kg PO.

Contraindications : Known hypersensitivity.

Special precautions : Hepatic impairment.

Adverse drug reactions : G.I. symptoms like nausea, vomiting, diarrhoea and abdominal cramps.

Status in

1. Pregnancy : Contraindicated
2. Lactation : Use with caution.

Pyrid Oral Paste	Cipla	26 gm Syringe	Pyrantel Embonate 11.41 gm / Syringe
PYRANTEL + FEBANTEL Combination			
Prantel Suspension	Cipla	50ml, 100ml Bottles	Pyrantel 14.4mg + Febantel 15.0mg/ml

RAFOXANIDE

Belongs to Salicylanilides. Prevents ATP synthesis in worms.

Indicated in adult and juvenile Fasciola, Haemonchus, Bunostomum infestation, Nasal bots and fly maggots.

DOSE: Cattle: 7.5 mg/Kg PO; repeat at 3 week interval. C/I in lactating animals.

- safe for pregnant and debilated animals.

RAFOXANIDE	USV	Powder 10 gm pack	powder 20% w/w
Flunide Suspension	Jeps Pharma	100 ml. Bottle 1 Lit. Bottle	Rafoxanide 3% w/v.
HEXANIDE	Medivet pharma	4 boli strip	Each bolus contains: Rafoxanide BP (Vet) : 750 mg
RANIDE	Glaxo	Powder 10 gm pack	powder 20% w/w
Rafocip Drench	Cipla	1 litre can	Rafoxanide 2.5% Drench
Rafocip 3 %	Cipla	1 litre can	Rafoxanide 3 % Drench
Rafocip 3% Gold	Cipla	1 litre can	Rafoxanide 3% Drench
RAFOXANIDE COMBINATION			
RANIZOLE suspension	Virbac	900 ml pack	Triclabendazole 14.6 % w/v + Rafoxanide 2.5 % w/v

FLUNIDE-LH FORTE suspension	Jeps	100 ml, 1 Ltr pack	Levamisole 1.5 % w/v + Rafoxanide 3.0 % w/v
TETRAMISOLE: Imidothiazole derivative. Action by spastic paralysis of parasite. Indicated in nematodal and filaroidal infection. **DOSE:** ➢ Cattle/Sheep/Goat/Horse/Pig: 7.5mg/kg BW Single dose oral. ➢ Poultry: 10gm/4 ltr water for 100 birds.			
NILVERM powder	Virbac	10 gm sachet, 100 gm tin	30 % w/w Tetramisole HCl
Tetramisole powder	Piya	100 gm	30 % w/w
INTAMISOL powder	Neovet	10 gm, 100 gm tin	30 % w/w
Tetracip bolus	Cipla	Pack of 48	Tetramisole 1.2gm Bolus
Tetracip 10%	Cipla	1/2kg , 1kg container	Tetramisole 10% Powder
Tetracip 30%	Cipla	1 kg container	Tetramisole 30% Powder
Tetracip Bolus	Cipla	48 Boli	Tetramisole 300 mg Bolus
Tetracip Bolus	Cipla	48 Boli	Tetramisole 600 mg Bolus
TRICLABENDAZOLE: Benzimidazole compound. Inhibits polymerization of tubulin in the parasite and blocks the glucose uptake. Interferes activity of enzyme fumarate reductase and blocks energy production in parasite, resulting death. Indicated for Trematodal infections. **Dose:** ➢ Cattle, Buffalo: 12 mg/kg BW Oral; ➢ Sheep/goat: 10 mg/KgBW oral.			
Fasinex 5% suspension	Novartis	HDPE bottle 1 lit, 500 ml, 250 ml	5 % w/w
Fasinex 900 mg bolus	Novartis	strip of 4 boli	250 mg / bolus; 900 mg / bolus
Trinex Bolus	Cipla	Pack of 50 boluses	Triclabendazole 1500mg
Trinex bolus	Cipla	50 boli	Triclabendazole 1500mg
Trinex bolus	Cipla	50 boli	Triclabendazole 600mg
Trinex Suspension	Cipla	1 Litre Can	Triclabendazole Suspension 10 %w/v
Trinex Suspension	Cipla	1 Litre Can	Triclabendazole Suspension 5 %w/v

TRICLABENDAZOLE COMBINATION			
FASIMEC suspension	Novartis	HDPE bottle 500 ml	Triclabendazole 5% + Ivermectin 0.1% w/v
ENDEX bolus	Novartis	4 x 4 boli	Triclabendazole + Levamisole
ENDEX 8.75% suspension	Novartis	HDPE bottle 60 ml, 250 ml	Triclabendazole 5% + Levamisole 3.75 %
ENDEX 19.5 % suspension	Novartis	HDPE bottle 30ml, 60 ml, 250 ml	Triclabendazole 12 % + Levamisole 7.5 %
RANIZOLE suspension	Virbac	900 ml pack	Triclabendazole 12 % + Rafoxanide 2.5 %
OLGARD suspension	Neovet	500 ml bottle	each ml contains Triclabendazole 50 mg + Ivermectin 1 mg
HELINO suspension	Neovet	250 ml, 500 ml bottle	Triclabendazole 5% + Levamisole 3.75 %
Trinex Plus 19.5 % w/v	Cipla	1 Litre Can	Triclabendazole 12 % + Levamisole HCL 7.5 % Suspension
Trinex Plus 8.75 % w/v	Cipla	1 Litre Can	Triclabendazole 5 % + Levamisole HCL 3.75 % Suspension
MISCELLANEOUS PREPARATION			
Paraherb Powder	Cipla	50gm, 100gm , 500gm & 1 kg Jar	Herbal de-worming formula

ECTOPARASITIC PRODUCTS				
AMITRAZ : Ectoparasiticide. Tick, mite, lice, keds infestation in animals. Prevent licking.				
RIDD soln. 12.5 %	PETCARE	60 ml bottle	2-4 ml solution /litre of water for spray/dip	each ml contains Amitraz 125 mg
TAKTIC 5 % EC	INTERVET	25 ml bottle	6-10ml solution /litre of water for spray/dip	each ml contains Amitraz 50 mg
TAKTIC 12.5 % EC	INTERVET	50 ml bottle	2-4 ml solution /litre of water for spray/dip	each ml contains Amitraz 125 mg
Vetraz Liquid	Cipla	250ml bottle	2-4 ml solution /litre of water for spray/dip	Amitraz 12.5% BP Vet

Vetraz 12.5 %	Cipla	50ml, 100ml, 250ml, 500ml, 1ltr, 5 ltr	2-4 ml solution /litre of water for spray/dip	Amitraz Liquid dip concentrate 125 mg / ml
Vetraz 5 %	Cipla	50ml, 100ml, 250ml, 500ml, 1ltr, 5 ltr	2-4 ml solution /litre of water for spray/dip	Amitraz Liquid dip concentrate 50 mg / ml
CARBAMATES/CARBARYL: external parasites				
Notix scrub liq	Petcare	15g, 150 gm	apply over affected area	Carbamates 10 % w/v
Notix talc liq	Petcare	150 gm	apply over affected area	Carbamates 5 % w/v
Carbacip 10 % Powder	Cipla	100 gms jar ; 250 gms jar	apply over affected area	Carbaryal 100 mg/gm
Carbacip 5 % Powder	Cipla	100 gms jar ; 250 gms jar	apply over affected area	Carbaryal 50 mg/gm
Ektocip Liquid	Cipla	50ml, 250ml, 1000ml	apply over affected area	Cypermethrin 100EC
COUMAPHOS: organophosphorus Ectoparasiticidal. Antidote is atropine sulfate.				
Asuntol WP 50 powder	Bayer	15 gm pack	dissolve 500mg - 3 gm /litre water for external application	coumaphos 50 % w/w
Asuntol medicated soap	Bayer	soap	for bathing purpose	coumaphos 10g/kg
CYPERMETHRIN: pyrethroids are contact poison. Ectoparasiticidal.				
ECTOMIIN 100 EC	Novartis	15ml, 50ml, 1 litre	1ml/litre water is dissolved.	Cypermethrin Hi-Cis 10 % w/v
CLINAR liquid	Virbac	5 ml, 15 ml, 50 ml, 1 litre	1-2 ml/litre water is dissolved and applied over animal body.	Cypermethrin Hi-Cis 10 % w/v
CLINAR PET Anti tick wash	Virbac	100 ml bottle	wet the animal body and apply sufficiently over animal body	Cypermethrin Hi-Cis 1 % w/v

CYPROL	INTAS	15ml, 50 ml spray	1ml/litre water is dissolved for body spray	Cypermethrin High Cis 100 gm/litre
PEKTOCIDE	Sarabhai zydus	Solution (15 ml & 50 ml)	1 ml/liter water for spray or as per directions	Cypermethrin :100gm/liter
TIKKIL	Indian Immunological	5 gm sachet	Backline spray: 5 gm powder in a litre water. @ 0.5 liter/animal	Cypermethrin - High CIS 100 EC
TIK-OUT	ALEMBIC LTD	Shrink-wrapped aluminium bottles of 15ml, 50ml and 1litre	Dog: 1ml / litre whole body spray wash. Cattle & Sheep: One host / Multi host ticks, Scab / Mites &Lice: 1ml / lit. of water: whole body spray, dip, initial charge & replenishment. Flies: 5ml / lit. of water. Backing spray: 0.5lit. / animal dip. Animal housing: 2oml / lit. of water 5 Litres of emulsion per 100sq. meter surface.	Cypermethrin - High CIS 100 EC.
Ektocip 10 % Liquid	Cipla	50ml, 100ml, 250ml, 500ml, 1ltr, 5 ltr	Dog: 1ml / litre whole body spray wash. Cattle & Sheep: One host / Multi host ticks, Scab / Mites &Lice: 1ml / lit. of water:	Cypermethrin HI - Cis 10 % [Hydro dispersible concentrate] 100 mg / ml
Ektocip 10 % Powder	Cipla	10 gm pouch ; 15 gm pouch	Dog: 1ml / litre whole body spray wash. Cattle & Sheep: One host / Multi host	Cypermethrin HI - Cis 10 % [Water dispersible powder] 100 mg / gm

			ticks, Scab / Mites & Lice: 1ml / lit. of water:	

DELTAMETHRIN

Mode of action: It is a pyrethroid. Produce muscular excitation and convulsion delaying depolarization leading to rapid paralytic action on insects. Acts on sodium channels in nerve membranes and causes membrane depolasization and subsequent death of the target arthropod. It is active against strains resistant to organophosphorus compunds and also has highly consistent action. Control of tick, mite, lice, flies of livestock, pets & poultry.

ADMINISTRATION AND DOSAGE

	Mixing rate	Ticks	Mites	Lice	Flies
Spray or dips	PPM	25	50	12.5	25
	Almethrin/Lit. of water	2 ml	4 ml	1 ml	2 ml
Topping up	PPM	37.5	75	18.75	37.5
	Almethrin/Lit. of water	3 ml	6 ml	1.5 ml	3 ml

Butox	Intervet	15ml, 50 ml, 250 ml, 1 litre bottle	for spray/dip, 2-4 ml per litre water or as per direction	each ml contains deltamethrin 12.5 mg
ALMETHRIN VET	Alved	**PACKING** 1 Litre	for spray/dip, 2-4 ml per litre water or as per direction	Each ml contains: Deltamethrin 12.5 mg
MEGACIDE VET	B V biologicals	50 ml liquid pack	for spray/dip, 2-4 ml per litre water or as per direction	each ml contains deltamethrin 1.75 % EC
DELTARIN LIQUID	Cadila	'50 ML	for spray/dip, 2-4 ml per litre water or as per direction	Deltamethrin - 12.5 mg. Solvent and Emulsifiers - q.s.
Deltrin 1.25 %	Cipla	50ml, 100ml, 250ml, 500ml, 1ltr, 5 ltr	for spray/dip, 2-4 ml per litre water or as per direction	Deltamethrin 1.25 % [Hydro dispersible concentrate] 12.5 mg/ml
Deltrin 1.75 %	Cipla	50ml, 100ml, 250ml, 500ml, 1ltr, 5 ltr	for spray/dip, 2-4 ml per litre water or as per direction	Deltamethrin 1.75 % [Hydro dispersible concentrate] 17.5 mg/ml

Deltrin Pour On	Cipla	50ml, 100ml, 250ml, 500ml, 1ltr, 5 ltr	for spray/dip, 2-4 ml per litre water or as per direction	Deltamethrin 10 mg/ml
Deltrin 0.7 % Shampoo	Cipla	50ml, 100ml, 250ml, 500ml, 1ltr, 5 ltr	for spray/dip, 2-4 ml per litre water or as per direction	Deltamethrin shampoo 0.7 mg/ml
DIAZINON: organophosphorus Ectoparasiticidal. Act as contact and stomach poison. Produce spastic paralysis. Antidote is atropine sulfate.				
Neocidal 20 EC	Novartis	30ml, 100 ml, 1 lt, 5 lt	60ml/20 lit water for spray or as per advice	Diazinon organophorus 20% w/v
Diazin 2 % w/w	Cipla	100 gms jar ; 250 gms jar	60ml/20 lit water for spray or as per advice	Diazinon 2 % w/w powder 20.00 mg/gm
Diazin 20 % w/w	Cipla	100 gms jar ; 250 gms jar	60ml/20 lit water for spray or as per advice	Diazinon 20 % w/w powder 200.00 mg/gm
Diazin 60 % solution	Cipla	50ml, 100ml, 250ml, 500ml, 1ltr, 5 ltr	20ml/20 lit water for spray or as per advice	Diazinon 600 mg / ml
DICHLORVAS: organophosphorus Ectoparasiticidal. Act as contact and stomach poison. Produce spastic paralysis. Antidote is atropine sulfate. **Dose rate**: Horse: 50 mg/kg Bwt by stomach tube in case of bots, Cattle: 30 – 60 ml of 1% soln as mist spray/day for Rx of horn and face flies. Dog: 8.9 % colloar or 20 % tag				
NUVAN liq	Novartis	100ml, 200 ml, 1 lit	Cattle: 30 – 60 ml of 1% soln as mist spray/day	dichlorvas 76% v/v
Dichlovet 76 %	Cipla	50ml, 100ml, 250ml, 500ml, 1ltr, 5 ltr	Cattle: 30 – 60 ml of 1% soln as mist spray/day	Dichlorovos 76 % w/v Hydro dispersible concentrate 760 mg/ml
FENVALERATE: pyrethroids are contact poison produce muscular excitation and convulsion delaying depolarization leading to rapid paralytic action on insects. Control of tick, mite, lice, flies of livestock, pets & poultry.				

SUMICIDIN 20% EC soln.	Novartis	100ml, 250 ml, 500 ml, 1 ltr., 5 ltr.	0.5 ml/Ltr water for topical application	20% w/v
TICOMAX EC	VETNEX	100ml	2-6 ml / Ltr Water	20% w/v
Fenvet 20 %	Cipla	50ml, 100ml, 250ml, 500ml, 1ltr, 5 ltr	2-6 ml / Ltr Water	Fenvelarate 20 % [Hydro Dispersible concentrate] 200 mg/ml
FIPRONIL It is phenylpyrazole group compound. Has insecticidal and acaricidal activity.				
Protektor Spray	Cipla	100ml,250ml	0.5 ml/Ltr water for topical application	Fipronil 0.25% w/v spray
Protektor Spot on	Cipla	3 applicators of 0.67 ml	0.5 ml/Ltr water for topical application	Fipronil Liquid 9.7% liquid
Protektor Spot on	Cipla	3 applicators of 1.34 ml	0.5 ml/Ltr water for topical application	Fipronil Liquid 9.7% liquid
Protektor Plus Spot On	Cipla	3 applicators of 0.67 ml	0.5 ml/Ltr water for topical application	Fipronil Liquid 9.7%w/v + (s) methoprene 11.8%
FLUMETHRIN AND COMBINATION fly repellant, effective against tick, fleas				
Kiltix dog collar neckband	Pfizer	neckband collar	neck collar effective for 7 month	Propoxur 10% + Flumethrin 2.25 %
PORON LIQ.	ALEMBIC LTD	50ml self-applicator bottle.	Apply PORON at the rate of 1ml / 10kg b.wt evenly along the mid line of back from the mid shoulder to the tail setting.	Each ml of solution contains 10mg of Flumethrin.
Cipticol 1 % Pour On	**Cipla**	**50ml, 100ml, 250ml,**	1ml / 10kg b.wt evenly along the mid line of back from the	**Flumethrin 1 %w/v Pour on solution 10.00 mg/gm**

		500ml, 1ltr, 5 ltr	mid shoulder to the tail setting.	
GAMMA BENZENE HEXACHLORIDE **Indications**: maggotted wounds, follicular mange. Fly repellant property.				
ECTOZIDE	Balloun	200 gm powder	apply over affected area	Gamma Benzene Hexachloride 0.6%w/w
Scabicip Lotion	Cipla	100ml bottle	apply over affected area	Gamma Benzene Hexachloride 20% w/w
Loraxane cream and spray				
GAMMA BEZENE HEXACHLORIDE AND COMBINATION: maggot, follicular mange				
Healall cream	Novartis	100 gm	apply over affected area	Y-BHC 0.1% + Proflavin Hemisulfate 0.1% + Cetrimide 0.45 % w/w
Cipexane Cream	Cipla	30gm tube	apply over affected area	Gamma BHC 0.1% w/w + Proflavine Hemisulphate 0.1% w/w + strong Cetrimide solution eq. to Cetrimide 0.45% w/w
Lorexane cream	Virbac	20gm, 100 gm	apply over affected area	Y-BHC 0.1% w/w + Proflavin Hemisulfate 0.1% w/w + Cetrimide 0.45 % w/w
Gabex emulsion	IPCL	50ml, 300ml, 4.5 lit	apply over affected area	Y-BHC 0.1%w/w + Proflavin Hemisulfate 0.1% w/v
D'MAG spray	Neovet Intas	50 ml & 100 ml spray	spray twice a day over affeted area	Y-BHC 0.1% w/w + Proflavin Hemisulfate 0.1% w/w + Cetrimide 0.45 % w/w + Eucalyptus oil + Turpentine oil
IMIDACLOPRID: It is a chloronicotinyl compound. Acts by binding to postsynaptic nicotinic acetylchloine. It has residual insecticidal action.				
Terminator	Cipla	6	Use applicator for	Imidacloprid 9.1 %

<table>
<tr><td>Spot on</td><td></td><td>Applicators of 0.8ml</td><td>spotting in dogs.</td><td>Spot On</td></tr>
<tr><td colspan="5">LUFENURON: Inhibits formation of chitin in insect. It acts systematically prevent feeding flea from producing viable eggs or larvae. Indicated in Flea control in dogs</td></tr>
<tr><td>Program</td><td>Novartis</td><td>strip of 6 tab</td><td>1 tab once in a month for large breeds of dogs</td><td>each tab contains Lufenuron 409.8 mg</td></tr>
<tr><td>Flease Suspension</td><td>Cipla</td><td>Pack of 6 ampoules</td><td>one ampoule per dog once in a month</td><td>Lufenuron (acylurea) 133.0mg</td></tr>
<tr><td>Flease Tablets(Dogs between 6.8kg & 20kg)</td><td>Cipla</td><td>6 tabs</td><td>1 tab once in a month for large breeds of dogs</td><td>Lufenuron (acylurea) 204.9mg</td></tr>
<tr><td>Flease Tablets(Dogs between 21kg & 40kg)</td><td>Cipla</td><td>6 tabs</td><td>1 tab once in a month for large breeds of dogs</td><td>Lufenuron (acylurea) 409.8mg</td></tr>
<tr><td>Flease Tablets(Dogs between 2.4kg & 6.7kg)</td><td>Cipla</td><td>6 tabs</td><td>1 tab once in a month for large breeds of dogs</td><td>Lufenuron (acylurea)67.8mg</td></tr>
<tr><td colspan="5">PERMETHRIN : It is a potent insectiside, it causes neurological paralysis of the insects by inhibiting Na+ influx. Less than 2% of the drug is absorbed systemically and residual drug action persists for 10 days after application.
Indications : Scabies, pediculosis.
Dosage : Scabies : 5% solution is applied all over the body below neck followed by a bath after 10-12 hours.
Pediculosis : 1% cream is applied to the affected area and left for 10 minutes, it is rinsed off throughly with warm water.
Contraindications : Hypersensitivity, calves
Special precautions : For External use only.
Adverse drug reactions : Mild and transient, burning, itching, tingling, erythema, rash, numbness, edema.</td></tr>
<tr><td>SOFTAS medicated dog soap</td><td>Neovet Intas</td><td>75 gm soap</td><td>apply to work up rich lather and allow to remain for 10 min followed by rinsing</td><td>permethrin 1 % + aloe vera 0.5 %</td></tr>
</table>

			with clean water. Avoid in nursing bitches and neonates.	
Advance Spot on	Cipla	3 applicators of 2-cc, 3 applicators of 1-cc	use applicator to apply over the skin	Permethrin 65%
POLYHERBAL ECTOPARASITIC / MULTIPURPOSE FORMULATIONS				
ERINA-EP shampoo	Himalaya	200 ml	weekly shampooing	Each ml has Tailparni 9 mg, Vacha 8 mg, Sarapunkha 6.5 mg, Nimba 6.5 mg
ERINA-EP powder	Himalaya	150 gm	weekly shampooing	Each ml has Tailparni 100 mg, Vacha 50 mg, Sarapunkha 75 mg, Nimba 75 mg
Maggacite lotion	Cattle remedies	50ml, 100ml, 450ml	apply over affected area	herbal
MELICON V OINTMENT	Cadila	15 GM, 100 GM	15 gm per day PO in cattle	Melia Azadirachta (G. Limbdo) - 10 %Colour – Amaranth, Combined extract of Lawsonia Inermis (G. Mahendipan) and Swertia Chirata (G. Kariyatu) - 15%, Cedrus Deodara (G. Devdar) - 3%, Gardenia Gummifera (G. Dikamali) - 2%, Absorption Base q.s. - 100%
CANIFUR AZ LIQUID	Cadila	120 GM	ECTOPARACITICIDAL Herbal Product Fur conditioner	Combined Extract of Melia Azadirachta (S. Nimba) - 17.5 % Lawsonia Inermis (S. Medika) - 17.5% Cocos nucifera (S. Sadapushpa) - q.s.

CANIFUR LIQUID	Cadila	120 GM	ECTOPARACITICIDAL Herbal Product Fur condition	Combined Extract of Melia Azadirachta (S. Nimba) - 17.5 % Lawsonia Inermis (S. Medika) - 17.5% Base - q.s.
PETMOSOL SOAP	ICI	75 gm Soap	ECTOPARACITICIDAL	monosulfirum 5 % w/w
Pestorid	Cipla	100 ml, 500ml	parasite repellant	Herbal repellant of parasites

ENDECTOPARASITICIDAL PRODUCTS

DORAMECTIN: increases permeability of membrane to chloride ions which inhibits electrical activity of nerve cells in neamtodes, resulting paralysis and death of parasites. Indicated in nematodal infection, ectoparasitic infestation, larval stage of Canine Heart Worm Disease.

DOSE: Cattle, Sheep, Goat, Horse, Pig, Dog: 200 mcg/kgBw SC.

Dectomax	Pfizer	20ml, 50 ml	200 mcg/kg bwt SC	Doramectin 10mg/ml
Doramax	Cipla	50ml ,250ml & 500ml Vials	200 mcg/kg bwt SC	Doramectin 1 % w/v injection

IVERMECTIN

Mechanism of action : Ivermectin is an extremly potent semisynthetic derivative of the antimetodal principle obtained from *Streptomyces avermitilis* that has nemotades develop tonic paralysis when exposed to ivermectin. It acts through a special type of glutamate gated Cl- channel found only in invertebrates. Potentiation GABAergic transmission in the worm has also been observed. Single dose cures most cases. Ivermectinis is well absorbed orally, widely distrubuted in the body, sequestrated in liver and fat and has a long elimination t½ of 48-60 hours. Ivermectin interferes with the neuronal synaptic junction in both ecto (arthropods) and endo (nematodes) parasites. It causes hyperpolarization, bringing about flaccid paralysis of the worms causing their immediate expulsion. Ivermectin also interferes with the reproductive mechanism of the ecto and endo-parasites.

Indications :

Endoparasites: Roundworms , nasal bots, heartworms and hookworms.

Ectoparasites: Ticks, lice, mites and warble fly larvae.

Ivermectin is the only drug effective orally in scabies and pediculosis. Infections with intestinal nematodes like strongyloidiasis, ascariasis, trichuriasis. .

DOSAGE

- Cattle and sheep: 0.2 mg/kg BW orally and injectable. 0.5mg/kgBW for pour on formulation (Effective more against Ectoparasites).

➢ Pigs: 0.3 mg/kg BW subcut. ➢ Horses: 0.2 mg/kgBW orally. Trichostrongylus sp., Parascaris sp., Oxyuris spp., Strongylus spp., Dictyocaulus spp., Strongyloides spp., Habronema spp. and bots (Gastrophilus spp.) ➢ Dogs: 6 µg/kg BW subcut, oral at interval of 1 month. Contraindications : Known hypersensitivity, meningitis. Adverse drug reactions : Mild-pruritus, giddiness, nausea, abdominal pain, constipation, lethargy and transient ECG changes. Rarely fever, tachycardia, hypotension, myalgia, arthralgia and edema may occur. **WITHDRAWAL PERIOD:** Slaughter : 35 days Status in 1. Pregnancy : Use with caution 2. Lactation : Use with caution 3. Neonates : Contraindicated Interactions : Sedation with CVS depressants and Sod. Valproate.			
G-WORM-100 tab	Genesis	2 tabs	Each tab contains 100 mg
HITEK	Virbac	Injection (1ml, 10 ml, 50 ml vial) Oral liquid: 1 litre, 500ml, 100 ml bottle Powder: 1 kg jar	➢ Injection contains Ivermectin B.P. 1% w/v ➢ Oral liquid contains Ivermectin B.P. 0.08 % w/v ➢ Powder contains Ivermectin B.P. 1% w/w
HITEK POUR ON	Virbac	50 ml HDPE pack	Ivermectin: 0.5 %W/V
IVECTIN	Indian Immuno logicals	1 ml, 7 ml, 10 ml vial	Ivermectin: 1%W/V
Iverin inj.	Alved	10 ml vial	Ivermectin: 1%W/V
Ivocip Drench	Cipla	500ml, 1 litre can	Ivermectin drench 0.08%
IVEXIN	Sushima	3 ml	Ivermectin: 1%W/V
Ivocip Compact Oral Paste	Cipla	6.42 gm Syringe	Ivermectin 120mg/6.42gm
Ivocip Pour On	Cipla	100ml bottle	Ivermectin 500mg /100ml
Ivocip Oral Paste	Cipla	25 ml	Ivermectin 4.8 mg /ml Oral Paste

IVOMEC inj	Virbac	1 ml, 7 ml, 20 ml vial	Ivermectin: 1%W/V
IVOMEC oral solution	Virbac	50 ml, 250 ml, 1 litre	0.08% w/v
MECTIN INJECTION	ALEMBIC LTD	Vial of 1ml, 7ml, 10ml & 20ml.	Ivermectin: 1%W/V Cattle & Sheep: 0.2mg / kg.b.wt (1ml / 50kg b.wt.) through SC route only. Dog: 0.05 – 0.1mg / kg b.wt. (0.4mg /kg b.wt. in case of Toxocara canis infection)
NEOMEC inj	Neovet	1 ml, 7 ml vial 10 ml, 20 ml vial	Ivermectin B.P. 1% w/v
NEOMEC tab	Neovet	1 x 2 tabs	Ivermectin 10 mg / tab
Remover inj.	Marc	1 ml, 10 ml vial	Ivermectin: 1%W/V
		IVERMECTIN & COMBINATION	
Equicip Forte Oral Paste	Cipla	10gm tube	Ivermectin 12mg + Praziquantel 150mg/gm Oral Paste
Alverin plus inj.	Alved	1 ml, 2, 5, 7, 10, 20, 30, 50, 100 ml pack	Ivermectin 10mg + Chlorsulon 100 mg per ml
Olgard suspension	Intas	500 ml	Ivermectin 0.1%w/v + Triclabendazole 5%w/v
Heartcare Chewable Tablets(medium)	Cipla	6 tabs	Ivermectin 136mcg + Pyrantel 114mg
Equicip oral paste	Cipla	6.42 gm Syringe	Ivermectin 18.7mg + Praziquantel 140.3 mg /gm Oral Paste
Heartz for large dogs [For dogs 23-45 kgs]	Cipla	6 Tab	Ivermectin 272 mcg + Pyrantel Pamoate 227 mg Tablet
Heartcare Chewable Tablets (large)	Cipla	6 tabs	Ivermectin 272mcg + Pyrantel 227mg

Ivocip plus Injection	Cipla	50ml, 100ml, 500ml vial	Ivermectin 1.0% +Clorsulon 10%
Heartz[For dogs up to 11 kgs]	Cipla	6 Tab	Ivermectin 68 mcg + Pyrantel Pamoate 57 mg Tablet
Heartcare Chewable Tablets(small)	Cipla	6 tabs	Ivermectin 68mcg + Pyrantel 57mg
Heartz for medium dogs [For dogs 12-22 kgs]	Cipla	6 Tab	Ivermectin 136 mcg + Pyrantel Pamoate 114 mg Tablet
MOXIDECTIN + PRAZIQUANTEL COMBINATION			
Equipar Gel	Cipla	12.2 gm Syringe	Moxidectin 20mg + Praziquantel 125mg/gm

CLOSANTEL

Closantel is a salicylanilide derivative. Broad spectrum ectoendoparasiticide. closantel disturbs phosphorylation in liver fluke mitochondria It can restrain insect body phosphation of mitochondria procedure, head off insect body adenosine triphosphate (ATP) and that is energy procreative. Metabolize energy of worm is effected so that its action is weaken rapidly till dead. can absolutely kill the parasites in and out of body for pig's sarcoptes scabiei, blood louse, roundworm, strongyloides, kidney insect, whipworn; oxen bloody spear nematode berghei, face upward nematode, radiation esophagus nematode, massive fluke, fasciola hepatica, capillaria and melophagus grub; sheep's nasal grub, melophagus, sarcoptes scabiei, itch, nematode, Fasciola hepatica; horse stomach fly, dog demodectica, and so on. Keeping the pigs' farm not infected by parasite. Please use of yearly drive insect procedure: that is all the pigs are used once at the same time and then used once every 3 months.

Indicated in nematode, flukes, cestode, ectoparasite infestation. Safe for pregnant animals and neonates.

Dose rate 7.5-10mg/kg bwt orally

Withdrawal time: Non toxin side-effect

EXINOT liq	Cadila pharma	30 ml	closantel 15% w/v
Zycloz soln. / bolus	Sarabhai zydus	Solution (30ml, 500 ml), Bolus (1 gm)	Closantel 150 mg/ml; 1000mg / bolus (dose rate 1 ml/10-15 kg Bwt PO 1 bolus/66-100 Kg Bwt PO)

ZENVET suspension	Neovet	30ml, 100 ml, 500 ml	closantel 15% w/v
CLOSANTEL + Levamisole :			
Anthelmect Injection	Cipla	50ml	Closantel [as HCL] 50mg/ml+ Levamisole [as HCL] 100mg/ml

Chapter 3

Drugs for Cardiovascular System

ANTIARRHYTHMICS

- AMIODARONE, ATENOLOL, ATROPINE SULPHATE
- DILTIAZEM
- DISOPYRMAIDE
- LIGNOCAINE
- METOPROLOL
- MEXILITENE HCl
- PHENYTOIN
- PROPRANOLOL
- QUINIDINE
- VERAMPAMIL
- RAMIPRIL

ANTIARRHYTHMICS

1. AMIODARONE: exerts a class III type of antiarrhythmic action. Prolongs duration of action potential and refractory period of cardiac fibre. Indicated in severe refractory atrial and ventricular arrhythmias.
DOSAGE: Dogs: 10-20 mg/kg BW BID orally. Contraindicated in severe sinus node dysfunction, 2nd and 3rd degree AV block.

Product	Company	Presentation	Composition
AMIODAR 100	Microlabs	strip of 10 tabs	each tab contains amiodarone 100 mg
EURYTHMIC	Troikaa	tab	each tab contains 100 mg and 200 mg

2. **ATENOLOL:** a cardio selective B1 adrenergic blockinig agent which reduces resting and exercise induced heart rate. Indicated in atrial and ventricular arrhythmia, hypertrophic cardiomyopathy, hypertension.
DOSAGE: Dogs: 0.25-1mg/Kg BW BID. Contraindicated in heart block 2nd / 3rd degree; uncopensated CHF, shock.

Product	Company	Presentation	Composition
Atecard	Dabur	strip of 14 tabs 25 mg, 50 mg, 100mg	each tab has 25 mg/ 50 mg / 100mg

<table>
<tr><td>Betacard</td><td>Torrent</td><td>strip of 14 tabs of 25 mg, 50 mg, 100mg</td><td>each tab has 25 mg/ 50 mg / 100mg</td></tr>
<tr><td colspan="4">3. ATROPINE SULPHATE: Abolishes Action Of muscarine and muscarinic actions of ACh, thus blocking cardiac vagus. Indicated in sinus bradycardia, cardiac arrhythmia, AV block, vagal syncope.
DOSAGE: Dog: 0.04 mg/kg BW TID IM, IV, SC. Overdosing may lead to atropine poisoning. Antidote is barbiturate.</td></tr>
<tr><td>Atropine Sulphate</td><td>Morvel</td><td>Injection 10 ml vial</td><td>0.6 mg/ml</td></tr>
<tr><td>Atropine Sulphate</td><td>Universal Medikit</td><td>Injection 10 ml vial</td><td>0.6 mg/ml</td></tr>
<tr><td>Tropine inj</td><td>Neon labs</td><td>Injection 1ml ampoule</td><td>0.6 mg/ml</td></tr>
<tr><td colspan="4">4. DILTIAZEM: Blocks L type calcium channel present in the heart and blood vessels. Indicated in supraventicular arrhythmias, hypertrophic cardiomyopathy, hypertension.
DOSAGE: Dogs: 0.1-1.5 mg/kg BW TID. Contraindicated in AAV block, hypotension, sick sinus syndrome.</td></tr>
<tr><td>Channel</td><td>Microlabs</td><td>strip of 10 tabs of 30 mg, 60 mg</td><td>30 mg and 60 mg in each tab</td></tr>
<tr><td>Dicard</td><td>Intas</td><td>strip of 10 tabs of 30 mg, 60 mg</td><td>30 mg and 60 mg in each tab</td></tr>
<tr><td colspan="4">5. DISOPYRMAIDE: depressant action on the heart. Indicated in ventricular tachyarrhythmia, supraventricular arrhythmias.
DOSAGE: Dogs: 10-20 mg/Kg BW BID oral. Contraindicated in diabetes mellitus, CHF, sick sinus syndrome, hypokalemia.</td></tr>
<tr><td>Norpace</td><td>Searle</td><td>pack of 10 caps of 100 mg, 150 mg</td><td>caps of 100 mg, 150 mg</td></tr>
<tr><td>Regubeat</td><td>Biddle Sawyer</td><td>strip of 30 tabs of 100 mg</td><td>tab of 100 mg</td></tr>
<tr><td colspan="4">6. LIGNOCAINE: local anesthetic with myocardial depressant action. Indicated in arrhythmia associated with gneral anesthesia and digitalis induced arrhythmia.
DOSAGE: Dogs: 1-2 mg/kg BW as bolus injection IV. CNS seizures may be evident follwing excess dosage.</td></tr>
<tr><td>Gesicain</td><td>S G pharma</td><td>30 ml vial injection</td><td>2 % w/v</td></tr>
<tr><td>Xylocaine</td><td>Astra IDL</td><td>30 ml vial injection</td><td>2 % w/v</td></tr>
</table>

<table>
<tr><td colspan="4">7. METOPROLOL: cardio selective B1 adrenergic blocking agent. Indicated in atrial and ventricular arrhytmia, hypertrophic cardiomyopathy.
DOSAGE: Dogs : 0.5 mg/kg BW TID oral. Contrindicated in heart block, uncompensated in CHF, shock.</td></tr>
<tr><td>Betaloc</td><td>Astra IDL</td><td>5x5 ml vial; strip of 10 tab of 50 mg, 100 mg</td><td>each tab contains 50 mg, 100 mg; Each ml has 1 mg/ml</td></tr>
<tr><td>Lopresor</td><td>Novartis</td><td>strip of 10 tab of 50 mg, 100 mg</td><td>each tab contains 50 mg, 100 mg;</td></tr>
<tr><td colspan="4">8. MEXILITENE HCl: class 1B antiarrhythmic. Indicated in ventricular arrhythmia.
DOSAGE: Dogs : 5-8 mg/kg BID oral. C/I in severe heart block, sick sinus syndrome.</td></tr>
<tr><td>Mexitil</td><td>German Remedies</td><td>pack of 10 caps of 50 mg, 150 mg</td><td>each cap contains 50 mg, 150 mg</td></tr>
<tr><td colspan="4">9. PHENYTOIN: class I antiarrhythmic agent with anticonvulsant action. Indicated in digitalis induced arrhythmia, status epilepticus. DOSAGE: Dogs : 2 mg / kg BW IV (max total dose upto 10 mg/KgBW). Infusion rate 25-50 mg/min; Oral dose : 15-40 mg / kg BW TID. C/I in severe heart block, sick sinus syndrome.</td></tr>
<tr><td>Epsolin</td><td>Cadila</td><td>inj 2 ml ampoule</td><td>each ml has 50 mg.</td></tr>
<tr><td colspan="4">10. PROPRANOLOL: Beta adrenergic blocker. Indicated in atrial and ventricular tachyarrhytmia, thyrotoxicosis. DOSAGE: Dogs : 0.2 -1 mg / kg BW TID increasing over 3-5 days to 1 mg/kg BW TID orally.</td></tr>
<tr><td>CORBETA</td><td>Sarabhai Zydus</td><td>strip of 10 tabs</td><td>each tab has 40 mg</td></tr>
<tr><td>INDERAL</td><td>ICI</td><td>strip of 10 tabs</td><td>each tab has 10 mg, 40 mg</td></tr>
<tr><td colspan="4">11. QUINIDINE: reduces rate of depolarisation of cardiac action potential, slows depolarisation and prolongs refractory period. Indicated in ventricular and supra ventricular arrhythmia, conversion of atrial fibrillation. DOSAGE: Dogs: 6-20 mg / kg QID orally. C/I in advanced heart block and sick sinus syndrome.</td></tr>
<tr><td>QUINIDINE</td><td>Burroughs Wellcome</td><td>strip of 100 tabs</td><td>each tab has 200 mg</td></tr>
<tr><td colspan="4">12. VERAMPAMIL: calcium channel blocker. Class IV papaverine derivative. Indicated in supraventricular tachycardia, sustained and paroxysmal tachycardia. DOSAGE: Dogs: 0.05 – 0.2 mg/kg BW slow IV as bolus injectionat 0.05 mg/kg in 10-30 min interval; 1-2 mg/kg BW TID oral.</td></tr>
<tr><td>CALAPTIN</td><td>Boehringer Mannheim</td><td>strip of 10 Tabs and injection of 2 ml ampoule</td><td>each tab has 40 mg and 80 mg; injection has 5 mg/2 ml.</td></tr>
<tr><td colspan="4">13. RAMIPRIL: It is vasodilator. Indicated in congestive heart failure.
Dose: 1.25 mg per adult large breed dog orally.</td></tr>
<tr><td>Heartsup 1.25 mg</td><td>Cipla</td><td>14 tablets</td><td>Ramipril 1.25 mg tablets</td></tr>
</table>

Heartsup 2.5 mg tablet	Cipla	14 tablets	Ramipril 2.5 mg tablets
Heartsup 5.0 mg tablet	Cipla	14 tablets	Ramipril 5.0 mg tablets

ANTIHAEMORRHAGIC/HEMOSTATICS

- ADRENALINE
- ADRENOCHROME MONOSEMI CARBAZONE
- ETHAMSYLATE/CYCLONAMINE
- HAEMOCOAGULASE
- MISCELLANEOUS PRODUCTS

ANTIHAEMORRHAGIC / HEMOSTATICS			
ADRENALINE: potent alfa agonist with a pressor action on smaller arterioles and precapillary sphincters. Indicated in epistxis, minor hemorrhage. Applied locally.			
ADRENOCHROME MONOSEMI CARBAZONE : reduces capillary fragility, effecting haemostatic action. Indicated in internal hemorrhages, hemogalactia.			
Product	**Company**	**Presentation**	**Composition**
ADCHROME	G. Loucatos	injection 10 ml vial.	5 mg/ml
STYPTOCHROME	Dr Reddy's	2 ml ampoule	750 mcg/ml
ETHAMSYLATE/CYCLONAMINE: action is attributed by stabilising capillary wall. Indicated in internal hemorrhages, hemogalactia. **DOSE** : 250-500 mg total QID IM, IV (cattle, dogs)			
DICYNENE	Dr Reddy's	2 ml ampoule	125 mg/ml
CLOTEX	Pranav Agro	20 ml vial	Ethamsylate 125 mg/ml
ETHAMSYL	Mejda	2 ml ampoule	125 mg/ml
HAEMOCOAGULASE: enzyme from venom of vipers Bothrops jacaraca or B. atrox. It acts on fibrinogen to produce a fibrin monomer which can be converted by thrombin into clot. **Dose** : 0.5-1.0 ml IM in dogs. C/I in thrombosis.			
BOTROPASE inj	Juggat	1 ml ampoule	1 unit per ml
REPTILASE inj	Troikaa	1 ml ampoule	1 unit per ml

MISCELLANEOUS PRODUCTS			
CADISPER-C inj	Cadila	strip of 2 tabs Dogs: 2 tabs TID orally	each tab contains hesperidin, rutin, vitamin C, adrenochrome semicarbazone, menadione, DCP
REIVICI inj	Kee pharma	5 ml vial. Dose: 5-10 ml IM, IV; local	each inj contains N-butanol, citric acid
Styplon Vet	Himalaya	strip of 4 bolus 1-2 bolus daily BID	Herbal
ERYTHROPOEITIC/HAEMATINIC PREPARATIONS			
FERITAS bolus	Neovet	1x5 boli	Each bolus has Ferrous Sulfate 1.5 gm + Vit B12 + Folic acid
IMFERON	Shreya	10x2ml Inj	Iron dextran equiv to 50mg elemental iron/ml
IMFERON F-12	Shreya	2x10x2ml	Fe dextran 50mg, Vit B12, Folic Acid/ml
IMFERON MD	Shreya	10ml Vial Inj	Fe dextran 50mg/ml
IRONA	Sayona	200ml Syr	Each ml contains Iron 250mg, Vit. B12 2.5mcg, Folic Acid 500mcg, L-Lysine Mono HCl 25mg
IRONA-P3	Sayona	10 Tab; 200ml Syr	Each tab/ml contains Elemental Iron 100mg, Folic Acid 350mcg

ANTIARRHYTHMICS

- AMIODARONE, ATENOLOL, ATROPINE SULPHATE
- DILTIAZEM
- DISOPYRMAIDE
- LIGNOCAINE
- METOPROLOL
- MEXILITENE HCl
- PHENYTOIN
- PROPRANOLOL
- QUINIDINE
- VERAMPAMIL

ANTIARRHYTHMICS

1. **AMIODARONE:** exerts a class III type of antiarrhythmic action. Prolongs duration of action potential and refractory period of cardiac fibre. Indicated in severe refractory atrial and ventricular arrhythmias. Dogs: 10-20 mg/kg BW BID orally. Contraindicated in severe sinus node dysfunction, 2nd and 3rd degree AV block.

Product	Company	Presentation	Composition
AMIODAR 100	Microlabs	strip of 10 tabs	each tab contains amiodarone 100 mg
EURYTHMIC	Troikaa	tab	each tab contains 100 mg and 200 mg

2. **ATENOLOL:** a cardio selective B1 adrenergic blockinig agent which reduces resting and exercise induced heart rate. Indicated in atrial and ventricular arrhythmia, hypertrophic cardiomyopathy, hypertension. Dogs: 0.25-1mg/Kg BW BID. Contraindicated in heart block 2nd / 3rd degree; uncopensated CHF, shock.

Product	Company	Presentation	Composition
Atecard	Dabur	strip of 14 tabs 25 mg, 50 mg, 100mg	each tab has 25 mg/ 50 mg / 100mg
Betacard	Torrent	strip of 14 tabs of 25 mg, 50 mg, 100mg	each tab has 25 mg/ 50 mg / 100mg

3. **ATROPINE SULPHATE:** Abolishes Action Of muscarine and muscarinic actions of ACh, thus blocking cardiac vagus. Indicated in sinus bradycardia, cardiac arrhythmia, AV block, vagal syncope. Dog: 0.04 mg/kg BW TID IM, IV, SC. Overdosing may lead to atropine poisoning. Antidote is barbiturate.

Product	Company	Presentation	Composition
Atropine Sulphate	Morvel	Injection 10 ml vial	0.6 mg/ml
Atropine Sulphate	Universal Medikit	Injection 10 ml vial	0.6 mg/ml
Tropine inj	Neon labs	Injection 1ml ampoule	0.6 mg/ml

4. **DILTIAZEM:** Blocks L type calcium channel present in the heart and blood vessels. Indicated in supraventicular arrhythmias, hypertrophic cardiomyopathy, hypertension. Dogs: 0.1-1.5 mg/kg BW TID. Contraindicated in AAV block, hypotension, sick sinus syndrome.

Product	Company	Presentation	Composition
Channel	Microlabs	strip of 10 tabs of 30 mg, 60 mg	30 mg and 60 mg in each tab
Dicard	Intas	strip of 10 tabs of 30 mg, 60 mg	30 mg and 60 mg in each tab

5. **DISOPYRMAIDE:** depressant action on the heart. Indicated in ventricular tachyarrhythmia, supraventricular arrhythmias. Dogs: 10-20 mg/Kg BW BID oral. Contraindicated in diabetes mellitus, CHF, sick sinus syndrome, hypokalemia.

Norpace	Searle	pack of 10 caps of 100 mg, 150 mg	caps of 100 mg, 150 mg
Regubeat	Biddle Sawyer	strip of 30 tabs of 100 mg	tab of 100 mg
6. **LIGNOCAINE:** local anesthetic with myocardial depressant action. Indicated in arrhythmia associated with gneral anesthesia and digitalis induced arrhythmia. **Dose :** Dogs: 1-2 mg/kg BW as bolus injection IV. CNS seizures may be evident follwing excess dosage.			
Gesicain	S G pharma	30 ml vial injection	2 % w/v
Xylocaine	Astra IDL	30 ml vial injection	2 % w/v
7. **METOPROLOL:** cardio selective B1 adrenergic blocking agent. Indicated in atrial and ventricular arrhytmia, hypertrophic cardiomyopathy. **Dose :** Dogs : 0.5 mg/kg BW TID oral. Contrindicated in heart block, uncompensated in CHF, shock.			
Betaloc	Astra IDL	5x5 ml vial; strip of 10 tab of 50 mg, 100 mg	each tab contains 50 mg, 100 mg; Each ml has 1 mg/ml
Lopresor	Novartis	strip of 10 tab of 50 mg, 100 mg	each tab contains 50 mg, 100 mg;
8. **MEXILITENE HCl:** class 1B antiarrhythmic. Indicated in ventricular arrhythmia. **Dose :** Dogs : 5-8 mg/kg BID oral. C/I in severe heart block, sick sinus syndrome.			
Mexitil	German Remedies	pack of 10 caps of 50 mg, 150 mg	each cap contains 50 mg, 150 mg
9. **PHENYTOIN:** class I antiarrhythmic agent with anticonvulsant action. Indicated in digitalis induced arrhythmia, status epilepticus. **Dose :** Dogs : 2 mg / kg BW IV (max total dose upto 10 mg/KgBW). Infusion rate 25-50 mg/min; Oral dose : 15-40 mg / kg BW TID. C/I in severe heart block, sick sinus syndrome.			
Epsolin	Cadila	inj 2 ml ampoule	each ml has 50 mg.
10. **PROPRANOLOL:** Beta adrenergic blocker. Indicated in atrial and ventricular tachyarrhytmia, thyrotoxicosis. Dogs : 0.2 -1 mg / kg BW TID increasing over 3-5 days to 1 mg/kg BW TID orally.			
CORBETA	Sarabhai Zydus	strip of 10 tabs	each tab has 40 mg
INDERAL	ICI	strip of 10 tabs	each tab has 10 mg, 40 mg
11. **QUINIDINE:** reduces rate of depolarisation of cardiac action potential, slows depolarisation and prolongs refractory period. Indicated in ventricular and supra ventricular arrhythmia, conversion of atrial fibrillation. **Dose :** Dogs: 6-20 mg / kg QID orally. C/I in advanced heart block and sick sinus syndrome.			
QUINIDINE	Burroughs Wellcome	strip of 100 tabs	each tab has 200 mg
12. VERAMPAMIL: calcium channel blocker. Class IV papaverine derivative. Indicated in supraventricular tachycardia, sustained and paroxysmal tachycardia. **Dose :** Dogs: 0.05 – 0.2 mg/kg BW slow IV as bolus injectionat 0.05 mg/kg in 10-30 min interval; 1-2 mg/kg BW TID oral.			

CALAPTIN	Boehringer Mannheim	strip of 10 Tabs and injection of 2 ml ampoule	each tab has 40 mg and 80 mg; injection has 5 mg/2 ml.

INOTROPIC DRUGS

- AMRINONE
- DIGOXIN
- DOBUTAMINE
- DOPAMINE

VASODILATORS

- CAPTOPRIL.
- ENALAPRIL
- ISO SORBIDE DINITRATE
- PRAZOSIN
- SODIUM NITROPRUSSIDE

INOTROPIC DRUGS

AMRINONE: positive inotropic agent. Inhibits phosphodiesterase with vasodilation. Indicated in short term management of severe myocardial failure.

DOSAGE: Dogs: 1-3 mg/kg bolus inj. Then 10-100 mcg/kg/min constant rate infusion.

Product	Company	Presentation	Composition
AMICOR inj	**Win Medicare**	20 ml vial	100 mg/20ml

DIGOXIN: cardiotonic glycoside. Increases intracellular concentration of free ions in the myocardial fibre, increases contractility of myocardium resulting positive inotropic effect. indicated in atrial tachycardia, CHF.

DOSAGE: Dogs: 5-10 mcg/kg BW BID oral maintenance dose. Loading dose: 0.02 mg/kg IV

CARDIOXIN	**Novartis**	strip of 10 tabs, injection 10 ml.	Each tab has 0.25mg. Inj has 0.5mg/2ml.
DIGOX	Cadila	strip of 10 tabs,	Each tab has 0.25mg.

DOBUTAMINE: sympathomimetic. Stimulates Beta-1 receptors of the heart, increases stroke volume and cardiac output. Used for short term management of severe myocardial failure, septic shock, cardiac surgery.

DOSAGE: Dogs: 5-20mcg/kgBW/min. C/I in hypertrophic cardiomyopathy.

Cardiject inj 250	Sun pharma	20 ml vial	each 20 ml has 250 mg.
Kardia inj	Panacea	5 ml vial	250 mg/5ml

DOPAMINE: antishock drug with positive inotropic and chronotropic action. Indicated in severe myocardial failure, shock, endotoxic septicemia, renal failure, chronic cardiac decompensation, trauma. **DOSAGE:** Dogs: 2-20 mcg/KgBW/min (titrate upto effect). C/I in tachyarrhythmia.

Dopamine inj	TTK	5 ml vial	200 mg/5 ml
DOPAPLUS	VHB	5 ml ampoule	200 mg/5 ml

VASODILATORS

1. **CAPTOPRIL:** inhibits angiotensin converting enzyme (ACE) reducing angiotensin II level and increasing bradykinin level; which reduces aldosterone and sodium water retention. Indicated in CHF and hypertension.

DOSAGE: Dogs: 0.5-1 mg/kgBW TID orally. C/I in hypotension.

Aceten	Wockhardt	strip of 10 tabs	each tab has 25 mg
Captopril	Lupin	strip of 10 tabs of 12.5 mg, 25 mg	each tab has 12.5 mg or 25 mg.

2. **ENALAPRIL:** ACE inhibitor. inhibits angiotensin converting enzyme (ACE) reducing angiotensin II level and increasing bradykinin level; which reduces aldosterone and sodium water retention. Indicated in CHF and hypertension. **DOSAGE:** Dogs: 0.25-0.5 mg/kgBW BID orally. C/I in hypotension.

BQL	Cadila	strip of 10 tabs	each tab has 2.5 mg, 5 mg, 10 mg, 20 mg.
Enapril	Intas	strip of 10 tabs	each tab has 2.5 mg, 5 mg, 10 mg, 20 mg.
Enpril	Wockhardt	strip of 10 tabs	each tab has 2.5 mg, 5 mg, 10 mg.
Vivipril	Sarabhai	strip of 10 tabs	each tab has 2.5 mg, 5 mg, 10 mg.

ISO SORBIDE DINITRATE: nitrovasodilator. Relaxes plain muscle, low dose dilates venous capacitance vessels thereby reducing venous return. At higher doses, arterioles are dilated reducing afterload. Indicated in CHF. **DOSAGE:** Dogs: 0.22-1.1 mg/kg BW BID orally. C/I in cerebral hemorrhage, increased intracranial pressure, severe anemia.

CARDICAP	Natco	strip of 100 tabs	each tab has 10 mg
SORBITRATE	Nicholas Piramal	strip of 50 tabs and 100 tabs	each tab has 5mg, 10 mg

PRAZOSIN: alfa-1 adrenoceptor blocker. Indicated in CHF, Hypertension.
DOSAGE: Dogs: 1mg/15 kg BW TID oral, titrate up to effect. C/I in CHF due to mechanical obstruction.

Minpress XL GITS	Pfizer	strip of 15 tabs	each tab has 2.5 mg, 5 mg.
Prazopress	Sun pharma	strip of 10 tabs	each tab has 1mg, 2 mg.

SODIUM NITROPRUSSIDE: relaxes vascular smooth muscle. Dilates peripheral arteries and veins. Reduces both preload and afterload which reduce work load on the heart. Indicated in severe CHF. **DOSAGE:** Dogs: 1-10 mcg /kgBW/min in dextrose 5%, titrate upto effect. C/I in hypertension.			
PRUSIDE	Troikaa	injection 5 ml amp	50mg/5ml
SONIDE	Gufic	injection 5 ml amp	50mg/5ml

Chapter 4

Drugs for Gastrointestinal System

ANTACIDS/ANTIBLOAT/ANTIZYMOTICS:

- ALUMINIUM HYDROXIDE COMBINATION;
- ACTIVATED DIMETHICONE,
- MISCELLANEOUS PREPARATION

ANTACIDS/ANTIBLOAT/ANTIZYMOTICS				
ALUMINIUM HYDROXIDE COMBINATION: Ruminal acidosis, grain overload, gastritis, peptic ulcer, dyspepsia. **Dose** rate: Ruminants: 1 gm/kg body weight oral; Dogs: 100-200 mg total dose, oral. Chronic ingestion may lead to hypophosphatemia, increased resorption of calcium.				
PRODUCT	COMPANY	PRESENTATION	DOSE RATE	COMPOSITION
Digene gel	Knoll pharma	200 ml suspension	Dogs: One tsf TID P.O.	Each 100 ml contains: Dried Al(OH) gel 830 mg, Methyl polysiloxane 25 mg, $Mg(OH)_2$ 185 mg, Na Carboxy methyl cellulose 100mg
Gelusil-MPS	Parke Davis	170 ml, 400 ml suspension	Dogs: One tsf TID P.O.	Each 5 ml contains: Dried Al(OH) gel 250 mg, Methyl polysiloxane 20 mg, $Mg(OH)_2$ 200 mg
Mucaine suspension	Wyeth Iederle	200 ml	Dogs: One tsf TID P.O.	Each 5 ml contains: Dried Al(OH) gel 291 mg, Oxethazine 10 mg, $Mg(OH)_2$ 98 mg
Siloxogene gel	RPG	180 ml gel	Dogs: One tsf TID P.O.	Each 10 ml contains: Dried Al(OH) gel 300 mg, Methyl polysiloxane 40 mg, $Mg(OH)_2$ 150 mg
ACTIVATED DIMETHICONE (SIMETHICONE): Bloat, Tympany. **DOSE:** Cattle/buffalo: 100 ml (1% w/v emulsion); Sheep/goat: 20 ml				

BLOTOSIL susp.	Wockhardt Limited	Liquid 100 ml	Oral: 100 ml of Bloatosil orally or as per direction of veterinarian	Simethicone B. P. : 1 % w/v
Blotocare	Neospark	Liquid 100 ml	Oral: 100 ml orally or as per direction of veterinarian	Simethicone B. P. : 1 % w/v
Blotonil susp	Jeps	Liquid 100 ml	Oral: 100 ml orally or as per direction of veterinarian	Simethicone B. P. : 1 % w/v
GASTINA liquid	Virbac	100 ml bottle	Oral: 100 ml orally or as per direction of veterinarian	Simethicone B. P. : 1 % w/v Dil oil : 0.5 %
Nobloat	Cipla	Bottle of 100ml	Oral: 100 ml orally or as per direction of veterinarian	Silica in Dimethicone suspension 1% + Dilloil 0.5%
MISCELLANEOUS PREPARATION:				
AFANIL	Dabur	100 ml liq.	50 ml bid orally/day	Herbal preparation
Blotinox	Cattle remedies	100 ml, 450 ml	100 ml oraliy/day	Herbal preparation
Bufzone	Intas	200 gm sachet	200 gm daily x 3 days in cows	Rumen alkaliser
Timpol	Natural remedies	100 gm, 1 kg bag	80 gm in water q 3-4 hrs orally	Herbal mixture
Tyrel	Natural remedies	100 ml pack	100 ml orally per day	herbal mixture
SODACARB	ICON BIOLOGICAL PVT. LTD.	10 ml Injection	30 - 50 ml at 12 hours interval by IV with normal saline(large animals)	Sodium Bicarbonate IP - 7.5 mg / ml
TYMPLAX	Balloun	100 ml emulsion	100-140 ml orally per day	Formalin 3%w/v, arachis oil 35%w/v
TYMPGO emulsion	Triveni	100 ml	100 ml Per os once	Flax oil, Terpene oil, Heeng emulsion

ANTIDIARRHEAL PRODUCTS				
Product	**Company**	**Presentation**	**Dose rate**	**Composition**
3-care bolus	Vetcare	1.5 g bolus	1-2 boli BID (cattle)	Halquinol: 1.5 gm/bolus
Band bolus	Panacea pharma	4 boli pack	2 boli per day	Each bolus contains: Norfloxacin 1200mg + Tiinidazole 1800 mg
Becknor bolus	Natural remedies	bolus	1 bolus BID in cattle	herbal
BOVISCORE bolus	Indus Healthcar e	10 x 2 Strips	Large Animals 2 boli per day	Halquinol 1500mg Loperamide 7.5mg
Catorrhea	Cattle remedies	100 g, 1 kg, tabs	25-50g BID or 3-4 tabs TID in cattle	herbal
Centrogyl LM	Century	Bolus	4-6 boli/day large animal	Each bolus contains : Metronidazole 1 g + Furazolidone 500mg + Loperamide 75 mg
CHQ-60 powder 12%w/w	Sarabhai zydus	1 kg polypack	250 – 500 gm/ton feed of poultry	Halquinol: 12% w/w
COLIDOX powder	Vetcare	500 gm, 25 kg pack	500 gm/ton feed in broilers daily	(Colistin SO_4: 1 g + Doxycycline 10 gm)/kg powder
CULEX bolus	Univet	8x4 boli	1 bolus / 50 kg bwt bid	Each bolus contains Furazolidone 200 mg + Metronidazole 1g
DIAREX	Himalaya	strip of 4 boli	2 boli twice daily in large animals	polyherbal
Diaroak	Dabur	dry suspension (30g, 400g, 1 Kg, 2.5 kg)	30 gm/day in cattle or as per direction	herbal

Laybro mix powder	Glaxo	1 kg, 5 kg	500 gm/ton feed in broilers daily	(Colistin SO4: 1 g + Doxycycline 10 gm)/kg powder
Lomotil	RPG	tabs	2-5 mg total dose in dogs	Diphenoxylate 2.5 g
Lopamide	Torrent	2 mg tab	100 mcg/kg bwt orally in dog	Loperamide 2mg / tab
MARCOGYL bolus	Marc India Ltd	Blister of 4 boli and Box of 10 blisters	Large animals: 2-4 boli/day for 3-5 day, Small animal : 1-2 boli/day for 3-5 days,	Each bolus contains: Quinolone :1,000mg Furazolidone : 500 mg Kaolin : 2 gm
MARCOGYL LM	Marc India Ltd	Blister of 4 boli and Box of 10 blisters	Large animals: 4-6 boli/day for 3-5 day, Small animal : 1-2 boli/day for 3-5 days,	Each bolus contains: Metronidazole:1,000mg Furazolidone : 500 mg Loperamide HCl : 7.5 mg
Marcogyl TZ bolus	Marc	4 boli pack	2 boli per day	Each bolus contains: Norfloxacin 1200mg + Tiinidazole 1800 mg
METRONOR	P.C.I.	30ml Syrup	Dogs: One tsf BID	Each 5 ml contains Metronidazole 100mg, Norfloxacin 100mg
METRONOR M	Modern Pharma	30ml Susp	Dogs: One tsf BID	Norfloxacin 100mg, Metronidazole 100mg/5ml
Neblon powder	Natural remedies	100 gm pack, 1 kg bag	30-50 gm BID in cattle orally	herbal preparation
PESULIN bolus	Cadila	Bolus	4-8 boli/day/cow	Each bolus contains pectin 75 mg; Phthalyl sulphathiazole 1g; light kaolin 2 g; KCl 15.6 mg; NaCl 38.7 mg; K citrate 67.9 mg; Na acid

				phosphate 26.5 mg
SVIFTA bolus	Sarabhai Zydus Animal Health Limited	Strip of 4 boli	Large Animals 4-8 boluses twice daily	Each bolus contains : Phthalysulphathiazole I.P. : 1 g Light Kaolin I.P. : 3 g Pectin I.P. : 75 mg Potassium Chloride : 15.6 mg Sodium Chloride : 31.8 mg Potassium Citrate : 67.8 mg Na Acid Phosphate : 26.4 mg
Statz Syrup	Cipla	100ml, 500ml pack	20-50 ml per day in cattle	Herbal anti-diarrhoeal preparation
Diasulf Suspension	Cipla	225ml	10 – 20 ml per day large animal orally	Each ML contains:Sulphadimidine 21.3mg + Sulphaquanidine 21 Sulphadimidine 21.3mg + Sulphaguanidine 21.3mg + Sulphadiazine 28.4mg + Streptomycin sulfate 7.6mg+Neomycin sulpfate 1.8mg+Hyoscine hydrobromide 0.02mg+Sodium chloride 11.33mg+Calcium gluconate 2.2mg+Magnesium sulphate0.6mg+Potassium sulphate-3.6mg+Kaolin 103.3mg+Pectin 7.1mg+Glycine 20.9mg
Neoplus	Cipla	Pack of 6	12 gm per day	Neomycin -2.4gm +

Powder		sachets x12gm	in cattle orally	Sulphaguanidine – 24gm+Kaolin –24gm +Pectin –2.4gm
Tripar Powder	Cipla	100gm sachet	10 gm bid orally in cattle	Sulfadimidine Sodium 180 gm + Pyrimethamine HCl 15 gm + Furaltadone HCl 50 gm + Tetracycline HCl 10 gm + Vitamin A palmitate 10,000,000 IU + Vitamin K3 5 gm

ANTIEMETIC/GIT SEDATIVE

- ATROPINE SULPHATE
- DICYCLOMINE
- DOMPERIDONE
- METOCHLOPRAMIDE
- PROCHLORPERAZINE
- PROMETHAZINE
- TRIFLUPROMAZINE
- CIMETIDINE
- RANITIDINE
- SUCRALFATE

ATROPINE SULPHATE blocks muscarinic receptors of smooth muscle, cardiac muscle, secretory glands. It is used as antidote in organophosphorus poisoning, preanaesthetic.

Dose (IM/SC) is 0.25 mg/kg BW in cattle; 0.05 mg/kg BW in pig, horses; 0.2 mg/kgBW in dogs; 0.3 mg/kgBW in cats. Contraindicated in glaucoma, chronic respiratory disease, pyloric nephritis. Antidote is barbiturates

Product	Company	Presentation	Composition
Atropine sulphate inj	Morvel	10 ml vial	Atropine sulphate 0.6mg/ml
Atropine sulphate inj	Universal Medikit	10 ml vial	Atropine sulphate 0.6mg/ml

Tropine inj	Neon labs	1ml ampoule	Atropine sulphate 0.6mg/ml
DICYCLOMINE: antispasmodic, antiemetic; produces nonspcific direct relaxant action on smooth muscles. Indicated in colic, irritable bowel syndrome, abdominal pain. **Dose** rate is 0.5 mg/KgBW IM in ruminants, horses; 0.1 mg/kg BW TID IM in dogs. Avoid use in neonates, old age animals, urinary retention and GIT obstruction cases.			
Spasmo-Proxyvon	Wockhardt	injection 2ml, 30 ml	each ml contains 10 mg/ml
Spasmovet	Wockhardt	injection 30 ml	each ml contains 10 mg/ml
DOMPERIDONE: antiemetic. Indicated in symptomatic relief of vomiting. **Dose:** Dogs: 5-10 mg total dose BID orally. Contraindicated in G.I. obstruction and GIT haemorrhage.			
Domstal	Torrent	Tab	each tab contains 10 mg domperidone.
Domstal	Torrent	suspension 30 ml bottle	each ml contains 1 mg domperidone.
Endopace	Themis pharma	Tab	each tab contains 10 mg domperidone.
Endopace	Themis pharma	suspension 60 ml bottle	each ml contains 1 mg domperidone.
METOCHLOPRAMIDE: antiemetic action is attributed by specific dopamine antagonistic activity by blocking dopamine receptors. Indicated in vomiting due to gastritis, oesophageal reflux, impaction. **Dose**: Dog: 0.01-0.2 mg/kg BW I/V, I/M; 0.2-0.4 mg/kg BW oral.			
Perinorm	IPCA	tab, inj., liq	Injection contains 5 mg/ml; oral preparation contains 1mg/ml; each tab contains 10 mg.
Emenil	Astra IDL	tab; inj.	Injection contains 5 mg/ml; each tab contains 10 mg.
PROCHLORPERAZINE: phenthiazine derivative, very potent antiemetic. **Dose**: Dogs : 0.5 mg/kg BW TID, I/M; 1 mg/Kg BW TID orally. Contarindicated in glaucoma, GIT obstruction, and administration with epinephrine.			
Stemetil	Rhone poulenc	tab 5 mg; 25 mg	5 mg tab contains 5 mg prochlorperazine 25 mg tab contains 25 mg prochlorperazine
Stemetil inj	Rhone poulenc	1 ml ampoule	each ml contains 12.5 mg
PROMETHAZINE: antihistamine with sedative and antiemetic action. Indicated in vomiting and allergic disorders. **Dose**: Ruminants: 1.5-2.0 mg/kg BW IM; Dogs : 1.5-2.5 mg/kg BW oral, IM, IV.			
Avomine	Rhone poulenc	25 mg tab	promethazine 25 mg/tab

Phenergan	Rhone poulenc	tab 10mg; tab 25 mg; elixir 60ml; inj 2 ml	see products injection 25mg/ml tab 10mg, 25 mg; elixir: 5mg/5 ml
TRIFLUPROMAZINE: neuroleptic agent. Antagonise central dopamine D2 receptors. Prominent antiemetic activity. **DOSE:** Dog: 2-4 mg/kg BW IM, 1-2 mg/kg BW IV. Administration with epinephrine is contraindicated.			
Siquil injection	Sarabhai zydus	5 ml vial	Each ml has Triflupromazine HCl: 20 mg
CIMETIDINE: histamine receptor antagonist. Inhibits secretion of gastric acid and output of pepsin. Indicated in peptic ulcer, gastritis. **DOSE:** Dog : 5-10 mg/kg BW 2-4 times a day. High dose has antiandrogenic effect.			
Cimetidine-CHC	Cadila health care	tab	each tab has 200 mg cimetidine.
LOCK-2	Cadila	tab	each tab has 200 mg cimetidine
RANITIDINE: H_2 antagonist. Indicated in gastritis, GIT ulcer. Avoid use in pregnancy, lactation, renal disorder. **DOSE:** Dogs: 0.5 mg/kgBW oral, IM, IV, SC			
Aciloc	Cadila	tab, inj 2ml ampoule	tab has 150 mg, 300 mg. Injection has 50 mg/ 2 ml
Histac	Ranbaxy	tab, 2ml inj	tab has 150 mg, 300 mg. Injection has 50 mg/ 2 ml
Zinetac	Glaxo	Tab, 2 ml Inj	tab has 150 mg, 300 mg. Injection has 50 mg/ 2 ml
SUCRALFATE: cryoprotectant. Produce unlceradherent complex with proteinaceous exudate, inhibiting pepsin activity. **DOSE:** Dogs: 1 gm BID orally			
RACOLAT E	Reckitt & Colman	strip of 4 tabs	each tab has 1 gm sucralfate.
Sucrase	Alidac	strip of 4 tabs	each tab has 1 gm sucralfate.
Ulcerfate	Sun pharma	strip of 4 tabs	each tab has 1 gm sucralfate.
OMPERAZOLE: Proton pump inhibitor. Indicated in gastric ulcer. **Dose**: Dog: 0.7 mg/kg/day orally.			
E-gard	Cipla	6.15 gm Oral Paste in the Syringe	Omeprazole 37% w/w paste [Each syringe contains 2.28 gm of Omeprazole]
MISCELLANEOUS			
Atrospaz injection	Cipla	10ml vial	Papaverine hydrochloride 300mg + Atropine sulfate 30mg

GROWTH PROMOTER			
Trenbolone is a steroid used by veterinarians on livestock to increase muscle growth and appetite. Trenbolone compounds have a binding affinity for the androgen receptor three times as high as that of testosterone. Once metabolised, the drugs have the effect of increasing nitrogen uptake by muscles, leading to an increase in the rate of protein synthesis. It also has the secondary effects of stimulating appetite, reducing the amount of fat being deposited in the body, and decreasing the rate of catabolism.			
Gromax C Pellets	Cipla	Pellets	Trenbolone acetate 140mg + 17 beta Estradiol 28mg/pellet
Gromax X Pellets	Cipla	Pellets	Trenbolon acetate 140mg + 17 beta Estradiol 8mg/pellet
Gromax A Pellets	Cipla	Pellets	Trenbolon acetate 40mg + 17 beta Estradiol 8mg/pellet
Vitalife Powder	Cipla	Sachet of 100gms	Herbal performance enhancer

LAXATIVE & PURGATIVE

- BISACODYL
- DOCUSATES
- LACTULOSE
- MISCELLANEOUS PRODUCTS

LAXATIVE & PURGATIVE

BISACODYL: It is newer diphenylmethane. They are partially absorbed and re-excreted in bile; entero hepatic circulation is more important in Phenolphthalein. Bisacodyl is activated in the intestine by deacetylation. Then primary site of action is in colon; It causes muscles in the colon to contract and stool to pass. One or two semiformed motions occurs after 6-8 hours.

Indications : It is used to treat all forms of constipation and to cause evacuation of the colon, pre and post operative hemorrhoids, preparations of rectum and colon for radiological investigations.

Dosage :

Dogs/cats: 10mg Oral total dose

Interactions : Do not use antacids within 1 hour of the drug (enteric coated) intake.

Product	Company	Presentation	Composition
DULCOLAX	German Remedies	Tab 10x 10's	each tab contains 5 mg

JULAX	Rallis	Tab 10x10's	each tab contains 10 mg

DOCUSATES:

Mechanism of action : It is an anionic detergent and acts on intestinal mucosa to decrease net absorption of water, emulsifies colonic contents and increases penetration of water into faeces. It is a mild laxative, also used for sofetening ear wax.

Indications : Simple constipation, and adjuant to anthelmentic.

Dosage -

Dogs: 15-120 mg total dose. Cattle, Horse: 5-15 gm total dose.

Contraindications : Hypersensitivity, Intestinal obstruction, undiagnosed abdominal pain.

Special precaution : ***It should not be used with liquid paraffin, in hepatic insufficiency.***

Adverse drug reactions : Nausea, cramps and abdominal pain. Rarely causes hepatotoxicity.

Status in

1. Pregnancy : Use with caution.
2. Lactation : Use with caution.
3. Old age : Can be used.

Interactions : It can disrupt the intestinal mucosal barrier and enhance absorption of non-absorbable drugs like liquid paraffin.

LAXICON	Stadmed	Tab	100 mg per tab

LACTULOSE:

Mechanism of action : It is a semisynthetic disaccharide of fructose and lactose which is neither digested nor absorbed in the small intestine. It retains water osmotically and distends the bowel, also increases peristalsis indirectly.

Indications : Functional constipation. Also used in hepatic encephalopathy to reduce intestinal ammonia levels.

Dosage

Dog: 5-10 gm BID total dose Oral.

Contraindications : History of peptic ulcers, sub acute or acute intestinal obstruction. Avoid in cases with undiagnosed abdominal pain or vomiting, abdominal malignancy and in constipation due to hypothyroidism or drug induced.

Adverse drug reactions : Nausea, cramps, flatulence.

Status in

1. Pregnancy : Use with caution.
2. Lactation : Use with caution.
3. Old age : Use with caution.
4. Neonates : Not recommended.

DUPHALAC	Duphar Interfran	Liq 100 ml, 200 ml, 450 ml pack	667 mg/ml

MISCELLANEOUS PRODUCTS			
CREMAFFIN	Knoll	emulsion 200 ml (@ 5-10 ml/day orally small animals)	Each 15 ml contains Milk of Magnesia 11.25ml + Liquid Paraffin 3.75 ml
CREMAFFIN -FS	Knoll	100 gm pack (Small animal: 5 gm BID, PO)	Isaphgula husk 3.5gm/14.25 gm
PURSENNID	Novartis	Tablets	Senna glycosides as Calcium salt 18 mg in each tab

RUMENOTORICS / DIGESTIVE / PROBIOTIC PREPARATIONS				
Improves rumen ecology and stimulates appetite Indigestion, Anorexia, Rumen stasis, Anorexia, simple indigestion, revival of rumen microflora, moderate ruminal atony				
Product	**Company**	**Presentation**	**Dose rate**	**Composition**
Amyst bolus	Tineta pharma	2 boli strip	2 boli per day	Enzymic, prebiotic and mineral preparation
Ecotas bolus	Intas	2 boli strip	2 boli per day	contains Saccharomyces cerevisiae, Lactobacillus, Soya bean rich in Ca, P, Proteins
BIOBOOST BOLUS	Lyka	bolus	1-2 boli daily	prebiotic appetite stimulant
BIOBOOST POWDER	Lyka	powder	10 gm daily	prebiotic appetite stimulant
BIOBLOOM POWDER	Sarabhai Zydus	powder 250 gm pack	5 -10 gm daily PO	contains Saccharomyces cerevisiae, Lactobacillus, Soya bean rich in Ca, P, Proteins
BOVIRUM BOLUS	Sarabhai zydus	Blisters of 4 boli	3-4 boli per day	Each bolus contains Antimony K tartarte: 2 g Ferrous sulphate : 2 gm Copper sulphate: 50 mg Cobalt chloride : 100 mg
DIGEPLEX LIQ	Rallis	100 ml, 200 ml pack	5-10 ml daily BID in dogs orally	Each ml contains diastase 62.5mg, Pepsin 20 mg
FEEDON bolus	Virbac	2 boli pack	2 bolus daily in	Each bolus contains Choline tartarte: 18.2 mg

			cattle	Vit B12 40 mcg Thiamine mononitrate 45 mg Ferrous sulphate : 200 mg Cobalt chloride : 100 mg
LEVUCELL SC	BV Biologicals	100 gm, 1 kg, 5 kg	cattle: 5 gm daily PO; Horses: 6.5-10 gm daily PO (250 gm – 1 kg per ton feed)	each gram contains Live yeast Saccharomyces cerevisiae CNCM I – 1077 : 2000 million CFU
N-ZYME BOLUS	Univet	4x12 boli	2 boli BID	Live yeast culture, Bacillus subtilis, B. licheniformis
RUMEN-FS BOLUS	Alembic ltd	Blister of 4 boli & Box of 15 Strips	Cattle & Buffaloes - 2 boli twice daily, orally for at least 5days.	Each bolus contains: Ferrous sulphate I.P.: 1g Cobalt Chloride: 200mg Copper sulphate: 50mg Vitamin B1: 25mg Vitamin B12: 20mcg Dried yeast: 300mg Rumen stable enzymes + probiotic: 500mg
RUMICARE	Intervet	125 gm sachet	125 gm twice daily orally	each 125 gm contains: Ca propionate 60 gm; Methionine 5 gm; Picrorhiza extract 250 mg; Cobalt gluconate 40 mg; Vit B6 40 mg
ONFEED BOLUS	Cadila	'4 B	2 boli BID	Each Bolus contains- Nicotinamide - 100 mg., Copper Sulphate - 250 mg., Cobalt Cholride - 40 mg., Ferrous Sulphate - 500 mg., Dibasic Sodium Phosphate - 100 mg., Sodium Bicarbonate - 600 mg., Magnesium Trisilicate - 800 mg., Piper Nigrum - 100 mg., Zingiber Officinale - 20 mg., Andrographis Paniculata - 220 mg., Apium Graveolens - 100

				mg., Dried Yeast Powder - 700 mg., Lysine - 20 mg., Methionine - 20 mg., Dextrose - 500 mg.
PROBIOTICS FEED SUPPLEMENT				
PROBLEND powder	Virbac	1 kg pack	3-5 gm daily in adult cattle orally with feed	Each 1000 gm contains: Lactobacillus acidophilus: 90,000 million CFU Lactobacillus acidophilus : 45 000 million CFU Bacillus subtillis 30,000 million CFU Bacillus licheniformis 30,000 million CFU Saccharomyces cerevisiae: 125,000 million CFU Sea weed extract 100 gm Amylase: 24,000 units Phytase: 22,00,000 units Protease: 400,00,000 units Cellulase: 150-250 units Beta Galactosidase: 800-1000 units Lipase: 50-100 units Vit C 35 gm Vit B1 – 1 gm Vit B6 – 1 gm Vit E- 5000 IU Na benzoate 6 gm
ALVIZYME-PLUS	Alembic Limited	1 kg pack	250 Gm / ton of poultry feed.	Each 500g contains: Lactobacillus acidophilus: 5,00,000 million CFU Saccharomyces cerevisiae: 5,00,000 million CFU Amylase: 2,50,000 units Protease: 3,50,000 units Lipase: 20,000 units Cellulase: 30,000 units Phytase: 45,000 units Galactosidase: 45,000 units Glucanase: 70,000 units Pectinase: 1,20,000 units Xylanase; 35,000 units

Prozyme –B Powder	Cipla	10 kg	250 Gm / ton of poultry feed. 3-5 gm daily in adult cattle orally with feed	Amylase 2800-3000 microns /gm,Cellulase 400 – 500 microns/gm,Xylanase 500–550 microns/gm,Protease 750–850 microns/gm,BG 100-150 microns/gm,Pectinase 400–500 microns/gm
Prozyme –L Powder	Cipla	10 kg	250 Gm / ton of poultry feed. 3-5 gm daily in adult cattle orally with feed	Amylase 5000-6000 microns /gm,Cellulase 500 – 600 microns/gm,Xylanase 600 – 700 microns/gm Protease 1000–1200 microns/gm,BG 50–200 microns/gm,Pectinase 600-700 microns/gm,Phytase 400–450 micron/gm
CTC 15% Powder	Cipla	1kg, 25Kg	1 kg per ton feed	Chlortetracycline 150gms /kg
Prozyme B	Cipla	25kgs HDPE Bags	250 Gm / ton of feed.	Cocktail Enzyme for Broilers Amylase 2800 – 3000 u/gm + Cellulase 400 – 500 u/gm + Xylanase 500 – 550 u/gm + Protease 750 –850 u/gm + BG 100 – 150 u/gm + Pectinase 400 – 500 u/gm
Prozyme L	Cipla	25kgs HDPE Bags	250 Gm / ton of feed.	Cocktail Enzyme for Layers Amylase 5000 – 6000 u/gm + Cellulase 500 – 600 u/gm +Xylanase 600 – 700 u/gm +Protease1000 – 1200 u/gm + BG 150 – 200 u/gm + Pectinase 600 – 700 u/gm + Phytase 400 – 450 u/gm
Vetzole	Cipla	500 gm,	500 gm per	Furazolidone 20% Feed

		1kg, 5 kg	ton feed	supplement
Enerzer Powder	Cipla	500 gm , 1 kg	500 gm per ton feed	Virginiamycin 2 % Feed Supplement
HERBAL PREPARATION: indigestion, anorexia, ruminal stasis, flatulance				
APPETONIC	Himalaya	strip of 4 bolus, 100 gm sachet, 1 kg powder	50 gm/2 boli twice daily in large animal	polyherbal formulation
APPETONIC forte	Himalaya	15 gm sachet, 1 kg powder	15 gm twice daily in large animal	polyherbal formulation
CATONE	Cattle Remedies	100 gm, 200 gm, 400 gm, 1 kg pack	as per directions	herbal
DIGYTON	Himalaya	30 ml drops pack	3-5ml BID in dogs or as per advice	herbal
DIGYTON DROPS	Himalaya	30 ml bottle	1-3 ml twice daily in dogs or as per advice	polyherbal formulations
LINTO LIQUID	Cadila	'50 ml and 1 ltr.	25 ml PO BID	Acacia Catechu - 25% Phyllanthus Niruri - 40% Andrographis Paniculata - 25% base q.s. to make - 100%
LINTO CONCENTRATE	Cadila	'50 gm.and 1 kg. Aluminium sachets	25 gm BID PO	Acacia Catechu - 25% Phyllanthus Niruri - 40% Andrographis Paniculata - 25% base q.s. to make - 100%
ZIG UP	Natural remedies	125 ml bottle	5-10 ml daily orally in dogs	herbal
RUMBION Bolus	Indian Herbs	2 boli pack	2 boli BID PO	herbal
RUMISTRONG POWDER	APPETISER	10 gms. and 100 gms.	10 gm per day PO	Sunthi (DGV) - 11.54% w/w; Amruta (DGV) -

		pouch packs		9.62% w/w Ugragandha (DGV) - 7.69% w/w; Dhanyak (DGV) - 7.69% w/w; Shatpushpa (DGV) - 7.69% w/w; Devkusum (DGV) - 5.77% w/w; Atmagupta (DGV) - 3.85% w/w; Ashwabala (AB) - 3.85% w/w ; Sauvarchal (AB) - 3.85% w/w; Yavani (DGV) - 3.85% w/w; Saindhav (AB) - 3.85% w/w; Haridra (DGV) - 3.85% w/w; Yashtimadhu (DGV) - 1.92% w/w ; Amalki(DGV)- 1.92% w/w; Jirak (DGV) - 1.92% w/w; Marich (AB) - 1.92% w/w; Bahula (DGV) - 1.92% w/w
Tefrosol - Forte Liquid	Cipla	1 ltr, 5 ltr	20 – 30 ml per day in cattle orally	Each 5 ml contains Tephrosia purpurea 1000mg+ Andrographis paniculata 400mg+ Terminalia chebula 750mg+ Oscimum sanctum500mg+ Mahasudarshan kadha 250mg+ Phyllantus neruri 200mg
Bioliv Powder	Cipla	100 gm jar	10-20 gm per day in cattle	Herbal digestive stimulant and bowel regulator

Chapter 5

Drugs for Galactopoeitic System

1. INTRAMAMMARY INFUSION/TOPICAL PREPARATION
2. GALACTOGOGUES
3. CALCIUM/MINERALS PREPARATIONS FOR HIGH MILK PRODUCTION

INTRAMAMMARY INFUSION/TOPICAL PREPARATION			
Product	**Company**	**Presentation**	**Composition**
COBACTAN LC	Intervet	syringe	each syringe contains 75 mg Cefquinone
FLOCLOX-L ointment	Vetnex RFCL	30 gm syringe	Cloxacillin Na 200 mg/syringe
MAMAL	ALEMBIC	5 gm disposable syringe	each 5 gm syringe contains erythromycin 300 mg + Neomycin 250 mg + Bacitracin 2000 IU
MAMMITEL ointment	Intas Neovet	10 gm syringe	Each syringe contains Colistin Sulfate: 5 lac IU; Cloxacillin Na 200 mg
MASTIJET FORT	Intervet	8 gm tube	each tube contains Tetracycline HCl 200 mg + Neomycin 250 mg+ Bacitracin 2000 IU + Prednisolone 10 mg
MASTILEP ointment	AYURVET	100 gm tube	Herbal
PENDISTRIN-SH ointment	Sarabhai Zydus	6 ml tube	Each tube has Procaine Penicillin 1 lac IU+ streptomycin SO_4 100 mg + Sulfamerazine 500 mg + Hydrocortisone 29 mg
TILOX oint	Wockhardt	5 gm tube	Each tube contains Ampicillin Na 75 mg + Cloxacillin Na 200 mg
VETIMAST suspension	Novartis	10 gm tube	Cephacetrile Na 235 mg/tube

WISPREC ointment	Natural Remedies	25 gm tube	Herbal ointment
Clavet LC Infusion	Cipla	3 gm disposable syringe	Amoxycillin (as amoxycillin trihydrate) 200mg + Clavulanic acid (as potassium clavulante) 50mg
Megaclox Infusion (LC)	Cipla	5gm disposable syringe	Ampicillin Sodium & Cloxacillin Sodium Intramammary Infusion (LC) BP (Vet) for Mastitis 5gm syringe contains Ampicillin 75mg (as Ampicillin Sodium IP) Cloxacillin 200mg (as Cloxacillin Sodium IP)
Cefaject Infusion	Cipla	7gm Disposable Syringe	Cefaperazone (as sodium) + Procaine penicillin G 150,000 iu / 7 gm
Cefamast Infusion	Cipla	8gm disposable syringe	Cefquinome 75mg/8gm
Megaclox Lente Infusion	Cipla	7 gms disposable syringes	Cloxacillin benzathine 500mg + Ampicillin sodium 100mg /7gm
Multibact	Cipla	5gm disposable syringe	Procaine penicillin G 100,000 iu + Streptomycin sulphate 100mg + Neomycin sulphate 100mg + Prednisolone 10 mg / 5 gm

GALACTOGOGUES			
Product	**Company**	**Presentation**	**Composition/dose**
DUGDHDAN tab	Cattle Remedies	6x8's tab	Herbal/ 4 tabs BID in cows
GALOG	Natural Remedies	300 gm, 1 kg powder	Herbal/ 40-50 gm in 2 divided doses; cows; oral.
GROMILK	Alembic	500 gm powder; 100's tabs	Herbal; Cows: 50 gm daily orally; 10-15 tabs BID daily.
PAYAPRO	Ayurvet	4's boli	Herbal; 4 boli daily in cows orally.
GALACTIN	Himalaya	strip of 4 boli	Herbal; 4-6 boli post calving for 10 days in cattle

Morolac tablet	Cipla	Pack of 100 tablets	Herbal galactogogue
HILAK	AYURVET	1 KG PACK	Rumen bypass fat (50-200 gm per day in feed)
Caldhan	Ayurvet	1 ltr, 5 ltr pack	Ca, P, Vit.B12, Vit D3 (50 ml bid)

CALCIUM/MINERALS PREPARATIONS FOR HIGH MILK PRODUCTION				
Product	**Company**	**Presentation**	**Dose rate**	**Composition**
CALBOROL inj	Novartis	450 ml Bottle	250-450 ml slow IV in cattle	Calcium 1.85 % w/v. proportion of boric acid to Calcium in the inj 2.26 to 1
MIFEX injection	Novartis	450 ml bottle	250-450 ml slow IV in cattle	Calcium 1.85 % w/v. proportion of boric acid to Calcium in the inj 2.26 to 1; Magnesium hypophosphite 5 % w/v, Dextrose 20 % w/v
CALPAR	Cadila	1 Ltr. & 5 ltr. HDPE Jar	50 ml per day PO per cattle	Each 20 ml. contains : Calcium - 350 mg. Phosphorus - 170 mg. Vitamin B12 - 20 mcg. Vitamin D3 -1600 I.U.
CAL-D-PLUS DS	Cadila	'100 ml., 500ml., 1000 ml., 5000 ml.	50 ml per day PO per cattle	Each 5 ml. contains : Calcium Gluconate - 416.5 mg. Cholecalciferol (Vit D3) - 800 'i.u. Stomach Extract - 1.65 mg. Ferric Ammonium Citrate - 83.5 mg. Vitamin B12 - 8.35 mcg. Colour - Amaranth
ASCAL LIQUID	Alembic Limited	1ltr, 500 ml, 5 lit.	Cattle and Horses : 50 ml/day orally	Each 5 ml contains : Calcium Phosphate 0.24 g (equivalent to 0.21 g of $Ca_3(PO_4)_2$ Cholecalciferol (Vitamin D3) I.P. 500 I.U. Vitamin B 12 I.P. 7.5 mcg
ASCAL-FS	Alembic Limited	Pet Bottle of 500ml,	Cattle &Horse:	Each 100ml contains: Tricalcium Phosphate -

		HDPE jars of 1lit & 5lits	100ml/day Calves, Goat & Pig: 10ml twice daily Dogs: 5-10ml twice daily	4800mg Eq.to elemental Calcium - 1867mg Elemental Phosphorous - 955mg Cholecalciferol (Vitamin D 3) - 10000 IU Cyanocobalamine (Vitamin B 12) - 150mcg Magnesium sulphate Eq.to elemental Magnesium - 200mg Calory contents- 80calories/100ml
KALZOL D3 powder	Virbac	5 kg bag	5 kg in 5 tonne poultry feed	Each 20 ml. contains : Calcium - 1250 mg. Phosphorus - 625 mg. Magnesium : 1.05 mg Cholecalciferol (Vitamin D3) - 2500 IU
METABOLIT E powder	Virbac	50 gm sachet	50 gm BID during last month of preganancy in cattle	BALANCED MINERALS AND VITAMINS
HYPORID powder	Intas	250 gm apck	250 gm per day or as per advice	Anionic feed supplement

Chapter **6**

Drugs for Musculoskeletal System

ANTIHISTAMINIC PRODUCTS			
CHLORPHENIRAMINE MALEATE: mechanism of action : It is an alkylamine derivative with potent histamine H_1- receptor antagonist activity. **Indications** : Various skin allergies like eczema, contact dermatitis, urticaria and drug reactions. Also used in allergic rhinitis, pruritis and angioedma due to insect bites. **Dosage** : Cattle: 30-50 mg total dose I/M; Dogs: 0.4-2 mg/kg BW BID I/M			
Product	**Company**	**Presentation Dose rate**	**Composition**
ANISTAMIN	Neovet	10ml, 30 ml, 50ml vial 3-5 ml IM (Large animal)	Chlorpheniramine maleate: 10 mg/ml
PHENIRAMINE MALEATE inj.	Intervet	30 ml vial Canine :0.5-1 ml; large animal: 5-10 ml, IM or IV	Each ml contains pheniramine maleate 22.75 mg
CADISTIN injection	Sarabhai zydus	30 ml vial 5-10 ml IM (Large animal)	Chlorpheniramine maleate: 10 mg/ml
CATLAN inj Vet	Cattle Remedies	10 ml, 30 ml 5-10 ml IM (Large animal)	Chlorpheniramine maleate: 10 mg/ml
CHLORIL	TTK Pharma	10ml, 30ml vial Dogs & Cats - 0.5 ml, Large Animals- 5-10 ml, I/M route only	Each ml contains : Chlorpheniramine maleate IP 10 mg
CROMINE	Icon Biological Pvt. Ltd.	10ml, 30ml vial Dogs & Cats - 0.5 ml, Large Animals- 5-10 ml, I/M route only	Each ml contains : Chlorpheniramine maleate IP 10 mg
ZEET INJECTION	ALEMBIC LTD	Vial of 10ml & 30 ml Large animals: 3 - 5ml Small animals: 0.5 - 2ml by IM route only.	Each ml contains: Chlorpheniramine maleate: 10mg

2. PHENIRAMINE MALEATE:
Mechanism of action : It is an alkylamine derivative with histamine H_1 receptor antagonist activity and antimuscarinic and central sedative properties. Duration of action of 4-6 hours (Terminal half-life after oral administration 19 hours).
Indications : Allergic rhinitis, urticaria, dermatoses with pruritis, angioedema.
Dosage
Large animal: 5-10 ml IM; small animals: 0.5-1.0 ml IM
Adverse drug reactions : Abuse potential because of CNS activity, vision and GI disturbances, parasthesia, tinnitus, hypotension, arrythmias, giddiness, urinary retention.

AVIL Vet inj	Intervet	10 ml vial 5-10 ml per large animal IM or IV	each ml contains Pheniramine maleate 22.75 mg
HISLOC	Cadila pharma	10 ml, 30 ml vial	each ml contains Pheniramine maleate 22.75 mg

PROMETHAZINE: Phenothiazine derivative with sedative and antiemetic action. Indicated in Vomiting, allergic disorder.
Dose: Large animals: 1.5 mg – 2.0 mg/kg BW, oral IM; Dog: 1.5 mg – 2.50 mg/kg BW, oral IM. C/I alongwith epinephrine.

PHENERGAN	Rhone poulenc	Tab, Syrup 60 ml, Elixir 400 ml, Injection 2 ml	Tab has 10 mg, 25 mg. Syrup/elixir has 5 mg/5ml; Inj has 25mg/ml
PROMETHAZINE	Biomedica	inj 10 ml vial	2.5 % W/V, 5 %w/v

MUCSLE RELAXANTS

- SUCCINYL CHOLINE

NON STEROIDAL ANTIINFLAMMATORY DRUGS

- ACECLOFENAC& COMBINATION
- ANALGIN COMBINATIONS
- ANALGIN/METAMIZOLE
- ASPIRIN
- DICLOFENAC
- DICLOFENAC + PARACETAMOL
- IBUPROFEN
- KETOPROFEN

- MELOXICAM
- MELOXICAM + PARACETAMOL COMBINATION
- MISCELLANEOUS COMBINATION PRODUCTS
- NAPROXEN
- NIMESULIDE
- NIMESULIDE + PARACETAMOL COMBINATION
- PARACETAMOL
- PHENYL BUTAZONE

NEUROMUSCULAR DRUGS

- NEOSTIGMINE

RUBIFACIENTS AND TOPICAL AGENTS

MISCELLANEOUS PREPARATION

MUCSLE RELAXANTS

SUCCINYL CHOLINE: Interfere with ACh mediated depolarization of post synaptic membrane to produce skeletal muscle paralyzing effect. Indicated in orthopaedic problem, surgical intervention. Dogs: 0.3 mg/kg BW IV (as bolus injection), Cattle/goat: 0.01-0.02 mg/kg BW IV, Pig: 2 mg/kg BW IV, Horse: 0.08 mg/kg BW IV.

Product	Company	Presentation	Composition
SUXOMIN inj	**Neon labs**	10 ml vial	50 mg/ml
SCOLINE inj	Glaxo pharma	**2 ml vial**	50 mg/ml

NON-STEROIDAL ANTI-INFLAMMATORY DRUGS

ACECLOFENAC

an orally administered phenyl acetic acid derivatives with effects on a variety of inflammatory mediators.

MOA: Aceclofenac is a potent inhibitor of the enzyme cyclooxygenase, which is involved in the production of prostaglandins. The Drugs inhibits synthesis of the inflammatory cytokines interleukin (IL)-1 and tumor necrosis factor and prostaglandin E_2 (PGE2) production.

DOSAGE:

100 mg/100 kg bwt PO per day

Drug Interactions

Aceclofenac may increase plasma concentrations of lithium, digoxin and methotrexate, increase the activity of anticoagulant, inhibits the activity of diuretics, enhance cyclosporin nephrotoxicity and precipitate convulsions when co-administered with quinolone antibiotics.

SAFE-A	ZIPP pharma	**2 boli strip**	Each bolus contains Aceclofenac 400 mg + paracetamol 1500 mg
ANALGIN/METAMIZOLE Imidopyrin analgesic. Indicated in pain, fever, spastic condition, colic, inflammation. **Dose : Dogs**: 0.5-2.5 g total IM/IV; **Cattle**: 10-20 g IM/IV; **Horse**: 10-30 g IM/IV; **Pig**: 5-15 g IM/IV; Sheep, **Goat**: 1-4 g IM/IV.			
ANAKGIN inj	KAPL	Vial of 30 ml (20-60 ml IM or IV in large animals)	each ml contains 0.5 gm analgin
Vetalgin	Intervet	Vial of 30 ml (20-60 ml IM or IV in large animals)	each ml contains 0.5 gm analgin
ANALGIN COMBINATIONS:			
Esgipyrin –N injection	Sarabhai zydus	5 ml ampoule (5-15 ml deep IM)	Each ml has Phenylbutazone:150 mg Analgin: 150 mg Lignocaine HCl: 10 mg
PETOFEN inj	Marc	Vial of 30 ml (20-60 ml IM or IV in large animals)	each ml contains 0.5 gm analgin, Petofenone HCl 2 mg, Fenpiverinum Bromide 0.02 mg
POLYGESIC inj	Unichem	Vial of 10 ml, 30 ml (20-60 ml IM or IV in large animals)	each ml contains 0.5 gm analgin, Petofenone HCl 2 mg, Fenpiverinum Bromide 0.02 mg
ASPIRIN (Acetyl salicylic acid) Inhibit prostaglandin synthetase and prevents synthesis of Prostaglandin. Indicated in inflammation, pain, pyrexia. Cats are highly susceptible to aspirin toxicity. **Dose :** Dogs: 10-30 mg/kgBW BID Oral, Pig: 10 mg/kgBW BID Oral.			
COLSPRIN tab	Rackitt & Colman	strip of 10 tabs	each tab contains 325 mg, 650 mg.
ECOSPRIN	USV	strip of 10 tabs	each tab contains 325 mg.
CARPROFEN It is nonpsychotropic analgesic. **Dose**: Dogs- 4 mg/kg IV or S/C sid.			
Care-O-Pet Tablets	Cipla	60's container	Carprofen 100 mg chewable tablets
Care-O-Pet Tablets	Cipla	60's, 100's container	Carprofen 25mg chewable tablets
Carprofen 50 mg chewable	Cipla	60's, 100's container	Carprofen 50 mg chewable tablets

<table>
<tr><td>tablets</td><td></td><td></td><td></td></tr>
<tr><td>Care-O-Pet Tablets</td><td>Cipla</td><td>60's container</td><td>Carprofen 75 mg chewable tablets</td></tr>
<tr><td colspan="4">DICLOFENAC & Combination
Anti-inflammatory, antipyretic, analgesic actions. Sodium and potassium salts of Diclofenac inhibit the synthesis of enzyme cycloxygenase in path way of prostaglandin (PG) Synthesis. It has potent analgesic - antipyretic antiinflammatory and lasting antiplatelet action. It is well absorbed orally, 90% protein bound, metabolized and excreted both in urine and bile. Plasma t½ is~2 hours.
Dose: 1 mg/kg BW oral, IM in all animals.
C/I in Elephants. May cause gastric disorders.
Status in
1. Pregnancy : Contraindicated in last trimester.
2. Lactation : Use with caution.
3. Old age : May be given in reduced dose.</td></tr>
<tr><td>3D vet Inj</td><td>Intas</td><td>30 ml,
100ml vial
1 mg/kg b.wt.
I/M</td><td>Each ml contains
Diclofenac Na: 25 mg</td></tr>
<tr><td>BUTAGESIC inj</td><td>Concept</td><td>10 ml, 30 ml vial</td><td>Each ml contains:
Diclofenac Na 25 mg;</td></tr>
<tr><td>CATLOFENAC inj Vet</td><td>Cattle Remedies</td><td>30 ml vial
1 mg/25 kg BW IM in cattle per day</td><td>Each ml contains:
Diclofenac Na 25 mg;</td></tr>
<tr><td><u>CICLOFEN BOLUS</u></td><td>Cadila</td><td>4 Boli pack</td><td>Each uncoated bolus contains :
Diclofenac Sodium - 200 mg.
(As Enteric Coated Granules);
Paracetamol I.P. - 1500 mg.
Excipient - q.s.</td></tr>
<tr><td><u>CICLOFEN - D INJECTION</u></td><td>Cadila</td><td>'30 ml.</td><td>Each ml. contains :
Diclofenac Sodium I.P. - 25 mg.</td></tr>
<tr><td>DICLOVET inj</td><td>Alembic</td><td>30 ml vial</td><td>Each ml contains:
Diclofenac Na 25 mg;</td></tr>
<tr><td>VERASTAN</td><td>Vetnex (Ranbaxy)</td><td>30 ml vial</td><td>Each ml contains:
Diclofenac Na 25 mg;</td></tr>
<tr><td colspan="4">FLUNIXIN
it is a nonpsychotropic analgesic.
Dose rate is 1-2 mg/kg PO, IV, IM, SC sid in dogs.</td></tr>
<tr><td>Flugesic injection</td><td>Cipla</td><td>50 ml Vial</td><td>Flunixin injection (as meglumine) 50mg /ml</td></tr>
<tr><td>Flunequin</td><td>Cipla</td><td>10 gm,30 gm</td><td>Flunixin paste (as</td></tr>
</table>

oral paste		syringe	meglumine) 1500mg /30 gm
MELOXICAM A COX-2 inhibitor. **Indications** : Osteoarthritis, rheumatoid arthritis. Pneumonia, musculoskeletal affections, pain, swelling, inflammation. **Dosage** Large animal: 100-200 mg/animal/day oral. 0.5mg/kgBW IM. Special precautions : Arthritis with cardiac disease. Status in 1. Pregnancy : Use with caution. 2. Lactation : Contraindicated 3. Old age : Use with caution. Interactions : Same as NSAIDS.			
QIK bolus	Sarabhai zydus	Blister of 4 boli 1-2 boli /large animal	Each bolus has Meloxicam: 100 mg
QIK injection	Sarabhai zydus	15 ml vial 1ml/10 kg bwt IM (large animal)	Each ml has Meloxicam: 5 mg
Zobid –M bolus	Sarabhai zydus	Blister of 4 boli 1-2 boli /large animal	Each bolus has Meloxicam: 100 mg
Zobid –M vet injection	Sarabhai Zydus	15, 30, 100 ml vial 1ml/10 kg bwt IM (large animal)	Each ml has Meloxicam: 5 mg
Melonex inj	Neovet Intas Pharmaceutical	Vials of 2 ml, 15 ml 30 ml,100 ml; strip of 4 boli Cattle/Buffalo: 15 ml /300 kg b.wt or as per advice.	Each ml contains Meloxicam 5 mg
Melonex bolus	Neovet Intas Pharmaceutical	4's x 10	each bolus contains 100 mg Meloxicam
X-FLAM inj	Univet	30 ml vial	each ml contains 5 mg meloxicam
MILLI inj	Marc	30 ml vial	each ml contains 5 mg

			meloxicam
Petcam Oral Suspension	Cipla	10ml, 32ml, 100ml, 2.5ml	Meloxicam 1.5mg/ml oral suspension
Equi-Melfam	Cipla	5ml, 10ml	Meloxicam 15mg/ml Oral Suspension
Petcam Injection	Cipla	10ml	Meloxicam 5mg/ml
Equi-Melflam	Cipla	4 tabs. In a strips 5 strips in a box	Meloxicam 60mg chewable tablets
MELOXICAM + PARACETAMOL COMBINATION			
FIP bolus	Univet	Bolus 2 boli BID PO	Each bolus contains Paracetamol 1.5 gm + Meloxicam 100 mg
Melonex Plus inj	Neovet Intas Pharmaceutical	Vials of 30 ml, 100 ml; Cattle/Buffalo: 15 ml /300 kg b.wt IM or as per advice.	Each ml contains Meloxicam 5 mg + Paracetamol 150 mg + Lignocaine 1 %
Melonex Plus bolus	Neovet Intas Pharmaceutical	4's x 30 strip / box (1 bolus/200 kg bwt PO)	Each bolus contains Meloxicam 100 mg + Paracetamol 1500 mg

NIMESULIDE

It is a weak inhibitor of PG synthesis and there is some evidence to indicate relative COX-2 selectivity. It has its antiinflammatory action due to TNF-a inhibition, histamine inhibition and reduction in superoxide formation. Hematuria is reported in few cases. Recently several instances of fulminant hepatic failure have been associated with nimesulide and it has been withdrawn in Spain, Finland and Turkey.

Indications : pyrexia, musculoskeletal affections, ENT affections, systemic infectious disease, post operative or surgical inflammation,

Dosage

Dogs: 3-5 mg/KgBW Intramuscular. **Ruminants**: 2-4mg/kgBW I/M,

Contraindications : Hepatic impairment.

Special precautions : Renal and hepatic impairment, decreased blood volume.

Status in

1. Pregnancy : Contraindicated.
2. Lactation : Use with caution.

Interactions : It reduces antihypertensive effects of b-blockers, diuretics and ACE inhibitors.

NIMOVET	Indian Immunological	1ml, 15 ml, 50 ml.	each ml contains 100 mg.
NIMESULIDE + PARACETAMOL COMBINATION			
Oxalgin-NP bolus	Sarabhai zydus	2 gm bolus 1-2 bolus (Large animal)	Each bolus has Nimesulide: 400 mg Paracetamol: 1500 mg
Oxalgin-NP injection	Sarabhai zydus	15 ml vial 2-4 mg/kg bwt (Large animal)	Each ml has Nimesulide: 100 mg Paracetamol

PARACETAMOL/ACETAMINOFEN

Mechanism of action : It acts by inhibiting cyclo-oxygenase (COX) enzyme in brain, thus inhibiting formation of prostaglandins. It is a poor inhibitor of PG synthesis in peripheral tissues. The central analgesic action of paracetamol is that, it raises pain threshold, but has weak peripheral anti-inflammatory component. Paracetamol is a good and promptly acting antipyretic. Analgesic action of aspirin and paracetamol is additive.

Indications : Pain and fever.

DOSE: Dog: 10-20 mg/kgBW IM, oral. Large animals: 10 mg/Kg BW IM, oral.

Interactions : Cholestyramine, activated charcoal: Reduces absorption of paracetamol. Domperidone and metoclopramide : Enhance absorption of paracetamol.

C/I in cats.

Paracetol injection	Sarabhai zydus	30 ml vial 10 – 30 ml deep IM	Paracetamol : 150 mg /ml
PYROXIN	Marc	Bolus	2 gm/bolus

DICLOFENAC + PARACETAMOL combination

indicated in inflammatory conditions like arthritis, myositis, bursitis, fibrositis, tenosynovitis, Pyrexia of unknown origin.

ALFENAC-P FORTE	Alved	5x4 bolus 1-2 boli BID	Each bolus contains Diclofenac Na 300 mg; Paracetamol 1500 mg
CATLOFENAC PLUS inj Vet	Cattle Remedies	30 ml vial 1 mg/25 kg BW IM in cattle per day	Each ml contains: Diclofenac Na 25 mg; Paracetamol 150 mg
CICLOFEN bolus	Cadila	2 boli pack 1-2 boli BID oral	Each bolus contains Diclofenac Na 200 mg; Paracetamol 1500 mg
INFLAVET bolus	Glaxo	2 boli pack 1bolus BID oral	Each bolus contains Diclofenac Potassium 500 mg; Paracetamol 1000 mg

INIGESIC inj	Indian Immunological	30 ml vial 1 mg/25 kg BW	Each ml contains: Diclofenac Na 25 mg; Paracetamol 150 mg
OXALGIN-DS	Sarabhai Zydus	4 boli; 30 ml 1-2 boli BID; 1 ml/25kg BW IM	Each ml contains: Diclofenac Na 25 mg; Paracetamol 150 mg Each bolus contains: Diclofenac Na 200 mg; Paracetamol 1500 mg
PROXYVET-DS	Wockhardt	2 boli; 30 ml 1-2 boli BID; 1 ml/25kg BW IM	Each ml contains: Diclofenac Na 25 mg; Paracetamol 150 mg Each bolus contains: Diclofenac Na 250 mg; Paracetamol 1500 mg
VERASTAN PLUS inj	Ranbaxy	10ml, 30 ml vial 1 mg/25 kg BW	Each ml contains: Diclofenac Na 25 mg; Paracetamol 125 mg
DICLOVET BOLUS	Alembic Limited	Blister of 4 boli & Box of 15 blisters. Large animals: 1-2 boli daily. Small animals: 1/2 bolus daily.	Each bolus contains: Diclofenac Na: 250mg Paracetamol : 1500mg
MISCELLANEOUS COMBINATION PRODUCTS			
PECOREX bolus	Pranav	Blister of 4 boli. Large animals: 1-2 boli daily.	Each bolus contains: Diclofenac Na: 250mg Paracetamol : 1500mg Dicyclomine HCl: 100 mg
DIPLUS Bolus	Raps Health Care	2 boli pack	Each bolus contains: Diclofenac Na: 250mg Paracetamol : 1500mg Dicyclomine HCl: 100 mg
SPASDIC inj	Sushima	10 ml vial	Each ml contains Piroxicam: 10 mg Pitofenac: 2 mg Fenpiv bromide 0.2 mg
BUDSU bolus vet	Sushima	4 boli pack	Each ml contains Piroxicam: 200 mg Paracetamol : 2500mg
SPANIS FORTE	Genesis Pharma	Bolus2 boli BID PO	Each bolus contains Paracetamol 1.5 gm + Nimesulide 250 mg + Serratiopeptidase 75 mg

MARCOGESIC inj	Marc	30 ml vial	Each ml contains Paracetamol 150 mg + Mefenamic acid 50 mg
IBUPROFEN analgesic, antipyretic, anti-inflammatory. Inhibit Cyclo-oxygenase in Prostaglandin synthesis pathway. Prevents formation of Thromboxane A2 by platelets. Indicated in pain, pyrexia, musculoskeletal inflammation. **Dosage**: 10 mg/kg BW oral.			
IBUGIN tab	Virbac	strip of 10 tabs	Ibuprofen 200 mg/tab, 400 mg/tab.
IBUPROFEN + PARACETAMOL COMBINATION			
SERI-D FORTE bolus	Marc India Ltd	Bolus 2 boli BID PO	Each bolus contains Paracetamol 1.5 gm + Ibuprofen 2000 mg + Serratiopeptidase 75 mg
KETOPROFEN PG and leucotriene synthesis inhibitor, stabilises lysosomal membrane. **Indications** : Simple rheumatoid arthritis, osteoarthritis, musculoskeletal disorders, soft tissue injuries, fractures, vasectomy, tooth extraction, postpartum, postoperatively suppress swelling and inflammation, Any musculoskeletal disorders, clinical and subclinical mastitis. **Dosage** Ruminants: 2-4mg / kg B. wt., I/M or I/V,Oid Horses : 2.2 mg/kg B.wt by I/V,Oid Dogs and Cats : 2 mg / kg B. wt. IM. Status in : 1. Pregnancy : Use with caution. 2. Lactation : Use with caution.			
KETOP injection	Alembic Ltd	15 ml Vial	Each ml injection contains: Ketoprofen USP 100mg
Flex-O-Pet Tablets	Cipla	10's strip	Ketoprofen 20 mg tablets
Flex-O-Pet	Cipla	10's strip	Ketoprofen 5 mg tablets
NAPROXEN analgesic, antipyretic, anti-inflammatory. Inhibit Cyclo-oxygenase in Prostaglandin synthesis pathway. Prevents formation of Thromboxane A2 by platelets. Indicated in pain, pyrexia, musculoskeletal inflammation. **Dose**: 2-5 mg/kg BW oral.			
ARTAGEN	Vetnex	strip of 10 tabs	250 mg/tab

<table>
<tr><td colspan="4">PHENYL BUTAZONE
pyrazolone derivative. analgesic, antipyretic, anti-inflammatory. Produces oxygen tension reduction. Inhibits Cyclo-oxygenase in Prostaglandin synthesis pathway. Prevents formation of Thromboxane A2 by platelets. Indicated in pain, pyrexia, musculoskeletal inflammation.
Dose: Dogs: 22 mg/kg BW total dose per day IV. Horse: 1-2 g/450 kg BW total dose per day IV.
C/I in cats.</td></tr>
<tr><td>ALGESIN</td><td>Alembic Limited</td><td>3ml ampoule 3-12 ml I/M Large Animals</td><td>Each ml contains : Phenylbutazone Sodium 200 mg</td></tr>
<tr><td>Butagesic Paste</td><td>Cipla</td><td>230 ml jar</td><td>Phenylbutazone 1 gm per 5 ml paste</td></tr>
<tr><td>Butagesic Injection</td><td>Cipla</td><td>100 ml, 50ml vial</td><td>Phenylbutazone 18.61 gm + Sodium Salicyclate 5.0gm /100ml</td></tr>
<tr><td>Butagesic Plus Injection</td><td>Cipla</td><td>100 ml vial</td><td>Phenylbutazone 200mg+Lidocaine 10mg</td></tr>
<tr><td>Butagesic Powder</td><td>Cipla</td><td>100 sachets</td><td>Phenylbutazone – 1gm</td></tr>
<tr><td>SAFE-P bolus</td><td>ZIPP</td><td>2 boli pack</td><td>Phenylbutazone+paracetamol +serratiopeptidase</td></tr>
<tr><td colspan="4">NEUROMUSCULAR DRUGS
NEOSTIGMINE: reversibly inhibits AChase and potentiates nicotinic and muscarinic effects of ACh. Indicated in myasthenia gravis, atonic constipation, urinary retention. C/I in GIT and Urinary tract obstruction. Avoid in later stage of pregnancy.
Dose: 0.5 mg/kgBW BID oral, IV</td></tr>
<tr><td>MYOSTIGMIN inj</td><td>Neon labs</td><td>1ml, 5 ml ampoule</td><td>0.5mg/ml, 2.5 mg/ml</td></tr>
<tr><td colspan="4">RUBIFACIENTS AND TOPICAL AGENTS</td></tr>
<tr><td>DICLOMAX GEL</td><td>Torrent</td><td>30 gm tube</td><td>Diclofenac Na 1 % w/w</td></tr>
<tr><td>Iodine ointment with Methyl salicylate</td><td>Universal Medikit</td><td>500 gm</td><td>Iodine 4 % w/w, Methyl salicylate 5 % w/w</td></tr>
<tr><td>MEDICARE oint</td><td>Rallis</td><td>30 gm tube</td><td>Adrenaline 0.03 % w/w, Mephensin 2.5 % w/w, Methyl nicotinate 1 % w/w, Methyl salicylate 8 % w/w, Chlorpheniramine maleate 0.2</td></tr>
</table>

			% w/w, Menthol 2 % w/w.
NIMEGESIC transgel	Alembic	30 gm	Nimesulide 1 % w/w
VOVERAN emulgel	Novartis	30 gm, 50 gm	Diclofenac Na 1 % w/w
Cooljoint Gel	Cipla	500 gm	Levomenthol 20mg + Camphor 6.26mg+Eucalyptus 2mg/gm Gel
Eqimax	Cipla	2.5 ltr pack	Liniment Containing Oil of Bay 0.50%+ Oil of Wormwood 1%+ Oil of Amber 0.50%+Menthol 1%+ Thymol 0.5%+ Chloroxylenol .50% Acetone 66%
MISCELLANEOUS PREPARATION			
AYURGESIC	Alembic Limited	Strip of 4 bolus adult animals : 1 bolus twice daily or as directed by the Veterinarian. (Pyrexia of unknown origin, Fever due to infections, Inflammatory conditions)	Each bolus contains : Gauri 520 mg Mrugandini 520 g Sinduvar 300 mg Varahkarni 280 mg Shelfalika 280 mg Elaparni 200 mg Padmapatra 200 mg Nahush 200 mg Pitabeej 200 mg Vyosh 100 mg Jatipatri 100 mg Jatikosh 100 mg Subhra 100 mg Godanti bhasma100 mg
HIMPYRIN liquid	Himalaya	30 ml. 1-3 ml twice daily in dogs or as per directions	each ml contains guduchi (12 mg), sunthi (8 mg), Vacha (8 mg), Yashtimadhu (8 mg), Mushta (4 mg)
HIMPYRIN bolus	Himalaya	strip of 4 boli. 2 boli twice daily in cows and buffaloes;	each bolus has extract of guduchi, sunthi, Vacha, Yashtimadhu, Mushta
RUMALAYA	Himalaya	Bolus, 50 gm lamitube, 1 bolus twice	polyherbal

		daily, apply cream over affected area	
INFLAMMIN	Himalaya	50 gm lamitube apply cream over affected area	polyherbal
Vetgesic Balm	Cipla	500 ml	Camphor oil 1.0%+Methyl salicylate 2.0%+Levomenthol 0.5%+Turpentine oil 2.0%
Care-O-Pet Tablets	Cipla	60's container	Carprofen 100 mg chewable tablets
Care-O-Pet Tablets	Cipla	60's, 100's container	Carprofen 25mg chewable tablets
Carprofen 50 mg chewable tablets	Cipla	60's, 100's container	Carprofen 50 mg chewable tablets
Care-O-Pet Tablets	Cipla	60's container	Carprofen 75 mg chewable tablets
Maxima	Cipla	4.54 kgs. pack	Each 3.3 gm contains Glucosamine HCL1800gm + Sodium Chondroitin sulphate 600mg + Manganese [as Manganese Sulphate]16mg + Ascorbic acid (as calcium ascorbate] 104mg
Cooljoint Gel	Cipla	500 gm	Menthol 20mg + Isopropyl alcohol 350mg + Camphor 6.26mg + Eucalyptus 2 mg/gm gel
Tobact ointment	Cipla	6x 14gm tubes, 225gm container	Nitrofurazone 0.09% +Neomycin 0.50% + Prednisolone 0.25%

STEROIDAL ANTI-INFLAMMATORY DRUGS

- BETAMETHASONE
- DEXAMETHASONE
- HYDROCORTISONE
- PREDNISOLONE
- TRIAMCINOLONE

STEROIDAL ANTI-INFLAMMATORY DRUGS

BETAMETHASONE: Prednisolone derivative. Enhances carbohydrate and protein metabolism, modify cell mediated immunity. Potent antiinflammatory effects. Indicated in pregnancy toxemia, ketosis, induction of parturition. Doses: cattle (10-30 mg IM, IV); Dogs (1-2 mg IM, IV; 5 mg orally); Use with precaution in late pregnancy, deep corneal ulcers, cardiac insufficiency, renal disease.

Product	Company	Presentation	Composition
BETNESOL tab	**Glaxo**	strip of 10 tabs; injections 1 ml amp	each tab contains 0.5 mg; inj contains 4 mg/ml

DEXAMETHASONE: Prednisolone derivative. Enhances carbohydrate and protein metabolism, modify cell mediated immunity. Potent anti-inflammatory effects. Indicated in acute inflammation, pregnancy toxemia, ketosis, induction of parturition (@ 40 mg IV total dose in large animals). Doses: cattle (10-30 mg IM, IV); Dogs (1-2 mg IM, IV; 5 mg orally); Use with precaution in late pregnancy, deep corneal ulcers, cardiac insufficiency, renal disease.

Product	Company	Presentation	Composition
CADEX inj Vet	Cattle remedies	5 ml amp	Dexamethasone Phosphate - 4 mg /ml
Curadex inj	Concept	2ml, 5 ml vial 4-20 mg daily IM or as per direction	Dexamethasone $NaPO_4$: 3.34 mg /ml
DEXASONE (VET) INJ.	Cadila	5 ML vial	Dexamethasone Sodium Phosphate B.P. (Vet) - 4.4 mg. Equivalent to Dexamethasone Phosphate - 4 mg. Equivalent to Dexamethasone - 3.34 mg.
DEXAVET	Wockhardt Limited	5 ml vial 4-20 mg daily IM or as per direction	Dexamethasone $NaPO_4$: 3.34 mg /ml
Dexona injection	Sarabhai zydus	5 ml vial 4-20 mg daily IM or as per direction	Dexamethasone $NaPO_4$: 3.34 mg /ml
KETOCORT	Intas Pharmaceuticals	5 ml vial 4-20 mg daily IM or as per direction	Dexamethasone $NaPO_4$: 3.34 mg /ml
Vet cort inj	Alembic	5 ml vial Large animals: 4 to 20 mg i.e. 1 to 5 ml daily by IM or IV route.	Dexamethasone $NaPO_4$: 3.34 mg /ml
Cipdex	Cipla	50ml, 100ml vial	Dexamethasone 4mg inj

HYDROCORTISONE: Enhances carbohydrate and protein metabolism, modify body immunity, sodium and water retention. Potent anti-inflammatory effects. Indicated in allergy, feline asthma, shock. **Dose:** Dogs: 2.2 mg/kgBW IM; Large animals: 1-1.5 g total dose IM. Use with precaution in late pregnancy, deep corneal ulcers, cardiac insufficiency, renal disease.			
WYCORT inj	Wyeth Iderle	5 ml vial	25 mg/ml
PREDNISOLONE: Enhances carbohydrate and protein metabolism, modify body immunity, sodium and water retention. Potent anti-inflammatory effects. Indicated in flea allergy, Hydrocephalus, canine atopy, persistent haematuria, inflammatory conditions. **Dose:** Dogs: 1-3 ml (1 % soln) IM; Large animals: 0.5 mg/Kg BW IM. Use with precaution in glaucoma, late pregnancy, deep corneal ulcers, cardiac insufficiency, renal disease.			
PREDNISOLONE	Wockhardt Limited	10 ml vial 5-20 ml / day. IM	Prednisolone 10 mg/ml
PREDNISOLONE ACETATE	Intervet India Pvt. Ltd	10 ml vial 5-20 ml / day. IM	Prednisolone acetate:10 mg/ml
TRIAMCINOLONE: synthetic glucocorticoid. Enhances carbohydrate and protein metabolism, modify body immunity, sodium and water retention. Causes suppression of pituitary adrenal axis, which may lead to corticosteroid deficiency. Potent anti-inflammatory effects. **Indicated** in arthritis, tendosynovitis, myositis, bovine ketosis (2.5mg to 10mg I/M); inflammatory conditions. **Dose :** Dogs: 1-3 ml (1 % soln) IM; Large animals/dogs: 12-20 mg total dose IM, SC; 6-18 mg Intrasynovially. Use with precaution in glaucoma, late pregnancy, deep corneal ulcers, cardiac insufficiency, renal disease.			
Vetalog injection	Sarabhai zydus	1ml, 5 ml vial	Each 5ml vial contains : Triamcinolone acetonide 6mg/ml Each 1ml vial contains : Triamcinolone acetonide 10mg/ml
VETALOG	Sarabhai Zydus	1 ml, 5 ml vial	each 1 ml inj contains 10 mg/ml; each 5 ml inj contains 6 mg/ml

Chapter 7

Drugs for Integumentary System

SKIN RELATED PRODUCTS			
COAT CONDITIONER/CLEANSER: mange, seborrhea, ectoparasitic infestation, dermatitis.			
Product	**Company**	**Presentation**	**Composition**
DERMEEZ soln.	Vetnex	100 ml bottle shampoo	Bronopol: 0.2 % + Dichlorobenzyl alcohol 0.05 %
SELEDRUFF shampoo	Petcare	120 ml bottle	Selenium sulfide 2.5% w/v
TETMESOL soln., cake	ICI	50 ml solution, 75 gm cake	Tetraethyl thiuram monosulfide 5% v/v
Cipetic Shampoo	Cipla	230 ml shampoo	Boric acid 2% + Acetic acid 2%
Sebo-derm shampoo	Cipla	250ml shampoo	Boric Acid 2% + Acetic acid 2%
ORAL PREPARATION			
NUTRICOAT	PETCARE	150 gm liquid	Each 5 gm contains Linoleic+Linolenic: 3000 mcg; Oleic acid 3000 mcg; Lecithin 50 mg; Vit B6: 400 mcg; Vit A 1000 IU; Vit E 10 IU; Vit D3: 100 IU; Zn 4.5 mg; Selenium 0.2 mcg; Biotin 45 mcg
INDIGENOUS TOPICAL PREPARATION			
CANIFUR AZ liq	Cadila	120 ml pack	herbal
ERINA	Himalaya	120 ml pack	herbal
FLURRY	Sarabhai zydus	120 ml pack	herbal
TOPICAL ANTIFUNGAL			
1. CLOTRIMAZOLE			
CANESTEN	Bayer	15 ml soln, cream 15 gm	soln. has 1 % w/v; cream has 10 mg/gm

IMIDIL	Lyka	15 ml soln, cream 15 gm; 30 gm	soln. has 1 % w/v; cream has 10 mg/gm
2. CLOTRIMAZOLE COMBINATION			
CANDID-B	Glenmark	5 gm, 15 gm ointment; 15 ml lotion	Clotrimazole 1%w/v; Beclomethasone dipropionate: 0.025 % w/v.
CANDID-TV	Glenmark	60ml Susp	Clotrimazole 1%, Selenium disulphide 2.5% w/v
CANDIDERM A	Glenmark	15g, 5g Cream	Beclomethasone dipropionate 0.025%, Clotrimazole 1%w/w, Gentamicin (as sulph.) 0.1%
CANESTEN-S	Bayer	10g Cream	Beclomethasone dipropionate 0.025%, Clotrimazole 10mg
3. MICONAZOLE: ringworm.			
MICOGEL	Cipla	15g Cream	Miconazole: 2%
4. MICONAZOLE COMBINATION: seborrhic dermatitis, pruritus, erythema, exudation, scaly, greasy skin.			
MICOCORT-G	Themis Medicare	15g Cream	Beclomethasone 0.025%, Miconazole 2%, Gentamicin 0.1% all w/w
MICOLON	Ethnor	15g Cream	Miconazole nitrate 2%, Triamcinolone acetonide 0.1%)
MICODIN medicated shampoo	Neovet Intas	100 ml flip top bottle	Chlorhexidine gluconate 2 % w/v + miconazole nitrate 2 % w/v
BETNOVATE-GM	GSK	20g Cream	Betamethasone valerate 0.12%, Gentamicin sulph. equiv. to gentamicin 0.1%, Miconazole nitrate 2%, all w/w
TENOVATE-M	GSK	15g Cream	Clobetasol propionate 0.05%, Miconazole nit. 2%, all w/w
5. NYSTATIN COMBINATIONS			
KENACOMB	Sarabhai	10g Oint	Triamcinolone acetonide 0.1%, Neomycin 2.5mg, Gramicidin 0.25mg, Nystatin 100,000 i.u./g
TOPICAL ANTIMICROBIALS **1. FRAMYCETIN COMBINATION**			
SOFRADEX-F	Aventis	15g Cream	Dexamethasone acetate 0.1%, framycetin sulph. 1%, clotrimazole 1%
SOFRADEX CREAM	Aventis	20g Cream	Dexamethasone acetate 0.1%, soframycin (framycetin sulph.) 1%

2. GENTAMICIN COMBINATION			
GENTAMICIN SULPHATE	Lyka Hetero	15g Cream	Gentamicin 0.1% w/w
EUMOSONE	GSK	15g Cream	Clobetasol propionate 0.05% w/w, Gentamicin 0.05% w/w
3. NEOMYCIN COMBINATION			
NEOSPORIN OINTMENT	GSK	5g Oint	Polymyxin B sulphate 5000 i.u., Neomycin sulphate 3400 i.u., Zn Bacitracin 400 i.u., per g
NEOSPORIN POWDER	GSK	10g Powder	Polymyxin B sulphate 5000 i.u., Neomycin sulphate 3400 i.u., Zn Bacitracin 400 i.u., per g
NEOSPORIN-H	GSK	5g Oint	Polymyxin B sulph. 5000iu, Neomycin sulph. 3400u, Zinc. bacitracin 400u, Hydrocotisone 10mg, per g
4. SILVER SULPHADIAZINE & COMBINATION			
SILVER SULPHADIAZINE	Solvay	25g, 500g Cream	Silver sulphadiazine 1%w/w
SILVEREX	Croslands	10g, 25g, 100g, 250g Cream	Silver sulphadiazine 1%w/w, Chlorhexidine gluconate 0.2%, w/w
SILVEREX powder	Croslands	10g Powder	Silver sulphadiazine 1% w/w, Chlorhexidine Hydrochloride 0.5% w/w
SILVEREX lotion	Croslands	100ml Lotn.	Silver sulphadiazine 1% w/w, Chlorhexidine Hydrochloride 0.5% w/w
SILVERINE	Bal Pharma	20g Cream	Silver sulphadiazine1%
5. CLOBETASOL + GENTAMICIN + MICONAZOLE : Eczematous dermatitis with mixed infection, pyoderma and ringworm.			
KISKIN cream and lotion	Neovet Intas	20 gm tube and 30 ml lotion	clobetasol proprionate 0.025 % w/w + gentamicin 0.1 % w/w + miconazole 2.0 % w/w
TOPICAL ANTISEPTICS			
POVIDONE IODINE & COMBINATION			
WOKADINE ointment	Wockhardt	15g 125g 250g Oint	Povidone Iodine 5% w/v
WOKADINE soln.	Wockhardt	100ml 500ml Sol	Povidone Iodine 5% w/v
WOKADINE	Wockhardt	10g Pod.	Povidone Iodine 5% w/v

WOKADINE	Wockhardt	15g Cream; 50g Spray	Povidone Iodine 5% w/v
POVICIDAL-M	Cadila Pharma	15g Oint.	Povidone Iodine 5% and Metronidazole 1% w/w
POVIDINE	Stadmed	15g Oint; 100ml, 500ml Sol.	Povidone Iodine 5% w/v
Cipladine 10% Solution	Cipla	250ml,1Ltr,5Ltr	Povidone Iodine 10%solution
Cipladine Ointment	Cipla	250gm jar	Povidone Iodine 5% ointment
Cipladine 5% Solution	Cipla	100ml,250ml,1 Ltr, 5Ltr	Povidone Iodine 5% solution
MISCELLANEOUS products			
BOROZIN	Klar Sehen	10ml Dps	Boric acid 2%, Sod. borate 0.5%, zinc sulphate 0.1%, chlorbutol 0.65%, glycerine 2%, phenylethyl alcohol 0.5%, all w/v
DETTOL	Reckitt	50ml, 100ml, 200ml, 500ml, 5 lt. Can Liq.	Choroxylenol 4.8%w/v, Terpineol 9%v/v, Absolute alcohol 13.1% v/v
DETTOL ANTISEPTIC	Reckitt	25g Cream	Choroxylenol 0.8%w/v
DERMAL OINT	Amrutanjan	10g Oint	Salicylic Acid 10%, Boric Acid 5%, Camphor 1%, perfumed base 84%
DERMASPAN	Bliss	5g, 15g Cream	Beclomethaaone dipropionate 0.025%, Gentamicin Sulphate equiv. to Gentamicin base 0.1%, Clotrimazole 1%
DERMINOL	Brown & Burk	5g, 15g Cream	Beclomethasone dipropionate 0.025%, Gentamicin sulph. 0.1%, clotrimazole 1%, Iodochlor hydroxyquin 0.1%
DERMIS-S	Sierra Pharma	10g Cream	Beclomethasone dipropionate 0.05%, Salicylic acid 3%, Urea 10%, Lactic acid 3%, Sodium Lactate eq. to Lactic acid 2%)
DERMITOP CREAM	Cream (Generic)	5g, 10g Cream	Betamethasone Valerate 0.6mg, Gentamicin 1mg, Tolnaftate 10mg, Iodochlorhydroxyquinoline 10mg, Chlorocresol 1mg

DERMOGAR D	Indi Pharma	10g, 20g, 100g, 250g Cream	Silver Sulphadiazine 1 %wlw, Chlorhexidine gluconate Solution equiv. to Chlorhexidine gluconate 0.2%w/w, Aloe 15%w/w, Allantoin 0.1%wlw
Atopex 100	Cipla	10 Capsules	Cyclosporin capsules 100mg
Atopex 10	Cipla	10 Capsules	Cyclosporin capsules 10mg
Atopex 25	Cipla	10 Capsules	Cyclosporin capsules 25mg
Atopex 50	Cipla	10 Capsules	Cyclosporin capsules 50mg
Equitop ointment	Cipla	500gm	Each gm contains + Cod liver oil 100mg+ Undecenoic acid 20mg+ Neomycin Sulphate 5 mg+ Prednisolone Acetate 2.5mg & Nitrofurazone 2mg Nitrofurazone 2mg
Micohex Shampoo	Cipla	100ml & 250 ml, 1ltr. bottle	Medicated Shampoo containing Chlorhexidine Gluconate 20mg + Miconazole nitrate 20mg /ml
Micohex Plus Medicated Foam	Cipla	250ml	Selenium sulfide 2.5mg + Chlorhexidene gluconate 20mg + Miconazole nitrate 20gm/ltr
Sulfatop ointment	Cipla	100 gm	Sulphadiazine 400mg/ gm ointment
Notiks Pour On	Cipla	100 ml	Solution of Phoxim

INDIGENOUS PREPARATION: Dryskin, Skin eruptions, Acne, Chapped skin, Craked nipples, Minor cuts, burns			
BOROTOTAL	Baidyanath	20 gms tube	Each 100gm contains Aloe vera, Shwetha sareeva, Chandana oil, Ushira oil each 3.125gms, Tila taila 2gms, Bees wax 3gms, Yashada bhasma 0.8gms, shuddha tankana, Sangajeeraka each 0.4gms, cream base q.s
DERMOTONE Syrup	Anjani	100ml, 200ml, 400ml	Each 5ml syrup contains Chirayata,Gorakmundi, Manjista, Shirisha, Pittapapda each 125mg, Kanchanar, Kantakari,

			Amrita, Nimba each 250mg, Sugar q.s
DRESSOL	Cattle remedies	100 ml, 450 ml lotion, 50 gm oint	Herbal
Charmil	Dabur	25 gm, 50 gm, 1 kg oint	Herbal
Canisep	Himalaya	30 gm cream	herbal
HIMAX	Natural Remedies	50 gm, 1 kg ointment, 100 ml lotion	Herbal
Maggacite	Cattle remedies	50 ml, 100 ml, 450 ml lotion	herbal
SCAVON	Himalaya	50 gm cream	herbal
TOPICURE	Natural remedies	250 ml spray	herbal
WISPREC	Natural remedies	25 gm ointment tube	herbal
Herbact Shampoo	**Cipla**	**Pack of 500 ml**	**Hebal anti-bacterial, deodrant bath shampoo**

Chapter 8

Otoocular Products

OCULAR/AURAL ANTI-INFECTIVE/ANTI-ALLERGIC PRODUCTS			
BETAMETHASONE & COMBINATION			
BETNESOL E/E DPS	GSK	5ml E/E Dps	0.1%w/v
BETNESOL EYE OINT	GSK	5gm Oint	0.1%w/v
BETNESOL-N E/E	GSK	5ml E/E Dps	Betamethasone Na Phosphate 0.1%, Neomycin Sulphate 0.5%
CHLORAMPHENICOL: infectious inflammation in eye/ear			
CHLOROMYCETIN aplicaps	Parke-Davis	50 Applicaps	Chloramphenicol 1% w/w
CHLOROMYCETIN ear drops	Parke-Davis	5ml Dps	Chloramphenicol 5% w/v, Benzocaine 1% w/v, Propylene glycol q.s.
PARAXIN EAR DROPS	Nicholas Piramal	5ml Dps	Chloramphenicol 5% w/v, Benzocaine 1% w/v, Butylane Glycol base
PARAXIN DPS	NPIL	5ml Dps, 5g Oint	0.4% w/v in Dps; 1% w/w in Oint
CIPROFOLOXACIN: infectious inflammation in eye/ear			
CIPLOX EYE	Cipla	5ml Dps, 5g Oint, 30 Caps	Dps has 0.3% w/v; Oint 0.3% w/v; Caps 0.3% w/w
CIPLOX-D	Cipla	5ml 10ml Dps; 5g Oint	Dexamethsone 0.1%, Ciprofloxacin 0.3%, Benzalkonium chloride 0.01% all, w/v
CIPLOX-D Dps	Cipla	10ml Dps (E/E)	Ciprofloxacin Hydrochloride eqv. to Ciprofloxacin 0.3% w/v, Dexamethasone 0.1% w/v, Benzalkonium chloride NF 0.01% w/w

CIPLOX- D Oint	Cipla	5 g Tube Oint	Ciprofloxacin HCL eqv. to Ciprofloxacin 0.3% w/w, Benzalkonium chloride NF 0.01% w/w
Ciplox Eye Ointment	Cipla	5 gm tube	Ciprofloxacin 0.3% Eye Ointment
FRAMYCETIN & COMBINATION			
SOFRACORT E/E DROPS	Sanofi Aventis	5ml E/E Dps.	Framycetin sulphate 5mg, Dexamethasone 0.5mg (as sodium metaulphobenzaote), Gramicidin 0.05mg, Benzalkonium Cl (as preservative) 0.02%, all as w/v
SOFRACORT	HMR	5ml Dps e/e drops	Framycetin, sulph. 1%, Dexamethasone sod. metasulphobenzoate 0.116% w/v
Canear Drops	Cipla	7.5ml, 15ml, 25ml, 100ml	Dethanolamine fusidate 5mg + Framycetin sulphate 5mg + Nystatin 100,000units + Prednisolone 2.5mg
GENTAMICIN			
GENTA SWIFT E/E	Ind Swift	10ml Dps (E/E)	Gentamicin Sulph. 0.3% w/v
GENTASPORIN E/E	PCI	5ml Dps (E/E)	Gentamicin sulph. 0.3%, Benzalkonium chl. soln. 0.04%, w/v
GENTASPORIN HC E/E	P.C.I.	5ml Dps	Gentamicin sulph. 0.3%, Hydrocortisone Acetate 1.0% Benzalkonium Chloride 0.04% all w/v
GENTA CIP-D	Cipla	10ml E/E Dps	Gentamicin Sulphate 0.3% w/v, Dexamethasone Na Phosphate 0.1%
GENTAMICIN + CLOTRIMAZOLE COMBINATION: acute and chronic otitis externa or otitis media with mixed etiology			
POMISOL ear drop	Neovet Intas	15 ml, 30 ml	Gentamicin sulph. 0.3% w/v, Clotrimazole 1.0 % w/v, Betamethasone dipropionate 0.025 % w/v, Lignocaine HCl 2 % w/v
Otivet Ointment	Cipla	15gm	Gentamycin 3 mg +Betamethasone 1 mg +Clotrimazole 10mg/Gm

NEOMYCIN & COMBINATION			
NEOSPORIN DROPS	Wellcome	10ml Sol	Polymixin B 5000i.u, Neomycin sulph. 1700i.u, gramicidin 25i.u, per ml
NEOSPORIN-H EAR DPS	GSK	5ml Dps	Neomycin sulph. 3400i.u., Hydrocortisone 10mg, Polymyxin B sulph. 10,000i.u. per ml
NORFLOXACIN			
NORFLOX eye/ear	Cipla	5ml,10ml Dps	Norfloxacin : 0.3%w/v
NORILET EYE/EAR DROPS	Dr. Reddy's Lab	5ml Dps	Norfloxacin : 0.3%w/v
SULPHACETAMIDE:			
ALBUCID	Allergan	10ml Dps	10%, 20%, 30%
SODIUM CROMOGLYCATE: acute allergic conjunctivitis			
ALLERCROM	FDC	5ml Dps	Sodium cromoglycate 2% w/v, 4% w/v
FINTAL EYE DPS	Rhone Poulenc	10ml Dps Eye	Sodium cromoglycate 2% w/v
MISCELLANEOUS PRODUCTS			
CHLORAMSONE E/E DROPS	Ranbaxy	5ml E/E Dps	(Chloramphenicol 0.2%, Prednisolone acetate 0.5%, Benzalkonium Cl 0.002%)
CHLORMET-DM	Milmet	5ml Dps	(Dexamethasone sodium phos. 0.1%, Chloramphenicol 0.5%,)
PROFENAC	Cipla	5ml Dps	Diclofenac Na: 0.1%
CL-Ear Cleansing Solution	Cipla	118ml	Acetic acid 2% + Boric acid 2% with surfactants
Opticare Ointment	Cipla	3.5gm	Cyclosporine 2mg/gm
Otibact Ear Drops	Cipla	15 ml Bottle	Enrofloxacin 5mg /ml& Silver Sulfadiazine 10mg/ml
Oticlear Liquid	Cipla	125 ml	Lactic acid 2.5% & Salicyclic acid 0.1% Liquid

Otikfree Ear Drops	Cipla	15 ml Bottle	Miconazole nitrate 23 mg/ml + Prednisolone acetate 5 mg/ml+ Polymyxin B sulphate 5500 IU/m l

Chapter 9
Toxicology

COMMON POISONS/TOXINS AND THEIR ANTIDOTES	
POISON/TOXIN	**ANTIDOTE/Rx**
Arsenic	Dimercaprol
Cyanide	Oxygen, Dicobalt edetate, Na nitrite, Na thiosulphate
Ethylene glycol	Ethanol
Organophosphorus insecticides (chlorpyriphos, coumaphos, diazinon, dichlorvos, Famphur, Dioxathion, malathion, parathion, phorate, Ronnel, Temephos, TEPP, Trichlorfon)	Atropine and Pralidoxime chloride
Carbamate (carbaryl, carbofuran, methomyl, propoxur)	Atropine sulfate + Alloxine
Beta blockers	Glucagon,
Digoxin	Digoxin specific antibody, Oxygen
Carbon monoxide	Vitamin K
Lead	Penicillamine, Dimercaprol
Inorganic mercury	Ethanol
Atropine	Activated charcoal
Cadmium	Atropine
Organochlorine insecticide/pesticide	Barbiturates, saline purgative
Copper	Dimercaprol
Formaline	Oxygen
Nitrate/nitrite	Methylene blue
Phosphorus (rodenticide)	Gastric lavage with $KMnO_4$ soln.
Selenium	Na arsenite
Urea	Acetic acid
Warfarin (rodenticide)	Oxygen, Vit. K
Zinc phosphide	Soda bicarb,
Bracken Fern	Ca borogluconate, DL-butyl alcohol, Thiamine
Horse tail	Thiamine
Lantana	Activated charcoal, Antihistamines

Poppy/morphine	Naloxone
Sorghum	Ca infusion
Sweet clover (dicoumerol)	Vit. K
Tobacco (Nicotine)	Caffeine, Oxygen
Aflatoxin	Activated charcoal, stanozolol, oxytetracycline,

TOXICOLOGY

DIMERCAPROL:

Mechanism of action: It is an oily pungent, viscous fluid. The two sulphydryl (SH) groups of dimercaprol bind the metals which produce toxicity by interacting with sulphydryl containing enzymes in the body.

Indications: Poisoning by arsenic, mercury, gold, bismuth, nickel and antimony. Adjuvant with calcium disodium edetate in lead poisoning. Adjuvant to penicillamine in copper poisoning, Wilson's disease.

Dosage: Dog/cat: 3 mg/kg as 5 % soln. in 10 % Benzylbenzoate soln. in arachis oil IM for 2 days q 4 hr.

Contraindications: Hepatic failure. Not to be given in iron and cadmium poisoning.

Adverse drug reactions: Rise in blood pressure, tachycardia, vomiting, tingling sensation, sweating, cramps, anxiety, and inflammation of mucus membranes.

DESFEROXAMINE:

It is isolated as the iron containing complex from *Streptomyces pilocus* and is treated chemically to obtain iron-free ligand. It thus has high affinity for ferric ions. It is poorly absorbed orally and is usually given parenterally. It enhances excretion of ferric iron forming a nontoxic complex with it.

Indications: Acute iron poisoning, chronic iron intoxication leading to siderosis. Aluminium poisoning in renal dysfunction.

Dosage

Dogs : 1-2 gm PO as 5 % soln.; 20 mg/kg/4hr IM; in shock, 40 mg/kg as a drip over 4 hr followed by 20 mg/kg/12 hr

Contraindications: Primary hemochromatosis. Known hypersensitivity. Renal failure.

Adverse drug reactions: Allergic reactions like wheels, rash, pruritis and even anaphylaxis. Loose motions, abdominal cramps, fever, dysuria, muscle cramps may occur. Occasionally cataract and neurotoxicity occur.

ATROPINE SULPHATE

Mechanism of action: They block muscarinic receptors in the iris and ciliary body of eye. This leads to pupillary dilatation (mydriasis) and paralysis of accomodation (cycloplegia). Mydriasis may last upto 10 days and cycloplegia upto 7-12 days.

Indications: Refraction. Atropine is extremely useful in the treatment of anterior uveal inflammation. Relieves the pain by relaxing the ciliary muscle spasm and helps prevent posterior synechiae by dilating the pupil, may prevent or slow the progression of myopia, treatment of amblyopia. Also useful in organophosphorus poisoning.

Dosage:

- Horse/cattle: 30-60 mg/kg SC;
- Pig: 20-40 mcg/Kg SC;
- Dog/cat: 30-100 mcg/Kg SC.

Contraindications: Known hypersensitivity.

Adverse drug reactions: Ocular reactions include direct irritation due to drug, allergic contact dermatitis, increase risk of angle-closure glaucoma and elevation of IOP. Allergic reaction is seen as erythema with pruritus and edema of eyelids, allergic conjunctivitis and keratitis. Adverse systemic reactions appears to be dose dependent. They include depression of salivation and drying of the mouth. Slightly higher dosage produce facial flushing and inhibit sweating.

Status in

1. Pregnancy : Use with caution.
2. Lactation : Use with caution.
3. Old age : Use with caution.

D-PENICILLAMINE:

Mechanism of action: It is dimethyl cysteine, obtained as a degradation product of penicillin. It selectively chelates Cu, Hg, Pb and Zn. The d-isomer is used therapeutically; it is adequately absorbed after oral administration, slowly metabolized in the body and excreted in urine and faeces. Penicillamine increases soluble collagen and is the preferred drug for stage II and III scleroderma.

Indications: mercury and lead poisoning.

Dosage: 40 mg/kgBW orally

Contraindications: Simultaneous gold therapy.

Special Precautions: Renal, haematological diseases.

Adverse drug reactions: Rash, proteinuria, kidney damage, bone marrow depression. SLE or myasthenia gravis may be precipitated.

Status in

1. Pregnancy : Contraindicated.
2. Lactation : Use with caution.
3. Old age : May be used in reduced dose.

Interactions: The pharmacologic and toxic effects of penicillamine may be increased by chloroquine, indomethacin. Pharmacologic effects of penicillamine may be attenuated by probenecid. Penicillamine may decrease the serum levels of digoxin.

PRODUCT	COMPANY	PRESENTATION	COMPOSITION
B.A.L. inj	Knoll pharma	2 ml	100 mg penicillamine /ml
ARTIN	Arvind Remedies	tablet	250 mg Penicillamine/tab
CILAMIN	Panacea	caps	250 mg Penicillamine /cap

ATROPINE SULPHATE	Samarth Pharma	1ml, 50ml Inj.	6mg/ml in 1 ml amp; 30mg/ml in 50 ml vial
ATROPINE Inj.	Life Pharma	1ml Amp	Atropine Sulphate 0.6mg/ml

Chapter 10

Nutritional Preparation

DOG FOOD

- Normal Growth & development of pet. Normal reproduction of both male and female dog;
- Facilitates normal development of skeletal & muscular system;
- To enrich the nutritionally incomplete traditional food;
- Promotes healthy development of skin & coat;
- To improve appetite & overcome pica;
- Alongwith any antibiotic prescribed in cases of gastritis, enteritis, URT infection, UTI, skin ailment , nephritis etc.;
- To restore the normal gut microflora ;

Product	Company	Presentation	Dose rate	Composition
Nutripet Supra	Pet Care	1 kg, 40 kg pack	15-20 gm/Kg BW PO	Protein 30% + Fat 20% + Fibre 4 % + Ca 2.8 % + Phosphorus 1.65 % + Energy 3250 Kcal/Kg pack
Regale Meal	Venky's Pet	40 kg pack	15-20 gm/Kg BW PO	Protein 30% + Fat 20% + Fibre 4 % + Ca 2.8 % + Phosphorus 1.65 % + Energy 3250 Kcal/Kg pack
Regale Pup	Venky's Pet	1 kg, 200 g	Dogs below 10 kg: 20gms/day	Multivitamin+ nutrients q.s.
Nutripet Food Booster	Pet Care	1 kg, 200 g	Growing puppies & pregnant bitches : 15 gms. twice daily Adult dogs below 10kg. : 20gms./day	Each 30gms. contains.: Live Yeast Culture 7.5 billion cells Vitamin A (Retinol) 1100.00 I.U. Vitamin B1(Thiamin 220.00 mcg. Vitamin B2(Riboflavine 480.00 mcg.

			Adult dogs above 10 kg : 30 gms./day	Vitamin B3(Niacin) 2500.00 mcg. Vitamin B5(Ca Pantothenate)2200.00 mcg. Vitamin B6 (Pyridoxine) 220.00 mcg. Vitamin B12(Cyanocobalamine) 5.00 mcg. Vitamin D3(Cholecalciferol) 220.00 I.U. Vitamin E(Tocopherol) 110.00 I.U. Vitamin H(Biotin) 22.00 mcg. Choline Chloride 260.00 mcg. Calcium 2419.00 mg. Copper 1.50 mg. Iron 13.00 mg. Sodium 45.00 mg. Zinc 12.27mg. Manganese 1.08 mg. Phosphorous 1876.00 mg. Potassium 680.00 mg. Selenium 2374.00 mcg. Iodine 336.00 mcg. Arginine 510.00 mg. Cystine 85.00 mg. Glycine 714.00 mg. Lysine 765.00 mg. Methionine 280.00 mg. Tryptophan 90.00 mg.

GROUP: VITAMINS/MINERALS/LIVER STIMULANTS				
PROHEPATIC PRODUCTS: Indicated in ascites, cirrhosis, metabolic stimulant, Neurological disorders, Anorexia, Anemia, Convalescence, Liver disorders, Blood protozoan diseases, Supportive therapy, Anorexia, Anaemia, Convalescence, Liver disorders, Blood protozoan diseases, Growth of young animals.				
Product	**Company**	**Presentation**	**Dose rate**	**Composition**
ANABOLITE liquid	Virbac	1 litre bottle	200 ml twice daily followed by 100 ml BID from second day for 3 days.	Gluconeogenic precurosors fortified with B-complex vitamin
BELAMYL INJECTION	Sarabhai Zydus	10, 30, 50 ml vials	5-10 ml on alternate day, Deep IM in Large animal	Each ml contains: Thiamin HCl I.P.: 10mg Riboflavin I.P: 3mg Niacinamide I.P.: 100mg Vitamin B 12 I.P.: 10mcg Liver injection crude 0.66ml having Vitamin B 12 acivity eq.to 2 mcg of Cyanocobalamin per ml.
BIVINAL FORTE INJECTION	ALEMBIC LTD	10, 30 ml vials	5-10 ml on alternate day, Deep IM in Large animal	Each ml contains: Thiamin HCl I.P.: 10mg Riboflavin I.P: 3mg Niacinamide I.P.: 100mg Vitamin B 12 I.P.: 10mcg Liver injection crude 0.66ml having Vitamin B 12 acivity eq.to 2 mcg of Cyanocobalamin per ml.
BIVINAL LIQUID	Alembic Limited	5 liter HDPE jar	10 - 20 ML /100 Birds in drinking water.	Each 5ml contains: Cholin chloride: 5mg Vitamin B2: 1.25mg Vitamin B6: 0.62mg Niacinamide: 37.5mg Dl- Panthenol: 1.25mg Vitamin B12: 6.25mcg Methionine: 5mg Lysine: 5mg
BOVOPLEX - CC	Indian Immunolo gicals	10, 30 ml vials	Large animal 5-10 ml small animal	Each ml contains: Thiamine HCl 25 mg Riboflavin 1.5 mg

			0.5 to 2.0 ml	Niacinamide 50 mg Cyono coblamine 50 mcg Liver injection crude having vit. B12 activity equivalent not less than 2 mg Pyridoxine HCl 5 mg Choline esterase 25 mg
BROTONE tonic	Virbac	120 ml, 500 ml bottle	dogs: 5-10 ml twice daily	Each 10 ml contains: Nicotinic acid 24 mg Yeast extract : 0.4 gm Liver fraction : 1.25 gm having vit. B12 activity equivalent not less than 7.5 mcg
Cureliv forte	Curevet	500 ml, 1 litre bottle	10-20 ml oid or apa	Each 5ml contains: Cholin chloride: 5mg Vitamin B2: 1.25mg Vitamin B6: 0.62mg Niacinamide: 37.5mg Dl- Panthenol: 1.25mg Vitamin B12: 6.25mcg Methionine: 5mg Lysine: 5mg
E-booster liq	Intas	1 litre bottle	250 ml twice daily for two days followed by 100 ml BID for 2 days.	Gluconeogenic precurosors fortified with B-complex vitamin
ENERBEE FDS	Cadila	1 kg. Polypack in 25 x 1 kg. HDPE Drums	25 gm BiD PO	Each gm. contains Vitamin B1 - 8 mg. Vitamin B6 - 16 mg. Vitamin B12 - 80 mcg. Vitamin E - 80 mg. Niacin - 120 mg. Folic Acid - 8 mg. Calcium D Pantothenate - 80 mg. Calcium - 125 mg. Phosphate - 300 mg. Carriers - q.s.
GENPLEX inj	Genesis	30 ml vial	5-10 ml IM	Each ml contains:

	pharma		large animal	Thiaminehydrocloride 10 mg Riboflavin 3 mg Niacinamide 100 mg
LIV-52 VET	Himalaya	30 ml, 110 ml, 60 tabs	10-15 drops daily twice or as per advice	polyherbal formulation
LIVADEX FORTE inj	Virbac	10 ml, 30 ml vial	5 ml daily IM in cattle; 2 ml IM in dogs	Each ml contains: Pyridoxine HCl I.P.: 5 mg Cyanocobalamin: 50 mcg Nicotinamide I.P.: 100mg Choline : 100 mg Ligoncaine HCl : 10 mg Folic acid: 10 mg Liver injection crude 0.66ml having Vitamin B 12 acivity eq.to 2 mcg of Cyanocobalamin per ml.
LIVAMYL INJ. VET	Cattle Remedies	10 ml, 30 ml	5-10 ml on alternate day, Deep IM in Large animal	Each ml contains: Thiamin HCl I.P.: 10mg Riboflavin I.P: 3mg Niacinamide I.P.: 100mg Vitamin B 12 I.P.: 10mcg Liver injection crude 0.66ml having Vitamin B 12 acivity eq.to 2 mcg of Cyanocobalamin per ml.
LIVOMARC bolus	Marc India Ltd	2 boli pack	2 boli per day	liver ext + Vit B1 and B12 + Dried yeast 700 mg + Methionine + Fe sulfate + $CoCl^2$ + $CuSO^4$ + Ginger Powder + Dextrose
MARCOSID inj	Marc India	10 ml	10 ml per animal IM	Each ml contains: Thiamin HCl : 100 mg Riboflavin I.P: 3mg Niacinamide I.P.: 100mg Pyridoxine 5 mg Panthenol 10 mg Vitamin B 12 I.P.: 100 mcg Liver injection crude 0.66ml having Vitamin B

				12 acivity eq.to 2 mcg of Cyanocobalamin
NEUROXIN-12V INJ	Sarabhai Zydus	10, 30 ml vials	5-10 ml IM x 5 days	Each ml contains: Thiamin HCl I.P.: 30mg Pyridoxine HCl : 13.75 mg Cyanocobalamin : 500 mg
RUMIS CC bolus	RFCL	4 boli pack	2 boli BID PO	Liver Ext + Lysine + Histidine + Lactobacillus + Mg trisillicate
START bolus	PAIL pharma	4 boli pack	2 boli BID PO	Liver Ext + Lysine + Histidine + Lactobacillus + Mg trisillicate
VENTRIBEE PLUS	Venky's India Ltd	1 kg	200 g per ton of feed for broiler and layer 200 to 300 g per ton of feed in stress or intense summer seasons	Each g contains Vitamin B1 4 mg Vitamin B12 40 mcg Ca-D pantothenate 40 mg Vitamin B6 8 mg Vitamin E 40 mg Niacin 60 mg
VENTRIPLEX-M	Venky's India Ltd	500 mL, 1 L and 5 L	Upto 2 weeks of age - 15 mL per 100 birds in drinking water Above 2 weeks of age - 20 mL per 100 birds in drinking water	Each 5 mL contains Vitamin B2 1.25 mg Vitamin B6 0.62 mg Vitamin B12 6.25 mg D-Panthenol 1.25 mg Niacinamide 37.5 mg DL-Methionine 5 mg
Vetliv fort liq	Current pharma	1 ltre pack	50 ml per cow per day	Each 5 mL contains Vitamin B2 1.25 mg Vitamin B6 0.62 mg Vitamin B12 6.25 mg D-Panthenol 1.25 mg Niacinamide 37.5 mg DL-Methionine 5 mg

VITAMIN A AND COMBINATION: Infertility associated with Vitamin A deficiency, Night blindness, Xerophthalmia, Keratomalacia. As a supportive therapy in Respiratory, Gastrointestinal & urogenital tract infections. Repeat breeding, Poor conception, Night blindness, Xerophthalmia, Muscular dystrophy, Alleviating stress, Body resistance, Infertility, To improve milk yield and egg production, Faster growth and proper bone formation, curled-toe paralysis, rickets, poor bone and egg shell quality, poor hatchability, embryonic mortality				
ALVITON LIQUID	Alembic Limited	500ml, 20 m, 1 lit.	Cattle and Horses : 10 ml twice daily/animal ; 5-10ml/100 birds	Each 5 ml contains : Vitamin A :2,50,000 IU Vitamin D 3 : 25000 IU Vitamin E : 150 IU Vitamin C : 500mg
ALVITON-PLUS	Alembic Limited	Bottle of 20ml, 100ml, 500ml & 1litre.	Cattle & Horse: 10ml twice daily. Dogs: 3-5 ml twice Poultry: Chicks: 2 -3 ml /100Birds Broilers: 4 - 6ml /100 Birds.	Each 5ml contains: Vitamin A: 2,50,000 I.U. Vitamin D3: 25,000 I.U Vitamin E: 150mg Vitamin C: 500mg Selenium: 0.5mg
MULTIVET INJ	Dosch Pharma	30 ml, 50 ml vial	1 ml/15kg bwt/day IM	Each ml contains: Vitamin A, Vitamin D3, Vitamin E, Niacinamide, Thiamine, Pyridoxin, Riboflavin, Biotin, Calcium pantothenate, Vitamin B12, Choline Chloride, Calcium.

PROWINSTRES	Cadila	'30 ML,500ML	1 ml / 15 kg body wt IM	Each ml. provides : Vitamin A - 12000 'i.u. Vitamin D3 - 6000 'i.u. Vitamin E Acetate - 50 mcg. Vitamin B12 - 20 mcg. Vitamin C - 25 mcg. Protein Hydrolysate - 25 mg.
VENTRIFORTE-A	Venky's India Ltd	100 mL	2 ml for 100 birds everyday in drinking water	Each mL contains Vitamin A 100,000 I.U
VENTRIMIN-17	Venky's India Ltd	5 kg	Layers: 250 g per 100 kg of feed Starters, Breeders and Broilers: 250 g per 50 kg of feed	Each 250 g contains Vitamin A 500,000 IU Vitamin D3 100,000 IU Vitamin B2 00.20 g Vitamin B12 00.60 mg Vitamin E 75.00 Units Vitamin K3 00.10 g Niacin 01.00 g Calcium D Pantothenate 00.25 g Choline Chloride 15.00 g Calcium 82.00 g Cobalt 0.045 g Copper 00.20 g Iodine 00.10 g Iron 00.75 g Manganese 02.75 g Zinc 01.50 g
VENTRIMIX	Venky's India Ltd	1 kg pack	100 g per ton of feed for broiler and layer 150 to 200 g per ton of feed in stress or intense summer seasons	Each g contains Vitamin A 82,500 IU Vitamin B2 50 mg Vitamin D3 12,000 IU Vitamin K 10 mg
VETADE INJ	Sarabhai	10 ml vial	Cattle : 6-10	Each ml contains:

	Zydus		ml IM Horses : 4 ml IM Pig : 3 ml IM	Vitamin A I.P.: 6,00,000 I.U. Vitamin D3 : 25000 IU Vitamin E : 100 IU
VITAMIN-A injection	Alembic ltd	Box of 2ml x 6 ampoules	Large animals: 12ml /week Small animals: 6 - 12ml /week Dog & Cat: 2 -6ml / week	Each 2ml ampoule contains: Vitamin A I.P.: 6,00,000 I.U. Chlorbutol I.P.: 1% W/V (as preservative), in an oily vehicle
VITAMIN-A injection	Virbac	Box of 2 ml x 6 ampoules	Large animals: 12 ml /week Small animals: 6 - 12 ml /week Dog & Cat: 2 -6 ml / week	Each 2ml ampoule contains: Vitamin A I.P.: 6,00,000 I.U. Chlorbutol I.P.: 1% W/V (as preservative), in an oily vehicle

CALCIUM (in combination) PREPARATION Hypocalcemia, Phosphorus deficiency, Hypomagnesemia, Growth promoter, High Milk Yield, Pregnant & Lactating Animals				
ASCAL LIQUID	Alembic Limited	1ltr, 500 ml, 5 lit.	Cattle and Horses : 50 ml/day	Each 5 ml contains : Calcium Phosphate 0.24 g (equivalent to 0.21 g of $Ca_3(PO_4)_2$ Cholecalciferol (Vitamin D3) I.P. 500 I.U. Vitamin B 12 I.P. 7.5 mcg
ASCAL-FS	Alembic Limited	Pet Bottle of 500ml, HDPE jars of 1lit & 5lits	Cattle &Horse: 100ml/day Calves, Goat & Pig: 10ml twice daily Dogs: 5-10ml twice daily	Each 100ml contains: Tricalcium Phosphate - 4800mg Eq.to elemental Calcium - 1867mg Elemental Phosphorous - 955mg Cholecalciferol (Vitamin D 3) - 10000 IU Cyanocobalamine

				(Vitamin B 12) - 150mcg Magnesium sulphate Eq.to elemental Magnesium - 200mg Calory contents- 80calories/100ml
AGRIMIN powder	Virbac	1 kg, 10 kg bags	1-2 kg per ton cattle feed; 30-35 gm daily in cattle	Each kg has Calcium – 24% Phosphorous – 12 % Cobalt – 150 mg Copper – 1200 mg Iodine – 325 mg Iron – 5000 mg Magnesium – 6000 mg Manganese – 1500 mg Potassium 100 mg Selenium 10 mg Sodium 5.9 mg Zinc- 9600 mg Methionine: 1920 mg L-Lysine monoHCl – 4400 mg Sulphur : 0.922 %
AGRIMIN Forte powder	Virbac	1 kg, 5 kg bags	1kg per ton cattle feed; 30 gm daily in cattle; Fish: 10 kg per ton feed	Each kg has Vitamin A 7,00,000 IU Vitamin D3 70,000 IU Vitamin E 250 mg Nicotinamide 1000 mg Cobalt – 150 mg Copper – 1200 mg Iodine – 325 mg Iron – 1500 mg Magnesium – 6000 mg Manganese – 1500 mg Calcium – 25.5 % Phosphorous – 12.75 % Potassium 100 mg Selenium 10 mg Sodium 5.9 mg Zinc- 9600 mg Sulphur : 0.72 %
CHELATED AGRIMIN	Virbac	500 gm, 1 kg, 5 kg	1kg per ton cattle feed;	Each kg has Vitamin A 7,00,000 IU

FORTE powder		bags	30 gm daily in cattle; Fish: 10 kg per ton feed	Vitamin D3 70,000 IU Vitamin E 250 mg Nicotinamide 1000 mg Cobalt – 150 mg Copper – 1200 mg Iodine – 325 mg Iron – 1500 mg Magnesium – 6000 mg Manganese – 1500 mg Calcium – 25.5 % Phosphorous – 12.75 % Potassium 100 mg Selenium 10 mg Sodium 5.9 mg Zinc- 9600 mg Sulphur : 0.72 %
ALVITE-M	Alembic Limited	1kg, 2.5kg	Layers : 250 g/ 100 kg feed Live stock : 25 g/day/ Adult animal	Each 250-g contains: Vitamin A: 5,00,000 I.U, Vitamin D3: 1,02,500 I.U. Vitamin B2: 0.13g, Vitamin E: 87.5 I.U., Vitamin K: 0.1g, Calcium pantothenate: 0.25g, Vitamin B12: 0.75mg, Cholin Chloride: 6% w/v, Manganese: 2.75 g, Iodine: 0.1g, Zinc: 1.5 g, Iron: 0.75 g , Copper: 2 g, Cobalt: 0.045 g, Calcium: 85 g, Antioxidant added
ALVIZYME-PLUS	Alembic Limited	1 kg pack	250G / ton of poultry feed.	Each 500g contains: Lactobacillus acidophilus: 5,00,000 million CFU Saccharomyces cerevisiae: 5,00,000 million CFU Amylase: 2,50,000 units Protease: 3,50,000 units Lipase: 20,000 units Cellulase: 30,000 units Phytase: 45,000 units Galactosidase: 45,000 units Glucanase: 70,000 units Pectinase: 1,20,000 units

				Xylanase; 35,000 units
SOLEX-M	Venky's India Ltd	100 gm	100 g powder B-Complex makes 5 L liquid B-Complex 20 mL per 100 birds	Each gm has Vitamin B2 12.5 mg Calcium D pantothenate 29 mg Vitamin B6 06.2 mg Niacin 375 mg Vitamin B12 63 mcg DL – Methionine 50 mg
BESTMIN GOLD	Vetcare	Powder	25g/day/animal as per direction	Mineral preparation
BUCOMIN E	Natural Remedies	Bolus	2 boli BID PO	Trace minerals with Vit E
CAL-D-PLUS DS	Cadila	'100 ml., 500ml., 1000 ml., 5000 ml.	50 ml per day PO per cattle	Each 5 ml. contains : Calcium Gluconate – 416.5 mg. Cholecalciferol (Vit D3) – 800 'i.u. Stomach Extract – 1.65 mg. Ferric Ammonium Citrate – 83.5 mg. Vitamin B12 – 8.35 mcg. Colour – Amaranth
CALPAR	Cadila	1 Ltr. & 5 ltr. HDPE Jar	50 ml per day PO per cattle	Each 20 ml. contains : Calcium – 350 mg. Phosphorus – 170 mg. Vitamin B12 – 20 mcg. Vitamin D3 -1600 I.U.
CalvitForte bolus	Marc	2 boli strip	2 boli bid	Ca and vit B, D preparation
DICIROL	Cadila	'5 gm. Sachet and 100 gm. Plastic bottle	5 gm per day PO	Each gram contains : Cholecalciferol (Vitmin D3) : 6,00,000 i.u.
MINTRUS bolus	Ayurvet	Bolus	2 boli bid	Each bolus has Fe + Mn + Se + Zn + Co + Cu + Iodine
LACTOFAT	Dosch	Powder 1	30 gm/day	Each Kg contains:

Nutritional Preparation

	Pharmaceutical	kg pack		Vitamin A: 10,000,00 I.U Vitamin E: 300 I.U. Calcium: 30 g Phosphorus: 9 gm Live yeast culture : 5 gm Live lactobacillus: 50 million CFU Amino acid : 5 gm Asparagus racemosus : 50 gm Leptadenia □eticulate : 30 gm Nardostachys jatamasi : 30 gm
Lactin bolus	Tineta	2 boli strip	2 boli per day	Ca and other minerals preparation
MINAL FORTE	Alembic Limited	Poly bag of 1kg &10kg.	28g/day/animal with jaggery or hay or mix one kg of Minal Forte in 1tonne of feed.	Each 100g contains: Calcium - 28g Phosphorous - 9g Manganese - 0.12g Iodine - 0.10g Iron - 0.60g Copper - 0.10g Cobalt - 0.02g Zinc- 0.215g Magnesium - 1.3g L-LysinemonoHCl - 0.45g DL - Methionine - 0.2g Fluorine - 0.05g
SHARKOFERRO L-VET	Alembic ltd	Bottles of 450g	Layers; 20g/100 Birds daily Broilers: 20g/100 Birds daily Cattle, Buffaloes & Horses: 30 - 50g daily Calves, Sheep & Goats: 10 - 15g daily	Each 21g contains: Malt extract I.P - 4.52 gm Calcium gluconate IP - 360mg Ferric ammonium citrate - 300mg (Eq.to 64.5 mg of Fe) Copper sulphate - 100mg Cobalt Chloride - 1.5mg Cholecalciferol IP- 3600IU Nicotinamide IP - 45mg Biotin B.P - 75mcg Folic acid IP - 1.5mg CyanocobalaminIP -

				15mcg (Vit B 12)
SELVIT-E DS	Venky's India Ltd	1 kg	0.1 g per kg of feed	Each gm contains Vitamin E 200 mg Selenium 400 mcg

SHARKOFERRO L-PET	Alembic ltd	Bottles of 200g	Dogs& Cats: 5 to 10g daily	Malt extract I.P - 4.52 gm Calcium gluconate IP - 360mg Ferric ammonium citrate - 100mg (Eq.to21.5 mg of Fe) Copper sulphate - 12mg Cobalt Chloride - 1.5mg Cholecalciferol IP- 400IU Nicotinamide IP - 45mg Biotin B.P - 75mcg Folic acid IP - 1.5mg Cyanocobalamin IP - 15mcg (Vit B 12)
INTACAL PET	Intas Pharmace utical	200 ml glass bottle	Pups: 5 ml twice daily Adult dogs/ Bitches: 10 ml twice daily	Each 20 ml provides Calcium gluconate 325.6 mg Phosphors: 162.8 mg Vitamin D3: 100 IU Vitamin B12: 20 mcg Potassium chloride 250 mcg Sodium chloride 250 mcg Magnesium sulphate 10 mg Managense sulphate: 1000 mcg Zinc sulphate 15 mg Iron 50 mg Folic acid 0.04 mg Flavoured base
TONOPHOSPH AN	Intervet	10 ml, 30 ml vials	5-15 ml in large animals, IM	each ml contains 4-d, 2-m phosphenic acid: 0.2 gm
CALBOROL	Novartis	450 ml Bottle	as per advice	Calcium 1.85 % w/v. proportion of boric acid to Calcium in the inj 2.26 to 1
MIFEX	Novartis	450 ml bottle	as per advice	Calcium 1.85 % w/v. proportion of boric acid to Calcium in the inj 2.26 to 1; Magnesium hypophosphite

				5 % w/v, Dextrose 20 % w/v
SODAPHOS	Vetnex	60 gm pouch powder	as per direction	Sodium acid phosphate 99 % w/w
ALVIMIX-FORTE	Alembic Limited	1kg	250 Gm / ton of poultry feed	Each 250g.contains: Vitamin A: 1,00,00,000 IU. Vitamin D3: 25,00,000 IU VitaminB1: 800mg VitaminB2: 6,000 mg VitaminB6: 1,600mg VitaminB12: 20,500mcg Vitamin K: 1,000mg Vitamin E: 8,000mg Niacinamide: 12,000mg Calcium D Pantothenate: 8,000mg Folic Acid: 800mg

HERBAL PREPARATION: For effective liver function, Immunity and metabolism, Supports optimal growth and in-time maturity, Counteract damaging effects of mycotoxins, chemicals & drugs, For improving livability, production, resistance and better FCR				
VENTRILIV PLUS	Venky's India Ltd	5 LITRE PACK	500 g/ton of feed continuously for broilers, layers and breeders.	20 Herbal combination
DUDHEX bolus	Sushima	1x5 boli	as per direction	Leptadenia sp., Shatavari, Jatamasi, Kalonj, Nakul, Ca, P, Vit A, Vit D3
IMMUNOL	Himalaya	100 ml bottle	2-3 ml daily twice orally in dogs	Each ml contains guduchi (14.5 mg), ashwagandha (7 mg), punarnava (7 mg), shatavari (7 mg), methika (4.8 mg), arkaparni (4.8 mg), haritaki (3.5 mg)
REGURIN	Himalaya	100 ml	2-3 ml twice daily	each ml contains amra (20.8 mg), amlaki (5.8 mg), grunjana (5.8 mg), yashtimadhu (3.6mg), lavanga (3.2mg), draksha

				(0.8mg)
TOXIN BINDER: protection against mycotoxins; Mould Inhibitors				
BANTOX	Venky's India Ltd	1 kg	500 g to 1 kg per ton of feed	Zeolites, Silicon dioxide; Propionate, Acetate, Citrate ; E.O.E ; 3-p Cymenol
CHECK-O-TOX	Ranbaxy	Powder	1-2kg/ton feed	organic salts with Hydrated Sodium Calcium Alumino Silicate
TOXIBIND	Cadila Pharmaceuticals	1 Kg	1-2 kg/ton Feed	Hydrated Sodium Calcium Alumino Silicate
TOXICARE	Cadila Pharmaceuticals	1 Kg	1-2 kg/ton Feed	Hydrated Sodium Calcium Alumino Silicate

ANIONIC FEED SUPPLEMENT

Dietary cation-anion difference (DCAD) typically includes two cations [potassium (K) and sodium (Na)] and two anions [chlorine (Cl) and sulfur (S)]. Anion sources to reduce DCAD include the so-called anionic salts such as ammonium chloride, calcium chloride, magnesium chloride, ammonium sulfate, calcium sulfate, and magnesium sulfate. Minimizing the incidence of hypocalcemia and milk fever reduces the incidence of other associated metabolic disorders such as retained fetal membranes, abomasal displacement, and metritis. A target DCAD of -5 to -10 meq may improve transition cow health and performance. In lactation rations, DCAD between +25 to +30 meq/100 grams of dietary DM is effective and sufficient to achieve maximum feed intake and milk yield.

HYPORID powder	Intas	250 gm pack	250 gm per day or as per advice	Contains anions balanced with other ions

GROUP: VITAMINS/MINERALS/LIVER STIMULANTS

Vitamin A: It occurs in nature in several forms. Retinol (Vit. A) is present in liver, fish, egg, milk; dehydroretinol (Vit A2) is present in fish; Carotenoids which splits to retinol in the body is present in green leafy vegetables. Vitamin A is important component of visual cycle. It promotes differentiation and maintains structural integrity of epithelia. Inhibits keratinizatron, improves local immunity, is needed for spermatogenesis and normal fetal development. Deficiency occurs only in chronic malmetritran and leads to dry eye, Bitot's spots, softening of cornea, opacificatran and night blindness, dry and hyperkeratinized skin, keratinizatran of bronchopulmonary and GIT epithelium leading to recrument infections. Also is associates with sterility and growth retardation.

Vitamin B1 (Thaimine): It is a colorless, crystalline compound containing a pyrimidine and a thiazole ring, present in the outer layers of cereals, pulses, nuts, green vegetables, egg and meat. It acts as a coenzyme in carbohydrate metabolism, decarboxylation of ketoacids, hexose monophosphate shunt. Deficiency of Vit. B, leads to neurological defects (dry beri-beri) or cardiac symptoms and failure (wet beri-beri).
Indicatrons : Prophylaxis in patients on parenteral nutrition, chronic diarrhoea, chronic alcoholics. Helps in hyperemesis gravidarum, anorexia neurosa.
VITAMIN B12 (CYANOCOBALAMIN): complex cobalt containing compounds present in diet and referred to as Vit. B12. Dietary sources are liver, kidney, sea fish, egg yolk, meat, cheese, legumes (pulses). VitB12 is instricately linked with folate metabolism in many ways. It is essential for the conversion of homocysteine to methionine, purine and pyrimidine synthesis and VitB12 is essential for cell growth and multiplication.Vit B12 is directly and completely absorbed after i.m. or deep s.c. injection. Vit B12 deficiency occurs due to pernicious anaemia, other causes of gastric mucosal damage, like gastritis, gastric carcinoma, gastrectomy etc, malabsorption, consumption of B12 by abnormaly flora in intestine (blind loops syndrome), nutritional deficiency and increased demand as in pregnancy and infancy. Manifestations of deficiency are megaloblastic anaemia, glossitis, g.i. damage, subacute combined degeneration of spinal cord; peripheral neuritis. Indications : Treatment and prophylaxis of B12 deficiency, mega doses of B12 have been used in neuropathies, psychiatric disorders, cutaneous sarcoid and as a general tonic to allay fatigue, improve growth, tobacco amblyopia.
VITAMIN B2 (RIBOFLAVIN): It is a yellow flavore compound found in milk, egg, liver, green leafy vegetables and grains. Flavin adenene dinucleotide (FAD) and flavin mononucleotide (FMN) are coenzymes for flavo proteins involved in many oxidation-reduction reactions. Deficiency leads to stomatitis, cheilosis, dry skin, hair loss, anemia and later neuropathy. Indications : Treatment of deficiency state, usually with other deficiecy states.
VITAMIN B3 (NIACIN): Also called nicotinic acid, is derived in body from tryptophan, which is an aminoacid, present in liver, fish, meat, cereals, pulses and nuts. Nicotinic acid forms nicotinamide which is a component of the coenzyme nicotinamide adenine-dinucleotide (NAD) and its phosphate (NADP). They are involved in various oxidation-reduction reactions. Deficiency leads to 'pellagra' characterised by dermatitis, diarrhoea, dementia, sensory disturbances.
VITAMIN B5 (CALCIUM PANTOTHENATE): It is an organic acid found in liver, mutton, egg yolk and vegetables. It is a component of Coenzyme A which functions in carbohydrate, fat, steroid and porphyrin metabolism. Indications : It is usually a part of multivitamin preparations. Calcium pantothenate is used in paralytic ileus.
VITAMIN B6 (PYRIDOXINE): Pyridoxine, Pyridoxal, pyridoxamine are the 3 forms of Vit. B6 found in liver, meat, egg, soyabean, vegetables and whole grains. They are readily oxidized in the body to pyridoxal phosphate which acts as a coenzyme for transaminases, decarboxylases in important reactions like formation

of 5HT, GABA, dopmine, aminolevulenic acid etc. Deiciency leads to Seborrheic dermatitis, glossitis, growth retardation, peripheral neuritis, anemia and convulsions.

VITAMIN C (ASCORBIC ACID): It is a 6-carbon organic acid, is a potent reducing agent. Citrus fruits like lemons and oranges, black currants are rich in ascorbic acid, other sources are tomato, potato, green chillies, cabbage and other vegetables. It plays a role in important reactions like hydroxylation of protine to hydroxyproline essentitial component of collagen, conversion of folic acid to folinic acid, synthesis of adrenal steroids, oxytocin, ADH and prostaglandins etc. Deficiency leads to scurvy with swollen bleeding gums, peticheal and subperiosteal hemorrhages, deformed teeth, brittle bones, impaired wound healing and anemia.

VITAMIN E : Alpha tocopherol present in wheat germ oil, cereals, nuts, spinarch, egg yolk, is most abundant in nature that has Vitamin E activity. It acts as an antioxidant protecting cell membranes and coenzyme Q. Deficiency of Vit E is associated with sterility, degenerative changes is spinal cord and skeletal muscles, haemolytic anemias. Indications : Deficiency is rare. Usually given as supplenent in G6PD deficiency, acanthocytosis, to enhance absorption of Vit. A, in premature neonates at risk of retrolental fibroplasia. Is empirically used in providing symptomatic relief in noctural cramps, fibrocystic breast disease, toxemia of pregnancy, coronary artery disease and other neuro degenerative disorders.

VITAMIN K : It is a fat soluble vitamin present in green leafy vegetables, cheese and liver. It acts as a cofactor in the gamma carboxylation of glutamate residues of coagulation proteins factor 2, 7, 9 and 10 which is necessary to make them capable of binding to calcium and further phospholipids needed in coagulation cascade. Its daily requirement is 50-100 mcg/day. Deficiency occurs in patients with liver disease, obstructive jaundice , malabsorption syndrome, usually in hospitalized patients on parenteral therapy or prolonged surgery and uremia on long term antimicrobial therapy, rarely it is due to deficient diet. Deficiency leads to bleeding disorder most commonly manifested as hematuria. Indications : Prophylaxis in high risk patients like with hepatic cirrhosis, chronic active diseases, it is routinely recommended for all newborns to prevent hemorrhagic newborn disease. Treatment of over dose of oral anticoagulants.

VITAMIN D : The primary active metabolite of the vitamin is calcitriol, the product of two successive hydroxylations of vitamin D, the initial step in activation of vitamin D occurs in the liver and the final activation to calcitriol occurs primarily in the kidney. The mechanism by which vitamin D acts to maintain normal concentrations of $Ca2+$ and phosphate in plasma are to facilitate their absorption by the small intestine, to interact with PTH to enhance their mobilization from bone, and to decrease their excretion by the kidney. **Indications** : Along with calcium in various calcium deficiency states, vitamin D resistant and vitamin D dependent rickets, renal rickets, hypoparathyroidism.

MULTIVITAMIN PRODUCTS Indicated in ascites, cirrhosis, metabolic stimulant, Neurological disorders, Anorexia, Anemia, Convalescence, Liver disorders, Blood protozoan diseases, Supportive therapy, Anorexia, Anaemia, Convalescence, Liver disorders, Blood protozoan diseases, Growth of young animals.				
Product	**Company**	**Presentation**	**Dose rate**	**Composition**
ANABOLITE liquid	Virbac	1 litre bottle	200 ml twice daily followed by 100 ml BID from second day for 3 days.	Gluconeogenic precurosors fortified with B-complex vitamin
BELAMYL INJECTION	Sarabhai Zydus	10, 30, 50 ml vials	5-10 ml on alternate day, Deep IM in Large animal	Each ml contains: Thiamin HCl I.P.: 10 mg Riboflavin I.P: 3mg Niacinamide I.P.: 100 mg Vitamin B 12 I.P.: 10 mcg Liver injection crude 0.66 ml having Vitamin B 12 activity eq.to 2 mcg of Cyanocobalamin per ml.
BIVINAL FORTE INJECTION	ALEMBIC LTD	10, 30 ml vials	5-10 ml on alternate day, Deep IM in Large animal	Each ml contains: Thiamin HCl I.P.: 10 mg Riboflavin I.P: 3mg Niacinamide I.P.: 100 mg Vitamin B 12 I.P.: 10 mcg Liver injection crude 0.66 ml having Vitamin B 12 activity eq.to 2 mcg of Cyanocobalamin per ml.
BIVINAL LIQUID	Alembic Limited	5 liter HDPE jar	10 - 20 ML / 100 Birds in drinking water.	Each 5ml contains: Cholin chloride: 5 mg Vitamin B2: 1.25 mg Vitamin B6: 0.62 mg

				Niacinamide: 37.5 mg Dl- Panthenol: 1.25 mg Vitamin B12: 6.25 mcg Methionine: 5 mg Lysine: 5 mg
BOVOPLEX - CC	Indian Immunologicals	10, 30 ml vials	Large animal 5-10 ml small animal 0.5 to 2.0 ml	Each ml contains: Thiamine HCl 25 mg Riboflavin 1.5 mg Niacinamide 50 mg Cyanocoblamin 50 mcg Liver injection crude having vit. B12 activity equivalent not less than 2 mg Pyridoxine HCl 5 mg Choline esterase 25 mg
BROTONE tonic	Virbac	120 ml, 500 ml bottle	dogs: 5-10 ml twice daily	Each 10 ml contains: Nicotinic acid 24 mg Yeast extract : 0.4 gm Liver fraction : 1.25 gm having vit. B12 activity equivalent not less than 7.5 mcg
ENERBEE FDS	Cadila	1 kg. Polypack in 25 x 1 kg. HDPE Drums	25 gm BiD PO	Each gm. Contains Vitamin B1 - 8 mg; Vitamin B6 - 16 mg, Vitamin B12 - 80 mcg., Vitamin E - 80 mg., Niacin - 120 mg, Folic Acid - 8 mg, Calcium D Pantothenate - 80 mg, Calcium - 125 mg. , Phosphate - 300 mg.
GENPLEX inj	Genesis pharma	30 ml vial	5-10 ml IM large animal	Each ml contains: Thiamine HCl: 10 mg Riboflavin 3 mg Niacinamide 100 mg
LIVADEX FORTE inj	Virbac	10 ml, 30 ml vial	5 ml daily IM in cattle; 2 ml IM in dogs	Each ml contains: Pyridoxine HCl I.P.: 5 mg Cyanocobalamin: 50 mcg Nicotinamide I.P.:

				100mg Choline : 100 mg Ligoncaine HCl : 10 mg Folic acid: 10 mg Liver injection crude 0.66ml having Vitamin B 12 acivity eq.to 2 mcg of Cyanocobalamin per ml.
LIVAMYL INJ. VET	Cattle Remedies	10 ml, 30 ml	5-10 ml on alternate day, Deep IM in Large animal	Each ml contains: Thiamin HCl I.P.: 10mg Riboflavin I.P: 3mg Niacinamide I.P.: 100mg Vitamin B 12 I.P.: 10mcg Liver injection crude 0.66ml having Vitamin B 12 acivity eq.to 2 mcg of Cyanocobalamin per ml.
LIVOMARC bolus	Marc India Ltd	2 boli pack	2 boli per day	liver ext + Vit B1 and B12 + Dried yeast 700 mg + Methionine + Fe sulfate + $CoCl^2$ + $CuSO^4$ + Ginger Powder + Dextrose
MARCOSID inj	Marc India	10 ml	10 ml per animal IM	Each ml contains: Thiamin HCl : 100 mg Riboflavin I.P: 3mg Niacinamide I.P.: 100mg Pyridoxine 5 mg Panthenol 10 mg Vitamin B 12 I.P.: 100 mcg Liver injection crude 0.66ml having Vitamin B 12 acivity eq.to 2 mcg of Cyanocobalamin
MULTIVET INJ	Dosch Pharma	30 ml, 50 ml vial	1 ml/15kg bwt/day IM	Each ml contains: Vitamin A, Vitamin D3, Vitamin E,

				Niacinamide, Thiamine, Pyridoxin, Riboflavin, Biotin, Calcium pantothenate, Vitamin B12, Choline Chloride, Calcium.
NEUROXIN-12V INJ	Sarabhai Zydus	10, 30 ml vials	5-10 ml IM x 5 days	Each ml contains: Thiamin HCl I.P.: 30mg Pyridoxine HCl : 13.75 mg Cyanocobalamin : 500 mcg
RUMIS CC bolus	RFCL	4 boli pack	2 boli BID PO	Liver Ext + Lysine + Histidine + Lactobacillus + Mg trisillicate
START bolus	PAIL pharma	4 boli pack	2 boli BID PO	Liver Ext + Lysine + Histidine + Lactobacillus + Mg trisillicate
SOLEX-M	Venky's India Ltd	100 gm	100 g powder B-Complex makes 5 L liquid B-Complex 20 mL per 100 birds	Each gm has Vitamin B2 12.5 mg Calcium D pantothenate 29 mg Vitamin B6 06.2 mg Niacin 375 mg Vitamin B12 63 mcg DL – Methionine 50 mg
TRIBIVET inj	Neovet Intas	2, 10, 30, 50 ml vials	Large animals : 5-10 ml IM x 5 days	Each ml contains: Thiamin hydrochloride I.P.: 50 mg Pyridoxine HCl : 50 mg Cyanocobalamin : 500 mcg
TROX – P powder	Virbac	5 kg bag	500 gm per ton layer feed from 17 th week of age	Tylosin phosphate 10% w/w
VENTRIBEE PLUS	Venky's India Ltd	1 kg	200 g per ton of feed for broiler and layer	Each g contains Vitamin B1 4 mg Vitamin B12 40 mcg

			200 to 300 g per ton of feed in stress or intense summer seasons	Ca-D pantothenate 40 mg Vitamin B6 8 mg Vitamin E 40 mg Niacin 60 mg
VENTRIPLE X-M	Venky's India Ltd	500 mL, 1 L and 5 L	Upto 2 weeks of age - 15 mL per 100 birds in drinking water Above 2 weeks of age - 20 mL per 100 birds in drinking water	Each 5 mL contains Vitamin B2 - 1.25 mg Vitamin B6 - 0.62 mg Vitamin B12 - 6.25 mg D-Panthenol 1.25 mg Niacinamide 37.5 mg DL-Methionine 5 mg
VITABEST tonic	Virbac	100 ml, 150 ml bottle	2 tsf in adult dogs daily	Cod liver oil 50% Soya oil 50 %

VITAMIN A AND COMBINATION				
Infertility associated with Vitamin A deficiency, Night blindness, Xerophthalmia, Keratomalacia. As a supportive therapy in Respiratory, Gastrointestinal & urogenital tract infections. Repeat breeding, Poor conception, Night blindness, Xerophthalmia, Muscular dystrophy, Alleviating stress, Body resistance, Infertility, To improve milk yield and egg production, Faster growth and proper bone formation, curled-toe paralysis, rickets, poor bone and egg shell quality, poor hatchability, embryonic mortality				
ADCELIN inj	Virbac	5 ml vial	10 ml per week in large animals for hypovitaminosis	Each 5 ml contains : Vitamin A : 2,50,000 IU Vitamin D 3 : 25000 IU Vitamin E : 150 mg
ALVITON LIQUID	Alembic Limited	500ml, 20 m, 1 lit.	Cattle and Horses : 10 ml twice daily/animal; 5-10ml/100 birds	Each 5 ml contains : Vitamin A :2,50,000 IU Vitamin D 3 : 25000 IU Vitamin E : 150 IU Vitamin C : 500 mg
ALVITON-PLUS	Alembic Limited	Bottle of 20ml, 100ml, 500ml & 1litre.	Cattle & Horse: 10ml twice daily. Dogs: 3-5 ml twice Poultry: Chicks: 2 -3 ml /100Birds Broilers: 4 -6ml /100 Birds.	Each 5ml contains: Vitamin A: 2,50,000 I.U. Vitamin D3: 25,000 I.U Vitamin E: 150 IU Vitamin C: 500 mg Selenium: 0.5 mg

HYBLEND powder	Virbac	1 kg pack	poultry: 1 kg in 10 tonnes of feed	Each gm contains: Vitamin A: 82,500 I.U. Vitamin D3: 12,000 I.U Vitamin B2: 50mg Vitamin K 10 mg
INTAVITA-H inj	Neovet Intas	5 ml vial	5 ml per buffalodeep IM	Each 5ml contains: Vitamin A: 2,50,000 I.U. Vitamin D3: 25,000 I.U Vitamin E: 100 IU Biotin 12.5 mcg
INTAVITA-H inj	Neovet Intas	10 ml vial	10 ml per buffalo deep IM	Each 5ml contains: Vitamin A: 2,50,000 I.U. Vitamin D3: 25,000 I.U Vitamin E: 100 IU
MULTIVET INJ	Dosch Pharma	30 ml, 50 ml vial	1 ml/15kg bwt/day IM	Each ml contains: Vitamin A, Vitamin D3, Vitamin E, Niacinamide, Thiamine, Pyridoxin, Riboflavin, Biotin, Calcium pantothenate, Vitamin B12, Choline Chloride, Calcium.
PROWINSTRES liquid	Cadila	'30 ML,500ML	1 ml / 15 kg body wt IM	Each ml. provides : Vitamin A - 12000 'i.u. Vitamin D3 - 6000 'i.u. Vitamin E Acetate - 50 mcg. Vitamin B12 - 20 mcg. Vitamin C - 25 mcg. Protein Hydrolysate - 25 mg.
VENTRIFORTE-A	Venky's India Ltd	100 mL	2 ml for 100 birds everyday in drinking water	Each mL contains Vitamin A 100,000 I. U.
VENTRIMIX	Venky's India Ltd	1 kg pack	100 g per ton of feed for broiler and layer 150 to 200 g per ton of feed in stress or intense	Each g contains Vitamin A 82,500 IU Vitamin B2 50 mg Vitamin D3 12,000 IU Vitamin K 10 mg

			summer seasons	
VETADE INJ	Sarabhai Zydus	10 ml vial	Cattle : 6-10 ml IM Horses : 4 ml IM Pig : 3 ml IM	Each ml contains: Vitamin A I.P.: 6,00,000 I.U. Vitamin D3 : 25000 IU Vitamin E : 100 IU
VIMERAL liquid	Virbac	30, 60, 120, 300, 500 ml	10 ml/100 layers; 10 ml in large animals daily; 2-3 ml in pets daily	Each ml contains: Vitamin A I.P.: 12,000 I.U. Vitamin D3 : 6000 IU Vitamin E : 48 mg Vitamin B12 - 20 mcg.
VITABLEND AD3 powder	Virbac	1 kg tin, 20 gm sachet	5 gm daily in large animals	Each gm contains: Vitamin A I.P.: 50,000 I.U. Vitamin D3 : 5,000 IU
VITABLEND WM FORTE liquid	Virbac	1 ltr pack	10 ml/100 layers for 10 days	Each gm contains: Vitamin A I.P.: 1,00,000 I.U.
VITAMIN-A injection	Alembic ltd	Box of 2 ml x 6 ampoules	Large animals: 12ml /week Small animals: 6 -12ml /week Dog & Cat: 2 - 6ml / week	Each 2ml ampoule contains: Vitamin A I.P.: 6,00,000 I.U. Chlorbutol I.P.: 1% W/V (as preservative), in an oily vehicle
VITAMIN-A injection	Virbac	Box of 2 ml x 6 ampoules	Large animals: 12 ml /week Small animals: 6 -12 ml /week Dog & Cat: 2 -6 ml / week	Each 2ml ampoule contains: Vitamin A I.P.: 6,00,000 I.U. Chlorbutol I.P.: 1% W/V (as preservative), in an oily vehicle

VITAMIN E PREPARATION

Alpha tocopherol present in wheat germ oil, cereals, nuts, spinarch, egg yolk, is most abundant in nature that has Vitamin E activity. It acts as an antioxidant protecting cell membranes and coenzyme Q. Deficiency of Vit E is associated with sterility, degenerative changes is spinal cord and skeletal muscles, haemolytic anemias. **Indications** : Deficiency is rare. Usually given as supplement to enhance absorption of Vit. A, in premature neonates at risk of retrolental fibroplasia. Is

empirically used in providing symptomatic relief in toxemia of pregnancy and other neuro degenerative disorders.				
STAR BLEND powder	Virbac	200 gm pack	75-125 gm per ton of feed	Each 100 gm has Vitamin E : 100 IU Selenium 20000 mcg

PHOSPHORUS : Indicated in post parturient haemoglobinuria (PPH), Pica, Infertility, Ketosis, Milk fever, Transit recumbency. Dose rate: 400-800 mg total in large animal I/M, I/V, S/C. In case of PPH, 4000 mg total dose IV.				
SODAPHOS	Vetnex	60 gm pouch powder	as per direction	Sodium acid phosphate 99 % w/w
TONOPHOSPHAN	Intervet	10 ml, 30 ml vials	5-15 ml in large animals, IM	each ml contains 4-d, 2-m phosphenic acid: 0.2 gm
URIMIN inj	Virbac	10 ml, 30 ml vial	Large animal: 10 ml IM; Dogs: 2 ml IM	Na acid phosphate: 40.3% w/v equivalent to elemental Phosphorus 80 mg/ml
ANTI-MILK FEVER FORMULA / CALCIUM PREPARATION				
CALBOROL inj	Novartis	450 ml Bottle	250-450 ml slow IV in cattle	Calcium 1.85 % w/v. proportion of boric acid to Calcium in the inj 2.26 to 1
MIFEX injection	Novartis	450 ml bottle	250-450 ml slow IV in cattle	Calcium 1.85 % w/v. proportion of boric acid to Calcium in the inj 2.26 to 1; Magnesium hypophosphite 5 % w/v, Dextrose 20 % w/v
CALPAR	Cadila	1 Ltr. & 5 ltr. HDPE Jar	50 ml per day PO per cattle	Each 20 ml. contains : Calcium - 350 mg. Phosphorus - 170 mg. Vitamin B12 - 20 mcg. Vitamin D3 -1600 I.U.
CAL-D-PLUS DS	Cadila	'100 ml., 500ml., 1000 ml., 5000 ml.	50 ml per day PO per cattle	Each 5 ml. contains : Calcium Gluconate - 416.5 mg. Cholecalciferol (Vit D3) - 800 'i.u. Stomach Extract - 1.65 mg. Ferric Ammonium Citrate -

				83.5 mg. Vitamin B12 - 8.35 mcg. Colour - Amaranth
ASCAL LIQUID	Alembic Limited	1ltr, 500 ml, 5 lit.	Cattle and Horses : 50 ml/day orally	Each 5 ml contains : Calcium Phosphate 0.24 g (equivalent to 0.21 g of Ca3(PO4)2 Cholecalciferol (Vitamin D3) I.P. 500 I.U. Vitamin B 12 I.P. 7.5 mcg
ASCAL-FS	Alembic Limited	Pet Bottle of 500ml, HDPE jars of 1lit & 5lits	Cattle &Horse: 100ml/day Calves, Goat & Pig: 10ml twice daily Dogs: 5-10ml twice daily	Each 100ml contains: Tricalcium Phosphate - 4800mg Eq.to elemental Calcium - 1867mg Elemental Phosphorous - 955mg Cholecalciferol (Vitamin D 3) - 10000 IU Cyanocobalamine (Vitamin B 12) - 150mcg Magnesium sulphate Eq.to elemental Magnesium - 200mg Calory contents- 80calories/100ml
KALZOL D3 powder	Virbac	5 kg bag	5 kg in 5 tonne poultry feed	Each 20 ml. contains : Calcium - 1250 mg. Phosphorus - 625 mg. Magnesium : 1.05 mg Cholecalciferol (Vitamin D 3) - 2500 IU
METABOLITE powder	Virbac	50 gm sachet	50 gm BID during last month of pregnancy in cattle	Balanced minerals and vitamin preparation
HYPORID powder	Intas	250 gm apck	250 gm per day or as per advice	Anionic feed supplement

MULTI-VITAMIN/MINERAL PREPARATION Hypocalcemia, Phosphorus deficiency, Hypomagnesemia, Growth promoter, High Milk Yield, Pregnant & Lactating Animals				
AGRIMIN Forte powder	Virbac	1 kg, 5 kg bags	1kg per ton cattle feed; 30 gm daily in cattle; Fish: 10 kg per ton feed	Each kg has Vitamin A 7,00,000 IU Vitamin D3 70,000 IU Vitamin E 250 mg Nicotinamide 1000 mg Cobalt – 150 mg Copper – 1200 mg Iodine – 325 mg Iron – 1500 mg Magnesium – 6000 mg Manganese – 1500 mg Calcium – 25.5 % Phosphorous – 12.75 % Potassium 100 mg Selenium 10 mg Sodium 5.9 mg Zinc- 9600 mg Sulphur : 0.72 %
AGRIMIN powder	Virbac	1 kg, 10 kg bags	1-2 kg per ton cattle feed; 30-35 gm daily in cattle	Each kg has Calcium – 24% Phosphorous – 12 % Cobalt – 150 mg Copper – 1200 mg Iodine – 325 mg Iron – 5000 mg Magnesium – 6000 mg Manganese – 1500 mg Potassium 100 mg Selenium 10 mg Sodium 5.9 mg Zinc- 9600 mg Methionine: 1920 mg L-Lysine monoHCl – 4400 mg Sulphur : 0.922 %
ALVIMIX-FORTE	Alembic Limited	1kg	250 Gm / ton of poultry	Each 250g.contains: Vitamin A: 1,00,00,000 IU. Vitamin D3: 25,00,000 IU

			feed	VitaminB1: 800mg VitaminB2: 6,000 mg VitaminB6: 1,600mg VitaminB12: 20,500mcg Vitamin K: 1,000mg Vitamin E: 8,000mg Niacinamide: 12,000mg Calcium D Pantothenate: 8,000mg Folic Acid: 800mg
ALVITE-M	Alembic Limited	1kg, 2.5kg	Layers : 250 g/ 100 kg feed Live stock : 25 g/day/ Adult animal	Each 250-g contains: Vitamin A: 5,00,000 I.U, Vitamin D3: 1,02,500 I.U. Vitamin B2: 0.13g, Vitamin E: 87.5 I.U., Vitamin K: 0.1g, Calcium pantothenate: 0.25g, Vitamin B12: 0.75mg, Cholin Chloride: 6% w/v, Manganese: 2.75 g, Iodine: 0.1g, Zinc: 1.5 g, Iron: 0.75 g , Copper: 2 g, Cobalt: 0.045 g, Calcium: 85 g, Antioxidant added
ALVIZYME-PLUS	Alembic Limited	1 kg pack	250G / ton of poultry feed.	Each 500g contains: Lactobacillus acidophilus: 5,00,000 million CFU Saccharomyces cerevisiae: 5,00,000 million CFU Amylase: 2,50,000 units Protease: 3,50,000 units Lipase: 20,000 units Cellulase: 30,000 units Phytase: 45,000 units Galactosidase: 45,000 units Glucanase: 70,000 units Pectinase: 1,20,000 units Xylanase; 35,000 units
ASCAL LIQUID	Alembic Limited	1ltr, 500 ml, 5 lit.	Cattle and Horses : 50 ml/day	Each 5 ml contains : Calcium Phosphate 0.24 g (equivalent to 0.21 g of Ca3(PO4)2 Cholecalciferol (Vitamin D3) I.P. 500 I.U.

				Vitamin B 12 I.P. 7.5 mcg
BESTMIN GOLD	Vetcare	Powder	25g/day/animal as per direction	Vitamin A 7,00,000 IU Vitamin D3 70,000 IU Vitamin E 250 mg Nicotinamide 1000 mg Cobalt – 150 mg Copper – 1200 mg Iodine – 325 mg Iron – 1500 mg Magnesium – 6000 mg Manganese – 1500 mg Calcium – 25.5 % Phosphorous – 12.75 % Potassium 100 mg Selenium 10 mg Sodium 5.9 mg Zinc- 9600 mg Sulphur : 0.72 %
BUCOMIN E	Natural Remedies	Bolus	2 boli BID PO	Trace mineral with Vit E
CALSHAKTI liquid	Neovet Intas	500 ml, 1 ltr bottle; 5 ltr and 7.5 ltr jar	100 ml daily / cattle PO	Each 100 ml contains: Calcium – 1700 mg Phosphorous – 850 mg Cholecalciferol (Vitamin D 3) - 8000 I U Cyanocobalamine (Vitamin B 12) – 100 mcg Shatavari 1000 mg Jivanti (Leptadenia reticulata) 1000 mg Piper longum 400 mg
CHELATED AGRIMIN FORTE powder	Virbac	500 gm, 1 kg, 5 kg bags	1kg per ton cattle feed; 30 gm daily in cattle; Fish: 10 kg per ton feed	Each kg has Vitamin A 7,00,000 IU Vitamin D3 70,000 IU Vitamin E 250 mg Nicotinamide 1000 mg Cobalt – 150 mg Copper – 1200 mg Iodine – 325 mg Iron – 1500 mg Magnesium – 6000 mg Manganese – 1500 mg Calcium – 25.5 %

				Phosphorous – 12.75 % Potassium 100 mg Selenium 10 mg Sodium 5.9 mg Zinc- 9600 mg Sulphur : 0.72 %
DICIROL powder	Cadila	5 gm. Sachet and 100 gm. Plastic bottle	5 gm per day PO	Each gram contains : Cholecalciferol (Vitmin D3) : 6,00,000 i.u.
Electrovet powder	Cipla	113.5 gms	10-15 gm per day orally	Each Pound (454gm)Contains : Synthetic Retinol Concentrate (Oily Form)BP (as Vitamin A Palmitate) 20,000,000IU + Vitamin D3 3,000,000IU + Vitamin E 10,000IU + Riboflavin BP 2,000 mg Menadione Sodium bisulphite complex 8000mg d-Pantothenic Acid 16,000 mg Thiamine Nitrate BP 1,000mg Folic acid BP 500 mg Potassium (as Potassium Chloride BP) 4% Sodium (as Sodium Chloride BP) 4% Sodium (as Sodium Chloride BP) 4%
GROBLEND powder	Virbac	2 kg bag	2 kg in 1.5 tonnes poultry feed	Each kg has Vitamin A 50,00,000 IU Vitamin D3 6,25,000 IU VitaminB2: 2,000 mg VitaminB6: 400 mg VitaminB12: 5600 mcg Ca pantothenate : 4 gm Vitamin E 800 mg Choline chloride 10.00 gm Copper – 2000 mg Iodine – 1000 mg Iron – 7500 mg Manganese – 2750 mg

				Calcium – 27.5 % Phosphorous – 7.45 % Zinc- 15.00 gm
GROVIPLEX liquid	Virbac	500 ml, 5 litre jar	20 ml / 100 birds daily in water, Pigs: 50 ml daily Cattle: 100 ml daily	Each 5 ml contains: Riboflavin 1.25 mg D- Panthenol: 0.65 mg Vitamin B6: 6.25 mg Vitamin B12: 6.25mcg Niacinamide: 18.75 mg Choline chloride: 10 mg Lysine: 10 mg
GROVIPLEX Water soluble powder	Virbac	100 gm pouch		Each 5 ml contains: Niacinamide: 18.75 mg VitaminB2: 1250 mg Vitamin B6: 0.620 gm Vitamin B12: 6.25 mcg Ca pantothenate : 1.51 gm Lysine HCl: 10 gm Choline chloride: 15.82 gm
INTACAL PET liquid	Intas Pharmaceutical	200 ml glass bottle	Pups: 5 ml twice daily Adult dogs/ Bitches: 10 ml twice daily	Each 20 ml provides Calcium gluconate 325.6 mg Phosphors: 162.8 mg Vitamin D3: 100 IU Vitamin B12: 20 mcg Potassium chloride 250 mcg Sodium chloride 250 mcg Magnesium sulphate 10 mg Managense sulphate: 1000 mcg Zinc sulphate 15 mg Iron 50 mg Folic acid 0.04 mg Flavoured base
LACTOFAT	Dosch Pharmaceutical	Powder 1 kg pack	30 gm/day	Each Kg contains: Vitamin A: 10,000,00 I.U Vitamin E: 300 I.U. Calcium: 30 g Phosphorus: 9 gm Live yeast culture : 5 gm Live lactobacillus: 50 million CFU Amino acid : 5 gm Asparagus racemosus : 50

				gm Leptadenia reticulata : 30 gm Nardostachys jatamasi : 30 gm
LACTOFAT powder	Dosch Pharmace utical	Powder 1 kg pack	30 gm/day	Each Kg contains: Vitamin A: 10,000,00 I.U Vitamin E: 300 I.U. Calcium: 30 g Phosphorus: 9 gm Live yeast culture : 5 gm Live lactobacillus: 50 million CFU Amino acid : 5 gm Asparagus racemosus : 50 gm Leptadenia reticulata : 30 gm Nardostachys jatamasi : 30 gm
MINADEX –C powder	Virbac	50 kg bag	Mix 2 kg in 100 kg cattle feed; 50 gm per day in milch animal	Nutritional value Calcium – 20 % Phosphorous – 12 % Magnesium – 5% Iron – 0.4% Iodine – 0.026% Copper – 0.10 % Manganese – 0.12 % Cobalt – 0.012 % Flourine 0.07 % Zinc 0.8 % Sulphur : 3.0 %
MINAL FORTE	Alembic Limited	Poly bag of 1kg &10kg.	28g/day/animal with jaggery or hay or mix one kg of Minal Forte in 1tonne of feed.	Each 100g contains: Calcium - 28g Phosphorous - 9g Manganese - 0.12g Iodine - 0.10g Iron - 0.60g Copper - 0.10g Cobalt - 0.02g Zinc- 0.215g Magnesium - 1.3g L-LysinemonoHCl - 0.45g DL - Methionine - 0.2g Fluorine - 0.05g

MINAL FORTE	Alembic Limited	Poly bag of 1kg &10kg.	28g/day/animal with jaggery or hay or mix one kg of Minal Forte in 1tonne of feed.	Each 100g contains: Calcium – 28g Phosphorous – 9g Manganese – 0.12g Iodine – 0.10g Iron – 0.60g Copper – 0.10g Cobalt – 0.02g Zinc- 0.215g Magnesium – 1.3g L-Lysinemonohydrochloride – 0.45g DL – Methionine – 0.2g Fluorine – 0.05g
MINFA powder	Neovet Intas	1 kg & 10 kg	50 gm per cattle	Each 1000 g contains: Calcium – 240 g Phosphorous – 120 g Magnesium – 2.114 g Iodine – 1.6 mg Iron – 979 g Copper – 312 mg Cobalt – 45 mg Zinc- 2.13 g L-Lysine monohydrochloride – 4.4g DL – Methionine – 1.9 g Chromium : 65 mg
MINOTAS bolus	Neovet Intas	4's x 7 strip	2 boli per day / cattle	each 5 gm contains Zn sulfate 280 mg Cu sulfate 700 mg Mn chloride 2000 mg Co sulfate 5 mg K Iodate 30 mg Na selenite 2 mg Fe sulfate 1400 mg Live yeast 500 mg
MINTRUS bolus	Ayurvet	Bolus	2 boli bid	Each bolus has Fe + Mn + Se + Zn + Co + Cu + Iodine
NUTRICH tab	Virbac	30 tab pack	2 tabs daily in adult dog	Each tab contains Vitamin A : 1100 IU Vitamin D 3 : 110 IU Vitamin E : 2.5 mg Vitamin B1 0.2 mg

				Vitamin B2: 0.5 mg Vitamin B6 0.22 mg Vitamin B12 4 mcg Folic Acid – 0.04 mg Ca-D pantothenate 2 mg Niacinamide 2.25 mg Calcium - 110 mg. Phosphorus - 80 mg. Iron – 6.75 mg Zinc- 2.5 mg
OSTOPET liquid	Virbac	150 ml bottle	5-10 ml BID in dogs	Each 100 ml provides Calcium - 1650 mg. Phosphorus - 850 mg. Vitamin D 3 : 8000 IU Vitamin B12 100 mcg Carbohydrates : 40000 mg
OSTOVET liquid	Virbac	500 ml, 1 ltr, 2 ltr, 5 ltr	100 ml in lactating cattle with vimeral	Each 100 ml provides Calcium - 1650 mg. Phosphorus - 850 mg. Vitamin D 3 : 8000 IU Vitamin B12 100 mcg Carbohydrates : 40000 mg
OSTOVET FORTE liquid	Virbac	500 ml, 1 ltr, 2 ltr, 5 ltr	100 ml in lactating cattle with vimeral	Each 100 ml provides Calcium - 3500 mg. Phosphorus - 1750 mg. Vitamin D 3 : 15000 IU Vitamin B12 200 mcg Carbohydrates : 40000 mg
SELVIT-E DS	Venky's India Ltd	1 kg	0.1 g per kg of feed	Each gm contains Vitamin E 200 mg Selenium 400 mcg
SHARKOFERROL-PET	Alembic ltd	Bottles of 200g	Dogs& Cats: 5 to 10g daily	Malt extract I.P - 4.52 gm Calcium gluconate IP - 360mg Ferric ammonium citrate - 100mg (Eq.to21.5 mg of Fe) Copper sulphate - 12mg Cobalt Chloride - 1.5mg Cholecalciferol IP-400IU Nicotinamide IP - 45mg Biotin B.P - 75mcg Folic acid IP - 1.5mg Cyanocobalamin IP - 15mcg (Vit B 12)

SHARKOFERR OL-VET	Alembic ltd	Bottles of 450g	Layers; 20g/100 Birds daily Broilers: 20g/100 Birds daily Cattle, Buffaloes & Horses: 30 - 50g daily Calves, Sheep & Goats: 10 - 15g daily	Each 21g contains: Malt extract I.P - 4.52 gm Calcium gluconate IP - 360mg Ferric ammonium citrate - 300mg (Eq.to 64.5 mg of Fe) Copper sulphate – 100 mg Cobalt Chloride - 1.5 mg Cholecalciferol IP- 3600 IU Nicotinamide IP – 45 mg Biotin B.P – 75 mcg Folic acid IP - 1.5 mg CyanocobalaminIP – 15 mcg (Vit B 12)
VENTRIMIN-17	Venky's India Ltd	5 kg	Layers: 250 g per 100 kg of feed Starters, Breeders and Broilers: 250 g per 50 kg of feed	Each 250 g contains Vitamin A 500,000 IU Vitamin D3 100,000 IU Vitamin B2 00.20 g Vitamin B12 00.60 mg Vitamin E 75.00 Units Vitamin K3 00.10 g Niacin 01.00 g Calcium D Pantothenate 00.25 g Choline Chloride 15.00 g Calcium 82.00 g Cobalt 0.045 g Copper 00.20 g Iodine 00.10 g Iron 00.75 g Manganese 02.75 g Zinc 01.50 g
Fatsup Liquid	Cipla	250ml	10-25 ml per day orally	Each ml contains Soyabean oil 868mg+Gamma Linolenic acid 1.34mg+Eicosapentaenoic acid 6.6mg+ Docosahexanoic acid 4.4 mg+ Retinyl palmitate 112.7IU+DL-Alphatocopheryl Acetate

				1.86 IU+ Biotin 0.0018mg+Pyridoxine HCL 0.1mg+Zinc sulphate Monohydrate 6.1 mg+ Inositol 0.33mg
Carni Paste	Cipla	250gm	5 – 10 gm per day orally	L-Carnitine 200mg + Panthenol (Vit B5) 20mg
Aminocip	Cipla	55 gms	5 – 10 gm per day orally	L-Leucine 10.73 g + L-Isoleucine 7.88 g + L-Valine 7.88 g + L-Glutamine 0.62 g + L-Carnitine hydrochloride 0.39 g /55 g
Cattle Licks	Cipla	1kg, 2kg, 5kg	place the lick before the animal for adlib licking	Sodium Chloride 88.00%,Iron min.0.13%,Iodine min.,Copper min-.035%,Manganese min.-0.20%,Cobalt min.-0.002%
Vetsupp C 50 powder	Cipla	100gm, 1kg	10- 50 gm BID per cattle orally	Ascorbic acid (vitamin C) 50% w/w
Calbro 32.8% Inj	Cipla	450ml bottle	450 ml IV in cattle	Calcium Borogluconate 32.8% inj
Dextrose	Cipla	500 ml	250-500 ml IV in cattle	Dextrose 5 /20% w/v Infusion
Electrovet powder	Cipla	113.5 gms, 1kg	50 -100 gm per day in cattle dissolved in water	Each Pound (454gm)Contains : Synthetic Retinol Concentrate (Oily Form)BP (as Vitamin A Palmitate) 20,000,000IU Vitamin D3 3,000,000IU Vitamin E 10,000IU Riboflavin BP 2,000 mg Menadione Sodium bisulphite complex 8000mg d-Pantothenic Acid 16,000 mg Thiamine Nitrate BP 1,000mg Folic acid BP 500 mg Potassium

				(as Potassium Chloride BP) 4% Sodium (as Sodium Chloride BP) 4%
Milksup Powder	Cipla	**3.5 kg**	20 -30 gm per day orally in cattle	**Milk products+Vitamin E products and by-products of sugar production+ minerals , oils & fatsOil 6.8% +Protein 14.1% +Ash 7.5% +Fibre 0% + Vitamin E 50000IU per kg +Selenium 12.5mg per kg**
Ractofeed Premix Granules	Cipla	**1 Kg**	1 kg per ton feed	**Ractopamine HCL 10mg/kg**
Cattle Lick Brick	Cipla	**2kg, 5kg bricks**	ad lib	**Sodium Chloride 88% + Iron(min.) 0.13% + Iodine(min.) 0.003% + Copper(min.) 0.035% + Manganese(min.) 0.20% + Cobalt(min.) 0.002%**
Vetphos Forte	Cipla	**30 ml Injection**	10 ml IM in cattle	**Toldimphos Sodium 200 mg / ml + Cyanocobalamin 50 mcg/ml Inj**
Ciplavet	Cipla	**1000 ml Bottle**	10 ml IM weekly in cattle	**Vit A 100,000 IU / ml + Vit D3 20,000 IU / ml + Vit E 40 IU / ml Liquid**
Vitavet Plus Liquid	Cipla	**30 ml Bottle1000 ml Bottle**	10-15 ml orally weekly in cattle	**Vit A 12,000 IU / ml + Vit D3 6,000 IU / ml + Vit E 48 mg + Vit B12 20 mcg / ml Liquid**
Vitavet Inj	Cipla	**30 ml Injection**	10 ml IM in cattle weekly	**Vit A 2,50,000 IU / ml + VitD3 25,000 IU / ml + Vit E 100 IU/ ml + Benzyl Alcohol 2.0 %**
Vetsupp AD3 liquid	Cipla	**1 Ltr**	10-20 ml orally in cattle	**Vitamin A 1,00,000IU + Vitamin D3 10,000IU/ml**
Vetsupp A liquid	Cipla	**1 Ltr**	10-20 ml orally in cattle	**Vitamin A 1,00,000IU/ml**
Vetsupp ABD3E liquid	Cipla	**1 Ltr**	10-20 ml orally in	**Vitamin A 12,000IU + Vitamin B12 20mcg+**

			cattle	**Vitamin D3 6,000IU+Vitamin E 50mg/ml**
Vetsupp AD3EC Oral Liquid	Cipla	**1ltr**	10-20 ml orally in cattle	**Vitamin A 250000 IU +Vitamin D3 25000IU+ Vitamin E 150 mg + Vitamin C 500mg**
Vetsupp ABCE plus liquid	Cipla	**1 Ltr**	10-20 ml orally in cattle	**Vitamin A 3,600IU + Vitamin B6 2mg+ Vitamin C 100mg+Vitamin E 30mg+Biotin 12.5mcg/ml**
Vetsupp AD3 powder	Cipla	**250gm**	10-20 gm orally in cattle	**Vitamin A 55,000IU/gm+Vit D3 5,000IU/gm**
Vetsupp ABD3K powder	Cipla	**250gm**	10-20 gm orally in cattle	**Vitamin A 82,500IU + Vitamin B2 50mg+ Vitamin D3 12,000IU+Vitamin K10mg/Gm**
Vitaforte Powder	Cipla	**100gm, 500gm sachet, 1kg container**	10-20 gm orally in cattle	**Vitamin A palmitate 20,000,000 IU +Vitamin D3 – 4,000,000 IU + Vitamin E -10,000mg + Vitamin B1 –2,000mg + Vitamin B2 – 2,500mg + Vitamin B6 –2,000mg + Vitamin B12 –5mg + Vitamin C –10,000 mg + Vitamin K3 –2,000mg + Nicotinic acid 10,000mg + Calcium pantothenate – 5,000mg + Folic acid – 20,000mg + dl-methionine –2,000mg + Tryptophane 10,000mg + Cystine – 3,000mg + Lysine – 30,000mg + Arginine – 20,000mg**
Vetsupp BE powder	Cipla	**25gm, 250gm, 1kg**	10-20 gm orally in cattle	**Vitamin B1 4mg+ Vitamin B6 8mg+ Vitamin B12 40mcg+Vitamin E 40mg+Calcium Pantothenate 40 mg+ Niacin 60mg**

Vetsupp E plus powder	Cipla	**50 & 200 gm, 1kg Sachet**	10-20 gm orally in cattle	**Vitamin E 10% +Selenium 100 ppm**
Vetsupp E Plus Liquid	Cipla	**500ml,1lt r,25ltr**	10-20 gm orally in cattle	**Vitamin E 100mg + Selenium 0.5mg/ml**
Vetsupp AE liquid plus	Cipla	**1 Ltr**	10-20 ml orally in cattle	**Vitamin H (Biotin)12.5mcg +Vitamin E 50mg +Vitamin A 20,000IU /ml**
Vetsupp AD3E Plus liquid	Cipla	**1 Ltr**	10-20 ml orally in cattle	**Vitamin H (Biotin)12.5mcg +Vitamin E 50mg+ Vitamin A 20,000IU+ Vitamin D3 10,000IU /ml**
Vitapet Powder	Cipla	**60 tabs**	1-2 tab daily in pets orally	**Vitamins :Ca lcium (min.).-2.5%+(max)- 3.5%+Phosporus – 2.5% + Potassium-0.4%+ Salt (min) – 0.1%+ (max0 – 0.6% + Chloride – 0. 1%+Magnesium 0.15%+Iron – 3.0mg+Cu- 0.1mg+Mn-0.25mg + Zn – 1.4mg Minerals: Vit A – 1,000 IU + Vitamin D 100 IU + Vitamin E 2 IU + Thiamine 0.81mg + Riboflavine 1.0mg+ Niacin 10 mg + Pyridoxine 0.1 mg + Vitamin B12 0.5mcg**

IRON PREPARATION (haematinic / anaemic)				
FERITAS bolus	Neovet Intas	5's x 2 strip	2 boli daily / cattle	each bolus contains Ferrous fumarate 1500 mg Vit B^{12} 75 mcg Folic acid 7500 mcg
Fe-Folate liq	Venky's	200 ml bottle	5 ml bid PO per dog	Each 5 ml contains elemental iron 50 mg + folic acid 175 mcg + vitB12 2.5 mg
FERITAS inj	Neovet	10 ml vial	1 ml per	Each ml contains Elemental

	Intas		50 kg bwt IM	Iron 50 mg Folic acid 500 mcg Hydorxycobalamin 50 mcg
Ferritone	Cipla	20 ml Vial	2 ml per 50 kg bwt IM	Ferric-Hydroxide Sucrose Compound Injection[Each ml contains Iron (Fe) 20 mg as the compound
Imferon inj	Shreya	ampoule	10 ml IM, IV per cow	Elemental iron 50 mg/ml
Haem-Up liq	Cadila	200 ml pack	5 ml bid PO per dog	Each 15 ml contains Haemoglobin 1 gm + Ferric NH4 citrate 100 mg + Cu sulphate 30 mcg + Zn sulphate 30 mcg

HERBAL PREPARATION: For effective liver function, Immunity and metabolism, Supports optimal growth and in-time maturity, Counteract damaging effects of mycotoxins, chemicals & drugs, For improving livability, production, resistance and better FCR				
VENTRILIV PLUS	Venky's India Ltd	5 LITRE PACK	500 g/ton of feed continuously for broilers, layers and breeders.	20 Herbal combination
DUDHEX bolus	Sushima	1x5 boli	as per direction	Leptadenia sp., Shatavari, Jatamasi, Kalonj, Nakul, Ca, P, Vit A, Vit D3
IMMUNOL	Himalaya	100 ml bottle	2-3 ml daily twice orally in dogs	Each ml contains guduchi (14.5 mg), ashwagandha (7 mg), punarnava (7 mg), shatavari (7 mg), methika (4.8 mg), arkaparni (4.8 mg), haritaki (3.5 mg)
LIV-52 VET	Himalaya	30 ml, 110 ml, 60 tabs	10-15 drops daily twice or as per advice	polyherbal formulation
REGURIN	Himalaya	100 ml	2-3 ml twice daily	each ml contains amra (20.8 mg), amlaki (5.8 mg), grunjana (5.8 mg), yashtimadhu (3.6mg), lavanga (3.2mg),

				draksha (0.8mg)
Tefrosol -Forte Liquid	Cipla	1 ltr	20 ml per day orally in cattle	Each 5 ml contains Tephrosia purpurea 1000mg+ Andrographis paniculata 400mg+ Terminalia chebula 750mg+ Oscimum sanctum500mg+ Mahasudarshan kadha 250mg+ Phyllantus neruri 200mg
Slimz	Cipla	100gm	5 gm per day in pets	Herbal anti-obesity powder for dogs
TOXIN BINDER Provides protection against mycotoxins; Mould Inhibitors				
BANTOX	Venky's India Ltd	1 kg	500 g to 1 kg per ton of feed	Zeolites, Silicon dioxide; Propionate, Acetate, Citrate ; E.O.E ; 3-p Cymenol
CHECK-O-TOX	Ranbaxy	Powder	1-2kg/ton feed	organic salts with Hydrated Sodium Calcium Alumino Silicate
TOXIBIND	Cadila Pharmaceuticals	1 Kg	1-2 kg/ton Feed	Hydrated Sodium Calcium Alumino Silicate
TOXICARE	Cadila Pharmaceuticals	1 Kg	1-2 kg/ton Feed	Hydrated Sodium Calcium Alumino Silicate
Toxirid Powder	Cipla	450gm	20 – 25 gm orally large animals BID	Sodium thiosulphate-10%+Magnesium sulphate(heptahydrate)-54%+Sodium sulphate-25%+Gentian-0.2%+Ginger -1.25%+Linseed 0.1%+Fenugreek -0.2%+Iron oxide-1.0%+Magnesium carbonate-5.25%+Calcium phosphate tribasic-1.0%+Ethylenediamene dihydrochloride-0.008%
A-Tox Powder	Cipla	1 kg, 5kg, 25 kg	1-2 kg/ton Feed	Propionic acid – 8.75% + Benzoic acid-1.50% + Sorbic acid - 0.63%+Acetic acid-10.00% + Hydrated Sodium Calcium Alumunium silicate – 79.12%

Chapter 11

Antineoplastic Preparations

ANTINEOPLASTIC AGENTS

- 5 - FLUOROURACIL
- BUSULPHAN
- CHLORAMBUCIL
- CYCLOPHOSPHAMIDE
- DOXORUBICIN
- MELPHALAN
- MERCAPTOPURIN
- METHOTREXATE
- VINCRISTINE

5 - **FLUOROURACIL**

Mechanism of action : 5 - Fluorouracil is converted in the body to the corresponding nucleotide, 5-fluoro2 deoxyuridine monophosphate, which inhibits thymidylate synthetase and blocks the conversion of deoxyuridilic acid to deoxythymidlic acid and thymine formation. Selective failure of DNA synthesis occurs.

Indications : Tumours of mammary glands, stomach colon, rectum urinary bladder and liver. Topical application in cutaneous basal carcinoma.

Dosage : DOGS: 150-200mg/m^2 BSA weekly or 5-10mg/kg BW weekly IV.

Topical application in cutaneous basal carcinoma. Apply the cream once a day for 4 weeks.

Contraindications : Bone marrow depression, poor nutritional status, potentially serious infections, prior major surgery within 1 month. Hypersensitivity, anaemia, leucopenia, cardiac, hepatic and renal dysfunction.

Special precautions : Avoid topical application on mucus membranes.

Adverse drug reactions : Nausea, vomiting, GI ulcereation, bleeding from any site,diarrhoea, myelosuppression, rashes, hyperpigmentation, alopecia, dermatitis, erythema-multiformae. Central neurotoxicity and myocardial ischemia can cause death.

Status in
1. Pregnancy : Contraindicated
2. Lactation : Discontinue nursing or the drug.
3. Old age : Use with caution.
4. Neonates : Use with extreme caution.
Interactions : It may reduce responce to vaccines and there is possibility of generalised infections with live vaccines. It may reduce effect of warfarin.

Product	Company	Presentation	Composition
FIVOFLO inj	DABUR	5 ml, 10 ml inj	250 mg
FURACIL inj	Biochem	5 ml inj	250 mg, 500 mg

BUSULPHAN

Mechanism of action : It acts by sulphur stripping of macromolecules and it is highly specific for myeloid elements.

Indications : Drug of choice for chronic myeloid leukemia. Also used in polycythemia vera, myeloid leukaemia, myelocytic leukaemia, essential thrombocythaemia.

Dosage

Dogs: 0.1 mg/kg BW daily oral.

Contraindications : Hypersensitivity.

Special precautions : Patient should be hospitalised during induction of therapy.

Adverse drug reactions : Nausea, vomiting. Hepatotoxicity, hyperuricaemia, pulmonary fibrosis and sterility, hemorrhages by decreased platelets.

Status in
1. Pregnancy : Contraindicated
2. Lactation : Contraindicated
3. Old age : Use with caution
4. Neonates : Use with extreme caution in low dose

Interactions : It may reduce response to vaccines and possibility of generalised infections with live vaccines. Phenytoin increases and itraconazole decreases its renal clearence. Combination with thioguanine results in deranged liver function tests and oesophageal varices.

MYLERAN	Burrough Wellcome	100's tabs	2 mg/tab

CHLORAMBUCIL

Mechanism of action : Very slow and shortest acting alkylating agent. It inhibits the cell cycle at premitotic (G2) stage, process cross linking of DNA strands, destroyed DNA and causes cell death.

Indications : First line drug for long term maintenance therapy of chronic lymphocytic leukaemia and primary (Waldenstrom's) macroglobulinaemia.

Dosage

Chronic lymphocytic leukaemia

Dogs: 0.1-0.2 mg/kgBW in 2-4 days a week orally.

Contraindications : Known hypersensitivity.

Special precautions : Haematological monitoring.
Adverse drug reactions : Nausea, vomiting, pulmonary fibrosis, interstitial pneumonia, dermatitis, amenorrhoea, hepatotoxicity, seizures, azoospermia, peripheral neurophathy and bone marrow depression, though less than others.
Status in
1. Pregnancy : Contraindicated
2. Lactation : Contraindicated
3. Old age : May be used.
4. Neonates : Not recommended.
Interactions : Other Myelosuppressive drugs : Side effects of these enhanced.

LEUKERAN	Burrough Wellcome	25's tabs	2 mg/tab

CYCLOPHOSPHAMIDE
Mechanism of action : It exerts its action by alkylation of DNA. After oral administration it is well absorbed. It is a produrg and converted in the blood and liver to its active form namely hydroxyphosphamide and aldophosphamide. It is excreted in urine. Not being a local irritant, it is advantageous as injection.
Indications: Multiple myeloma, Leukemias, Retinoblastoma, Carcinoma of the mammary gland and lungs.
Dosage
Dogs: 2.2 mg/kg BW in 4 days a week orally. 10mg/kgBW/week as IV.
Contraindications : Bladder haemorrhage. Special precautions : Diabetics, old age, liver, heart or kidney impairment, blood dyscrasias. Important to maintain hydration during therapy. Mesna can counter act its urinary side effect.
Adverse drug reactions : Vomiting, myclosuppresion (not effecting platelet), CHF and alopecia are common. Mucosal ulceration, interstitial pulmonary fibrosis, hemorrhagic cystitis can occur. Syndrome of inappropriate ADH secretion occurs at high doses.
Status in
1. Pregnancy : Contraindicated
2. Lactation : Contraindicated
3. Old age : May be used in reduced dose.
4. Neonates : Use with extreme caution in reduced dose.
Interactions : Chloramphenicol : Retards the metabolism of cyclophosphamide.

CYCLOXAN	Biochem	tab, inj.,	50mg/tab; inj contains 100mg, 200mg, 500mg, 1 gm/vial
LEDOXAN	Dabur	tab, Injection	50mg/tab; inj contains 100mg, 200mg, 500mg, 1 gm/vial

DOXORUBICIN
Mechanism of action : Is capable of causing breaks in DNA strands by activating topoisomerase-II and generating free radicals besides interacting in DNA strands. Has mutagenic and carcinogenic potential. Maximum action is exerted at S phase, toxicity is usually exhibited in G2 phase.

Indications : Acute lymphoblastic leukemia, acute myeloblastic leukemia, Thyroid carcinoma, Lymphosarcoma, Mammary tumor

Dosage

Dogs: 30mg/m^2 BSA as IV in 150 ml 5 % Dextrose soln.

Contraindications : Severe myelosuppression, cardiac disease.

Special precautions : Heart and liver impairment.. Doxorubicin should not be mixed with 5-FU.

Adverse drug reactions : Myelosuppression with leucopenia, headache, seizures, confusion, stomatitis, GI disturbances, rashes, alopecia, cardiomyopathy with abnormal ECG, CHF.

Status in

1. Pregnancy : Contraindicated
2. Lactation : Contraindicated
3. Old age : May be used in reduced dose.
4. Neonates : Use with extreme caution.

Interactions : Mercaptopurine : Hepatotoxicity of mercaptopurine is enhanced. Co-administration of streptozocin enhances its toxicity.

ADRIM	Dabur	5 ml vial	2 mg/ml
CARDIA	Zydus cadila	vial	10mg/vial
DOXORUBICIN inj	Biochem	vial	10 mg/ml

MELPHALAN

Mechanism of action : It is active against both resting and rapidly dividing cells and is effective against some malignancies.

Indications : Very effective in multiple myeloma. Also used in advanced ovarian cancer and in mammary cancer.

Dosage : Oral

Multiple myeloma

Dogs: 0.1mg/kgBW x 10 days followed by 0.05-0.1 mg/kgBW daily.

Contraindications : Known hypersensitivity, severe mylosuppression.

Special precautions : Monitor blood counts.

Adverse drug reactions : Myelosupression is common, nausea, vomiting can occur. Alopecia, rash, itching, allergic reactions, liver and kidney damage are unusual and it is an advantage over other antineoplastic agents.

Status in

1. Pregnancy : Contraindicated
2. Lactation : Use with caution.
3. Old age : Use with caution.
4. Neonate : Use with caution.

Interactions : Co-administration with nalidixic acid in children produces fatal hemorrhagic enterocolitis. Cyclosporin enhance

ALKERAN	Burrough Wellcome	tablets	2mg/tab, 5 mg/tab

MERCAPTOPURIN

Mechanism of action : Mercaptopurine (6-MP) and thioguanine (6-TG) are highly effective antineoplastic drugs. They inhibit the conversion of inosine monophosphate to adenine guanine nucleotides.

Indications : Acute lymphatic including lymphocytic and lymphoblastic leukemias, acute myelogenous and myelomonocytic leukemia.

Dosage : (Oral) Dogs: 2 mg/kgBW oid

Contraindications : Hypersensitivity, severe bone marrow suppression, severe hepatic impairment and resistance to mercaptopurine.

Special precautions : Impaired kidney function and liver function.

Status in

1. Pregnancy : Contraindicated
2. Lactation : Contraindicated
3. Old age : Use with caution.
4. Neonates : Use with extreme caution.

Interactions : Delayed catabolism of mercaptopurine by allopurinol results in severe toxicity.

EMPURINE	Dabur	10's tab	50 mg/tab
PURI-NETHOL	Burrough Wellcome	tabs 25's	50mg/tab

METHOTREXATE

Mechanism of action : Inhibits dihydrofolate reductase (DHFRase) blocking the conversion of dihydrofolic acid (DFHA) to tetrahydrofolic and (THF) which is an essential coenzyme in denovo purine synthesis and amino acid interconversion. Methotrexate has cell cycle specific action and kills cells in S phase. It acts mainly on rapidly multiplying cells such as bone marrow, foetal cells, malignant cells, cells of buccal, intestinal and urinary bladder mucosa.

Indications : Choriocarcionoma. Useful in maintaining remission in acute lymphoblastic leukemias, but not good for inducing remission. Transmissible venereal tumor. Rh arthritis, Osteosarcoma.

Dosage : Dogs/cat: 0.3-0.8mg/kgBW weekly IV; 2.5 mg/m^2 BSA daily oral.

Contraindications : Severe liver and kidney dysfunction and bone marrow depression.

Special precaution : Monitor hematological, renal and hepatic functions regularly.

Adverse drug reactions : It exerts major toxicity on bone marrow causing megaloblastic anaemia and pancytopenia. Desquamation and bleeding may occur in g.i.t. Pneumonitis, hepatic cirhosis on long term use.

Status in

1. Pregnancy : Contraindicated
2. Lactation : Contraindicated
3. Old age : Use with caution.
4. neonates : Use with extreme caution.

Interactions : Salicylates, phenylbutazone, sulfonamides, dicoumerol : Displace it from protein binding sties; Aspirin, sulfonamides: decrease its renal tubular secretion, increase toxicity.			
ZEXATE	Dabur	tab, inj 2 ml, 3 ml	2.5 mg/tab, 25 mg/ml in 2 ml inj; 5 mg/ml in 3 ml inj
BIOTREXATE	Biochem	tab, inj 2 ml, 3 ml	2.5 mg/tab, 5 mg/ml in 2 ml inj; 15 mg/ml in 3 ml inj; 50 mg/ml in 2 ml inj

VINCRISTINE:

Mechanism of action : These are mitotic inhibitors, bind to microtubular protein-tubulin, prevent its polymerization and assembly of microtubules, cause disruption of mitotic spindle and interfere with DNA, RNA and protein synthesis

Indications : Transmissible Venereal Tumor, Lymphosarcoma, Immune thrombocytopenia.

Dosage

Dogs/cats: 0.025 mg/kg BW once weekly IV

Special precautions : Impaired liver functions, bronchospasm and preexisting neuromuscular diseases.

Adverse drug reactions : Peripheral neuropathy, convulsions. Alopecia and bone marrow depression, bronchospasm, azospermia, amenorrhoea, nausea, vomiting, diarrhoea, abdominal cramps, constipation, paralytic ileus, leucopenia.

Status in

1. Pregnancy : Contraindicated
2. Lactation : Use with caution.
3. Old age : Use with caution.
4. Neonates : Use with caution.

Interactions : Digoxin and phenytoin : Decreased plasma digoxin and phenytoin levels ; L-asparaginase : Hepatic clearance of vincristine is reduced if L-asparaginase is administered first; It has synergistic action with methotexate.

CYTOCRISTIN	Cipla	1 ml ampoule inj	1mg/ml
VINCRISTINE	Biochem	1 ml ampoule inj	1 mg/ml

Chapter 12

Biosecurity Products

ANTISEPTICS/DISINFECTANTS
➢ **Acids**: HCl, H_2SO_4 in concentration of 0.1N is used for disinfection. Benzoic acid is used as food preservative. Boric acid, Acetic acid (1% for surgical dressing, 0.25% for irrigation of urogenital tract, 5% is bactericidal and used for Rx of otitis externa) are antiseptic. Salicylic acid, Benzoic acid is fungicidal. Acetic acid, lactic acid are spermatocidal. Strong mineral acids are used as cauterizing agents. 2.5% HCl can kill anthrax spores in skin/hides.
➢ **Alkalies:** OH ion inhibits most of bacteria and viruses at pH >9. NaOH & $Ca(OH)_2$ are commonly used disinfectants.
➢ **Alcohols:** Ethyl alcohol, Isopropyl alcohol in 30-90% concentration. Rubbing alcohol is mixture of alcohols and used for skin disinfectants and rubefacient.
➢ **Biguanides**: Chlorhexidine (0.1% aqueous soln.) has potent activity against most gram positive and some gram negative bacteria. 4% emulsion of Chlorhexidine gluconate is used as a skin cleanser, 0.5% w/v in 70% Isopropanol as general antiseptic, 0.5% w/v in 70% Isopropanol with emollients as a hand rinse. 1% Chlorhexidine acetate ointment is used as a topical antiseptic.
➢ **Oxidizing agents**: PEROXIDES: H_2O_2 (3 % soln. for cleaning and deodorising tissue, superficial antimicrobial action); Na perborate (mouthwash), Benzoyl peroxide (antiseptic specially for pyoderma); $KMnO_4$ (1 ppm kills microbes in 1 hour).
➢ **Halogens/related compounds**: Chlorine and Iodine are bactericidal, fungicidal, virucidal and protozoacidal. Iodine is sporicidal and cysticidal too. Iodine tincture contains 2% iodine, used for skin disinfection. Strong Iodine solution (Lugol's Iodine, 5% I_2 + 10% NaI) is used in cases of cervicitis as intrauterine infusion. Povidone Iodine (combination of Iodine and polyvinylpyrrolidone detergent) is applied on wound (as 10% soln) and to clean ear canal (as 5% soln) in otitis externa and as teat dip.
➢ **Heavy metals:** silver nitrate (0.1%) is potent antiseptic and stimulates healing of indolent ulcers when applied topically. Toughened silver nitrate is applied for cauterisation of wounds and ulcers. **Zinc sulfate** is used as astringent, styptic, mild antiseptic, reticular groove closing agent. 10% Zn SO^4 is used as foot bath; 0.25 % soln. for conjunctivitis and 0.4 % with silver nitrate for corneal ulcers.

- **Phenols/related compounds: Thymol** is used for Rx of mycotic otitis externa. 5% **carbolic acid** (phenol) soln. kills anthrax spores. Phenol is bactericidal/fungicidal at 1-2%. Phenol has good penetration power into organic material. Used for disinfection of inorganic equipment and organic materials, for cauterization of infected umbilicus of neonates, incorporated in cutaneous application for pruritus, stings, bites, burns. **Cresol (cresylic acid)** is used as disinfectant (2% soln. of saponated cresol or lysol in hot water) for inanimate objects. **Hexachlorophene** (bacteriostatic) is used in medicated soap. Pine tar is used for antiseptic bandaging of wounds of hoof and horn. **Chloroxylenols** are bactericides and active in alkaline pH and used as skin sterilization (5% soln with water as 1:4) and for wound cleansing and irrigation of uterus and vagina.
- **Reducing agents:** Formaldehyde, Gluteraldehyde are potent germicides including spores. Both are used as disinfectants. Formalin (40% formaldehyde gas in aqueous soln.) is used for room disinfection. Glutaral (1-2% gluterladehyde alkaline soln.) is used to sterilize surgical and endoscopic instruments and plastic and rubber apparatus. SO_2 (gaseous fumigant) is batericidal and used for indoor disinfection.
- **Surface active compounds(Detergents):** soaps (anionic detergents) removes bacteria suspended in their lather. Cationic surfactants include Benzalkonium chloride, Benzethonium chloride (1 ppm soln. for preoperative disinfection of mucous membrane, irrigation of eye and vagina), cetylpyridinium chloride; act as detergnets, keratolytics, emulsifiers.
- **Vapor phase disinfectants: Ethylene** and **Propylene oxides** are gaseous fumigants for sterilizing animal feed, human food, surgical equipment, lab equipment.
- **Miscellaneous agents: Acriflavine** impregnated bandages and gauze; acriflavine jelly is used for Rx of burns. **Azo** dyes (scarlet red and phenazopyridine) are effective against gram negative organisms. Scarlet red is used on sores, ulcers, wounds as 5% ointment. Phenazopyridine is used as analgesic with sulfonamides for Rx of Urinary tract infection.

Product	Company	Presentation	Dose rate	Composition	Remark
ATTAK	VHPL	Lotion	Recommended Dilutions in Water Empty sheds 4 % Incubator Tank 4% Plastic Equipments 2%	Each 100 ml contains : Benzalkonium Chloride sol. I.P. 5 ml Glutaraldehyde Solution B.P. 7.5 ml Formaldehyde Solution I.P.	For the control of germs in and around poultry shed.

			Incubators/Hatchers 2% Vehicle Dip 2% Metal Equipments 1% Visitor Shoes 3% Livestock in Sheds 0.4%	7.5 ml Aqueous base q.s.	
BETADINE SCRUB	Win Medicare	50ml Sol. 500ml Sol.	apply locally for general disinfection	Povidone Iodine 7.5%	general antiseptic
BIO-QUAT-20	BV Biologicals	1 litre	1 ml/20-40 ltr water	20 % B. K. C.	Water disinfection
BROMOSEP T-50	Sarabhai Zydus	1, 5 ltr can	2.5 ml over the hand and rub well over hands for 30 seconds	Didecyl dimethyl ammonium bromide 50 gm/100 ml	Hand disinfection
CANISEP cream	Himalaya	30 gm	apply over affected area daily	each gram contains oils of Atasi (50 mg), Tailparna (30 mg), Karpura (25 mg), Tulasi (12 mg), Vacha (8 mg), Tankara (18 mg)	antimicrobial, antipruritic, antimaggot action; Useful in moist eczema, dermatitis, burns and wounds.
DETTOL	Reckitt	50ml Liq., 100ml, 200ml, 500ml, 5 lt. Can	apply superficially for local disinfection	Choroxylenol 4.8%w/v, Terpineol 9%v/v, Absolute alcohol 13.1% v/v	general antiseptic
DIPIN	BV Biologicals	1 litre	10 ml/ltr water for teat dipping	Benzalkonium chloride 50%v/v; Chlorhexidine Gluconate soln. I.P. 05 % v/v	Teat/udder disinfection

DISFECT-S	Pfizer Limited	100 ml, 1 ltr, 5 ltr	spray weekly	PAM phenols 40 % w/w; Dodecyl benzene sulphonic acid 24 % w/w; 40 % Metacresol 5% w/w	general purpose indoor disinfectants
DRESSOL	Cattle remedies	ointment 50 gm	apply locally over affected area as required	Herbal	antiseptic dressing
DRESSOL lotion	Cattle Remedies	100 ml, 450 ml	apply locally over affected area as required	Herbal	broad spectrum antiseptic fly repellent gel
DRESSOL-FR gel	Cattle Remedies	50 gm gel	apply locally over affected area as required	Herbal	broad spectrum antiseptic fly repellent gel
ERINA coat cleanser	Himalaya	120 ml	apply locally over affected area as required	each ml has oils of Nimba (5µl), Satahva (5 µl)	antibacterial, antidandruff, antipruritic, deodorant
GAMA BENZENE Hexachlorid e	Agrawal Pharma	50ml Lot., 100ml, 400ml	apply locally as required	Gama Benzene hexachloride 1%	infected and maggot wound
GAMID	Medicot Plus	100mI Lot.	apply over affected area	Gama Benzene 1%w/v, Cetrimide 0.1%w/v	wound
HPS1000	BV Biologicals	100 ml, 500 ml	30 ml/ltr water	H_2O_2 solution 10% w/v; Silver nitrate 0.01% v/v	surface and water channel disnifection
KOHRSOLI N-TH Liquid	Virbac	100 ml, 500 ml, 5 litre	10 ml/litre water for spray to 25 sq ft area	Each 100 ml has Gluteraldehyde 10 gm, Dihydroxy diohexane 10.4 g, Polymethyl	indoor disinfection

				urea derivative 7.2 gm	
ICHGON Liquid	Virbac	100 ml bottle	apply over wet skin and rinse thrice with water	Dichlorobenzyl alcohol 0.05%, Bronopol 0.2%	Anti itch wash for pets
LOREXANE Cream	Virbac	30 gm,100 gm tube	apply over affected area daily	Gamma Benzene Hexachloride: 0.1% w/w; Proflavin Hemisulfate: 0.1% w/w; Cetrimide soln. 0.45% w/w	broad spectrum antiseptic fly repellent
MAGGACI TE	Cattle Remedies	50 ml, 100 ml	apply over affected area daily	herbal	maggot killer
OXICLEAN -30	Kumaran	1 kg, 30 kg	10 gm /ltr water power spray	Hydrogen Peroxide with noble metals and stabilizers	dairy farm disinfection, general biosecurity purpose
OXICLEAN -50	Kumaran	1 kg, 30 kg	5 gm /ltr water power spray	Hydrogen Peroxide with noble metals and stabilizers	dairy farm disinfection, general biosecurity purpose
OXICLEAN -P	Kumaran	1 kg, 30 kg	water spray	Hydrogen Peroxide with noble metals and stabilizers	dairy farm disinfection, general biosecurity purpose
QUALITRO L	Vetnex	500 ml, 5 ltr	5 ml/litre water	Ortho-Phenylphenol 12%, Ortho-benzyl para chlorophenol 10%, para tertiary amyl phenol 4 %	general disinfection
RESILLIUM	BV	100 ml,	2.5 ml	Each ml	hygienic and

-EA	Biologicals	500 ml	dilution for hand disinfection	contains Ethanol 70% v/v, Didecyl Dimethyl Ammonium Chloride 1 % v/v	surgical hand disinfection
RES-Q	BV Biologicals	100 gm, 500 gm	5 gm/ltr water spray @ 1 ltr / 25 sqr ft carpet area	each gram contains stabilized blend of peroxygen compound, organic acids	dairy farm general disfection
SAFEGARD	BV Biologicals	1, 5, 30, 35 ltr can	8 ml/ltr water	Titrable Iodine 1.75%	foot and hand disinfection; dairy equipment disinfection
SAVLON	J & J	50ml Liq., 100ml, 250ml, 5 lt. Can	apply superficially for local disinfection	Chlorhexidine Gluconate soln. I.P. 0.3%, Stong Ceteramide I.P. Soln. BP Equiv to Cetrimide I.P. 0.6% w/v	general antiseptic
SAVLON	J & J	50ml, 100ml, 250ml Liq., 1 ltr	apply superficially for local disinfection	Chlorhexidine Gluconate soln. I.P. 0.3%, Strong Cetramide I.P. Soln. BP Equiv to Cetrimide I.P. 0.6% w/v	foot and hand disinfection; dairy equipment disinfection
SCAVON vet spray	Himalaya	120 ml spray	apply over affected area	each ml contains tailpatra 60 mg, Nimba 50 mg, Bhutrina 40 mg, Devadaru 28 mg, Haridra 2 mg	useful in surgical wounds, dermatomycosis, ringworm, pruritis, mange, alopecia
SOKRENA-WS Liquid	Virbac	500 ml, 5 litre	1 ml/ ltr drinking	Didecyl dimethyl	water sanitizer

			water daily. For fish: 2-4 litre/acre pond with depth of 1 meter	ammonium chloride 7 gm/100 ml	
TH 4+	Solvay	1,5,25 ltr pack	1 ml/ltr water	Didecyl dimethyl NH_4Cl, Dioctyl dimethyl NH_4Cl , octyl decyl dimethyl NH_4Cl, alkyl Didecyl dimethyl NH_4Cl, Gluteraldehyde , Pine oil, Terpinol	farm housing disinfection
VETBACIN ointment	Virbac	20 gm tube	Use ointment over wound after proper cleaning.	Each gram contains Neomycin sulfate 5 mg, Bacitracin 500 IU	Wound dressing, yoke gall, ulcers
Virkon S	Pfizer Limited	50 g, 500 g	5 gm/ltr water	Sodium Chloride 1.5%w/w, K monopersulphate, K hydrogen sulphate, K sulphate 49.8 % w/w	Farm housing disinfection
WOKADINE	Wockhardt Limited	50ml Sol. 500ml Sol.	apply locally for general disinfection	Povidone Iodine 7.5%	general antiseptic
Cipladine 10% Solution	Cipla	100ml, 250ml, 1Ltr, 5Ltr	apply locally for general disinfection	Povidone Iodine 10%solution	general antiseptic
Cipladine Ointment	Cipla	250 gm jar	apply locally for general	Povidone Iodine 5%	general antiseptic

			disinfection	ointment	
Cipladine 5% Solution	Cipla	100ml, 250ml, 500ml, 1 Ltr, 5Ltr	apply locally for general disinfection	Povidone Iodine 5% solution	general antiseptic
Cipladine Plus	Cipla	1 ltr, 5 ltr, 30 ltr	apply locally for general disinfection	Alkyl Aryl Poloxyethylene Iodine Complex + Quaternary Ammonium Compounds	general antiseptic
Cipladine	Cipla	1 ltr, 5 ltr, 30 ltr	apply locally for general disinfection	Alkyl aryl polyoxyethylene iodine complex which provides 1.6% iodine	general antiseptic
AQ4 Disinfectant	Cipla	1litre bottle, 5 litre jar	apply locally for general disinfection	Alkyldimethyl ammonium chloride+ Octyldecyldimethylammonium chloride+ Didoctyldimethylammonium chloride+ Didecyldimethylammonium chloride+Glutaraldehyde+Terpineol Pine oil, Terpineol	general antiseptic
BFG Vet	Cipla	1 ltr, 5 ltr, 30 ltr	apply locally for general disinfection	Benzalkonium Chloride + Glutardialdehyde+Formaldehyde Stabiliser in suitable aqueous Base	general antiseptic
Enviro Spray	Cipla	500ml	spray weekly indoor and	Cyromazine(triazine) –	Farm housing disinfection

			outdoor housing	31.2g/kg, Permethrin(40:60 cis:trans) (pyrethroid)-6.2g/kg	
Oxypure Powder	Cipla	125gm sachet	apply locally for general disinfection	Oxytetracycline Hcl-5.5gm,Myristalkonium chloride-5.5gm	general antiseptic
Clenz-Pond	Cipla	1 ltr, 5 ltr, 30 ltr	apply locally for general disinfection	Pond Sanitizer	general antiseptic
AQ2	Cipla	1 ltr, 5 ltr, 30 ltr	apply locally for general disinfection	Quaterinary Ammonium Compounds + Aldehydes	general antiseptic
AquaSan	Cipla	1 ltr, 5 ltr, 30 ltr	apply for water disinfection in fishery	Quaternary ammonium compounds with stabilizers in suitable solvent	water sanitizer
Bromocare	Cipla	1 ltr, 5 ltr, 30 ltr	apply locally for general disinfection	Tetradecyltrimethyl ammonium bromide + Alkylbenzyldimethyl Ammonium chloride + Nonyl Phenol Ethoxylates + Stabilizers and Diluents	general antiseptic
Herbact Cream	Cipla	50 g, 100 g	apply locally over the wound	Herbal anti-bacterial and anti-fungal cream	excellent antiseptic action

DISINFECTANTS/ANTISEPTICS PRODUCTS			
CHLOROXYLENOL is a chlorinated phenolic antiseptic, which is bactericidal against most gram positive bacteria but less active against staphylococci and gram negative. Acts by denaturing proteins. Indications : Disinfecting for minor wounds, surgical antiseptics and abstetric cream. Dosage : Use as required. Contraindications : Hypersensitivity, avoid use on the brain meninges, middle ear and other sensitive tissues. Special Precautions : Aqueous solution should be freshly prepared at the recommended concentration and appropriate measures must be taken to prevent contamination during storage of dilution. Syringes and needles immersed in chloroxylenol must be throughly rinsed. Adverse drug reactions :Irritation of the conjuctivae and other sensitive tissue.			
Product	**Company**	**Presentation**	**Composition**
ATTAK	Ventri	1, 5, 30, 35 ltr can	Benzalkonium chloride, Gluteraldehyde, Formaldehyde, Surface active agent
BROMOSEPT-50	Sarabhai Zydus	1, 5 ltr can	Didecyl dimethyl ammonium bromide 50 gm/100 ml
DETTOL	Reckitt	50ml Liq., 100ml, 200ml, 500ml, 5 lt. Can	(Choroxylenol 4.8%w/v, Terpineol 9%v/v, Absolute alcohol 13.1% v/v)
DISFECT-S	Pfizer Limited	100 ml, 1 ltr, 5 ltr	PAM phenols 40 % w/w; Dodecyl benzene sulphonic acid 24 % w/w; 40 % Metacresol 5% w/w
KOHRSOLIN-TH Liquid	GLAXO SMITH KLINE	100 ml, 500 ml	Each 100 ml has Gluteraldehyde 7 gm, Dihydroxy diohexane 9.5 g, Polymethyl urea derivative 16.3 gm
OXICLEAN-30	Kumaran	1 kg, 30 kg	Hydrogen Peroxide with noble metals and stabilizers
OXICLEAN-50	Kumaran	1 kg, 30 kg	Hydrogen Peroxide with noble metals and stabilizers
OXICLEAN-P	Kumaran	1 kg, 30 kg	Hydrogen Peroxide with noble metals and stabilizers
QUALITROL	Vetnex	500 ml, 5 ltr	Ortho-Phenylphenol 12%, Ortho-benzyl para chlorophenol 10%, para

			tertiary amyl phenol 4 %
SAFEGARD	Ventri	1, 5, 30, 35 ltr can	Iodine 1.6 % w/v
SAVLON	J & J	50ml, 100ml, 250ml Liq., 1 ltr	Chlorhexidine Gluconate soln. I.P. 0.3%, Stong Ceteramide I.P. Soln. BP Equiv to Cetrimide I.P. 0.6% w/v
SOKRENA-WS Liquid	Virbac	100 ml, 500 ml	Didecyl dimethyl ammonium chloride 7 gm/100 ml
TH 4+	Solvay	1,5,25 ltr pack	Didecyl dimethyl NH_4Cl, Dioctyl dimethyl NH_4Cl , octyl decyl dimethyl NH_4Cl , alkyl Didecyl dimethyl NH_4Cl, Gluteraldehyde, Pine oil, Terpinol
Virkon S	Pfizer Limited	50 g, 500 g	Sodium Chloride 1.5%w/w, K monopersulphate, K hydrogen sulphate, K sulphate 49.8 % w/w

Chapter 13

Drugs for Nervous System

ANTICONVULSANT

- DIAZEPAM
- PHENOBARBITONE
- PHENYTOIN
- PRIMIDONE
- SODIUM VALPROATE:

SEDATIVE/TRANQUILIZERS

- CHLORPROMAZINE
- KETAMINE
- TRIFLUPROMAZINE:
- XYLAZINE
- POLYHERBAL FORMULATION
- DICYCLOMINE
- DOMPERIDONE
- METOCHLOPRAMIDE
- PROCHLORPERAZINE
- PROMETHAZINE
- TRIFLUPROMAZINE

ANTICONVULSANT

DIAZEPAM:

Blocks spinal polysynaptic reflexes. Indicated in status epilepticus, convulsions due to poisoning. Dogs: 2-5 mg TID total dose, oral, IV.

Product	**Company**	**Presentation**	**Composition**
CALMOD	**IDPL**	**strip of 10 tabs**	each tab had 5 mg.
CALMPOSE	**Ranbaxy**	strip of 10 tabs, liq 60 ml, inj 2 ml amp.	each tab has 5 mg, 10 mg, syrup has 2 mg/5 ml; inj has 10 mg/2 ml.
DIZEP	**Intas**	strip of 10 tab	each tab has 5 mg, 10 mg

PHENOBARBITONE:

depresses the motor centres of cerebral cortex by potentiation of synaptic inhibition on GABA receptor, which inhibits epileptic seizures. Drug of choice in convulsive

seizures. Dogs/cats: 1.5 mg – 5 mg/kgBW BID IV; 1-1.5 mg/kg BW IM; 2.2-6.6 mg/kg BW Oral.			
Gardenal	Rhone Poulenc	strip of 10 tabs	each tab has 30 mg, 60 mg.
Phenobarbitone Na	Rhone Poulenc	inj 1 ml amp	200 mg/ml
PHENYTOIN: depresses motor are of cortex. No sedation. Effective antiarrhythmic property. Indicated in status epilepticus. Dogs: 8-17.6 mg/kg BW TID oral. Do not use with chlormaphenicol.			
EPSOLIN	Cadila	strip of 100 tabs; inj 2 ml ampoule	each tab has 100 mg; Inj has 50mg/ml.
PRIMIDONE: phenobarbital derivative. Potent anticonvulsant. Dogs: 50 mg/kg BW total daily in equal parts at 12 hr interval, orally. Ataxia may be seen 2-3 days after administration.			
MYSOLINE	ICI	strip of 10 tabs	each tab has 250 mg
SODIUM VALPROATE: interact with GABA metabolism in brain. Used in status epilepticus. Dogs: 60 mg/kg BW TID orally.			
EPILEX	Reckitt & Colman	tab and syrup	each tab has 200 mg; syrup has 200 mg/5 ml.

SEDATIVE/TRANQUILIZERS

CHLORPROMAZINE: Phenothiazine derivative. Blocks alfa adrenoceptors. Indicated for nervous and aggressive animals, as pre anaesthetic. Dogs: 1-2 mg/kg BW IV, IM, 3 mg/kg oral; Swine: 1.1 mg/kg BW IV; 2-4mg/Kg BW IM; Cattle: 1 mg/kg BW IM. C/I in equines. Do not use with adrenalin. Avoid in o-p poisoning and very weak animals.			
CHLORPROMAZINE	Rhone poulenc	Strip of 10 tabs, injection of 2ml amp.	each tab contains 10 mg; 25mg, 50 mg, 100 mg; Injection has 2.5 %
MEGATIL	Intas	Strip of 10 tabs, injection of 2ml amp.	each tab contains 25mg, 50 mg, 100 mg, 200 mg; Injection has 50mg/2ml.
DETOMIDINE : alfa agonist. Has sedative, analgesic and muscle relaxation action. Indicated of for sedation in equine. Dose: 10-20 mcg/kg IM			
Equi-Sed Injection	Cipla	10ml	Detomidine hydrochloride 10mg/ml
KETAMINE: potent inhibitor of GABA which enhance CNS inhibitory maechanisms. It inhibits GABA reuptake at synapses where it is normally liberated. Indicated in immobilisation and surgery. C/I in head injuries, status epilepticus. Dogs: 10 mg/kg BW IM; Pig: 15-20 mg/kgBW IM, SC; Horse: 2.2 mg/kgBW IV; Goat: 22-44 mg/kgBW IM, SC.			
KETALAR	Parke	injection 10 ml,	Inj contains 10 mg/ml, 50 mg/ml

	Davis	2 ml	
KETMIN	Themis	injection 2ml 10 ml, 20 ml	Inj contains 10 mg/ml, 50 mg/ml
TRIFLUPROMAZINE: neuroleptic agent. Antagonise central dopamine D2 receptors. Prominent antiemetic activity. Dog: 2-4 mg/kg BW IM, 1-2 mg/kg BW IV. Administration with epinephrine is contraindicated.			
Siquil injection	Sarabhai zydus	5 ml vial	Each ml has Triflupromazine HCl: 20 mg
Siquil tab	Sarabhai zydus	Strip Of 10 Tabs	Each tab has Triflupromazine HCl: 10 mg
ANICALM	**Intas**	Strip Of 10 Tabs, inj of 5 ml vial	Each tab has Triflupromazine HCl: 5 mg, 10 mg; injection has 20 mg/ml
SUGIL	**Biomedica**	inj of 5 ml vial	injection has 20 mg/ml
XYLAZINE: activates alfa-2 adrenoceptors with potent antinociceptive/analgesic action. Indicated for sedation, analgesia, muscle relaxation, immobilisation of animals. Horse/dog/cat: 1-2mg/kgBW IM, 0.5-1.1 mg/Kg BW IV; Cattle: 0.1-0.2 mg/kg BW IM, 0.05 mg/kg BW IV. C/I in GIT obstruction, stomach torsion, hernia, later stage of pregnancy. Antidote : Yohimbine HCl, 4-aminopyridine.			
Xylodac injection	Sarabhai zydus	2 ml & 10 ml vials	Each ml has Xylazine HCl: 23.32 mg
XYLAXIN	Indian Immunologicals	2 ml & 10 ml, 30 ml vials	Each ml has Xylazine HCl: 23.32 mg
XYLOCAD INJ	Cadila Pharmaceuticals Limited	5 ml vial	Each ml has Xylazine HCl: 23.32 mg
POLYHERBAL FORMULATION			
ANXOCARE liquid	Himalaya	100 ml (2-3 ml twice daily orally)	polyherbal formulation having Brahmi, mandukparni, ashwagandha, shankhpushpi,
DICYCLOMINE: antispasmodic, antiemetic; produces nonspcific direct relaxant action on smooth muscles. Indicated in colic, irritable bowel syndrome, abdominal pain. Dose rate is 0.5 mg/KgBW IM in ruminants, horses; 0.1 mg/kg BW TID IM in dogs. Avoid use in neonates, old age animals, urinary retention and GIT obstruction cases.			
Spasmo-Proxyvon	Wockhardt	injection 2ml, 30 ml	each ml contains 10 mg/ml
Spasmovet	Wockhardt	injection 30 ml	each ml contains 10 mg/ml

DOMPERIDONE: antiemetic. Indicated in symptomatic relief of vomiting. Dogs: 5-10 mg total dose BID orally. Contraindicated in G.I. obstruction and GIT haemorrhage.			
Domstal	Torrent	Tab	each tab contains 10 mg domperidone.
Domstal	Torrent	suspension 30 ml bottle	each ml contains 1 mg domperidone.
Endopace	Themis pharma	Tab	each tab contains 10 mg domperidone.
Endopace	Themis pharma	suspension 60 ml bottle	each ml contains 1 mg domperidone.
METOCHLOPRAMIDE: antiemetic action is attributed by specific dopamine antagonistic activity by blocking dopamine receptors. Indicated in vomiting due to gastritis, oesophageal reflux, impaction. Dog: 0.01-0.2 mg/kg BW I/V, I/M; 0.2-0.4 mg/kg BW oral.			
Perinorm	IPCA	tab, inj., liq	Injection contains 5 mg/ml; oral preparation contains 1mg/ml; each tab contains 10 mg.
Emenil	Astra IDL	tab; inj.	Injection contains 5 mg/ml; each tab contains 10 mg.
PROCHLORPERAZINE: phenthiazine derivative, very potent antiemetic. Dogs : 0.5 mg/kg BW TID, I/M; 1 mg/Kg BW TID orally. Contarindicated in glaucoma, GIT obstruction, and administration with epinephrine.			
Stemetil	Rhone poulenc	tab 5 mg; 25 mg	5 mg tab contains 5 mg prochlorperazine 25 mg tab contains 25 mg prochlorperazine
Stemetil inj	Rhone poulenc	1 ml ampoule	each ml contains 12.5 mg
PROMETHAZINE: antihistamine with sedative and antiemetic action. Indicated in vomiting and allergic disorders. Ruminants: 1.5-2.0 mg/kg BW IM; Dogs : 1.5-2.5 mg/kg BW oral, IM, IV.			
Avomine	Rhone poulenc	25 mg tab	promethazine 25 mg/tab
Phenergan	Rhone poulenc	tab 10mg; tab 25 mg; elixir 60ml; inj 2 ml	see products injection 25mg/ml tab 10mg, 25 mg; elixir: 5mg/5 ml
TRIFLUPROMAZINE: neuroleptic agent. Antagonise central dopamine D2 receptors. Prominent antiemetic activity. Dog: 2-4 mg/kg BW IM, 1-2 mg/kg BW IV. Administration with epinephrine is contraindicated.			
Siquil injection	Sarabhai zydus	5 ml vial	Each ml has Triflupromazine HCl: 20 mg

Chapter 14

Intravascular Infusion Fluid

INFUSION FLUID PREPARATIONs

- CALCIUM BOROGLUCONATE
- CALCIUM & MAGNESIUM BOROGLUCONATE
- DEXTROSE
- DEXTROSE SODIUM CHLORIDE
- MISCELLANEOUS INFUSIONS
- MANNITOL
- RINGER LACTATE
- SODIUM CHLORIDE
- AMINOACID INFUSION

INFUSION FLUID PREPARATIONs				
CALCIUM BOROGLUCONATE: Hypocalcemia or Milk fever. General rule for dosing Ca gluconate is 1 gm calcium per 45 Kg Body weight intravenous slowly. Ca is cardiotoxic. Cardiac auscultation is must during I/V infusion of calcium. Oral administration of calcium soln. avoids risks of cardiotoxicity. Oral administration of 50 gm of soluble calcium results in 4 gm calcium being absorbed into circulation.				
Product	**Company**	**Presentation**	**Dose rate**	**Composition**
BOROCAL	Sarabhai Zydus Animal Health Limited	200 ml, 450 ml	Horse/cattle: 200-400 ml; I/V, S/C	Ca borogluconate 25% w/v
CALBOROL	Novartis	450 ml	Horse/cattle: 200-400 ml; I/V, S/C	Ca borogulconate 25 % w/v
CALCIUM BOROGLUCONATE 25 %	Wochardt	450 ml	Horse/cattle: 200-400 ml; I/V, S/C	Ca borogulconate 25 % w/v

CALCIUM BOROGLUC ONATE INJ. BP(VET)	Cadila	450 ml	Horse/cattle: 200-400 ml; I/V, S/C	Ca borogulconate 25 % w/v
CALGONAT E	Indian Immunolog icals	450 ml	Horse/cattle: 200-400 ml; I/V, S/C	Calcium 1.86 %w/v, Boric acid 4.2 %w/v
CALMEX inj	Ranbaxy	450 ml	Horse/cattle: 200-450 ml; I/V, S/C	Calcium 1.86 %w/v, Boric acid 4.2 %w/v
CALVIB IV infusion	Virbac	450 ml	Horse/cattle: 200-450 ml; slow I/V, S/C	Calcium 1.86 %w/v, Boric acid 4.2 %w/v
INTACAL	Neovet Intas Ltd	450 ml	Large animals: 200-450 ml; slow I/V, S/C	Calcium Gluconate (equivalent to 1.86% w/v of calcium), Proportion of Boric acid to calcium 2.26:1
CALCIUM & MAGNESIUM BOROGLUCONATE Hypocalcemia or Milk fever complicated with Hypomagnesemia, Hpoglycemia and hypophosphatemia, Bovine Ketosis and pregnancy toxemia in sheep				
LACTOMA G	Neovet Intas Pharmaceut ical	450 ml Packing	Heavy Animals : 450 ml; Cow, mare, She buffalo : 200 – 300 ml Slow I/V and S/C Route	Each ml contains: Calcium Gluconate 20.75 %w/v (Proportion of Boric acid to Calcium 2.26 : 1) Magnesium hypophosphite 5 %w/v Anhydrous Dextrose 20 % w/v
CALMEX-M	Ranbaxy	450 ml Packing	Heavy Animals : 450 ml; Cow, mare, She buffalo : 200 – 300 ml Slow I/V and S/C Route	Calcium 1.86 %w/v, Boric acid 4.2 %w/v, Magnesium hypophosphite 5 %w/v, Anhydrous Dextrose 20 % w/v
CALBIM IV infusion	Virbac	450 ml glass bottle	250 – 450 ml by slow IV	Each ml contains: Calcium Gluconate 16.6 % w/v; Calcium

				hypophosphite: 2.14 %w/v; Boric acid 3.4% w/v, Magnesium chloride 1.33 % w/v, Anhydrous Dextrose 20 % w/v
BOROMAG	Sarabhai Zydus Animal Health Limited	450 ml Packing	Heavy Animals : 450 ml; Cow, mare, She buffalo : 200 – 300 ml Slow I/V and S/C Route	Each ml contains: Calcium Gluconate 20.75 %w/v (Proportion of Boric acid to Calcium 2.26 : 1) Magnesium hypophosphite 5 %w/v Anhydrous Dextrose 20 % w/v
MAGICAL (VET) INJ.	Cadila	Inj 450 ml pack	Heavy Animals : 450 ml; Cow, mare, She buffalo : 200 – 300 ml Slow I/V and S/C Route	Each ml contains: Calcium Gluconate 20.75 % w/v (Proportion of Boric acid to Calcium 2.26 : 1) Magnesium hypophosphite 5 %w/v, Anhydrous Dextrose 20 % w/v
MIFEX	Novartis	Inj 450 ml pack	Heavy Animals : 450 ml; Cow, mare, She buffalo : 200 – 300 ml Slow I/V and S/C Route	Each ml contains: Calcium Borogluconate 25 % w/v, Magnesium hypophosphite 5 %w/v, Anhydrous Dextrose 20 % w/v
MIPHOCAL	Indian Immunologicals	450 ml pack	Heavy Animals : 450 ml; Cow, mare, She buffalo : 200 – 300 ml Slow I/V and S/C Route	Calcium 1.86 %w/v, Boric acid 4.2 %w/v, Magnesium hypophosphite 5 %w/v, Anhydrous Dextrose 20 % w/v
THIACAL	Wockhardt	450 ml pack	Heavy	Calcium Gluconate 1.86

			Animals : 450 ml; Cow, mare, She buffalo : 200 – 300 ml Slow I/V and S/C Route	%w/v, Boric acid 4.2 %w/v, Magnesium hypophosphite 5 %w/v, Anhydrous Dextrose 20 % w/v

DEXTROSE

Indicated in Bovine Ketosis, Hypoglycemia, Cachexia. For prevention of starvation ketosis and protein catabolism in fasting, preoperative or post operative patients or in patients with restricted oral intake. Parenteral nutrition is provided by infusing dextrose 5%, 10% or 20% through intravenous route. Dextrose solution is ideal for providing adequate calories to needy patients. Solutions of dextrose in concentration of 10% or more can be used for mild osmotic diuresis resulting in temporary relief from cerebral edema.

DEXTROSE 25%	Wockhardt Limited	540 ml	cattle: 400 -500 ml IV or as per condition	Dextrose 25%
DEXTROSE 5%	Alembic	540 ml	cattle: 2000 ml IV or as per condition	Dextrose 5%
DEXTROSE INJ	Alb.David	540 ml	cattle: 400 -500 ml IV or as per condition	250 mg/ml
Dextrose 20%	Cipla	500 ml	cattle: 400 -500 ml IV	Dextrose 20% w/v Infusion
Dextrose 5%	Cipla	500 ml	cattle: 400 -500 ml IV	Dextrose 5 w/v Infusion

DEXTROSE SODIUM CHLORIDE

Indicated in Hypoglycemia, dehydration, trauma, surgery, burns.

DOSAGE: Large animal: 500 – 2000 ml per day IV

DEXTROSE 5% & SODIUM CHLORIDE 0.9 %	Alembic	540 ml	Dextrose 5% & Sodium Chloride 0.9 %
DEXTROSE 5% & SODIUM CHLORIDE 0.9 %	Wochardt	1000 ml inj IV	Dextrose 5% & Sodium Chloride 0.9 %
DEXTROSE -C	Alb.David	1000ml Inj	Dextrose Anhydrous 50mg, NaCl 9mg

RINGER LACTATE ELECTROLYTE INFUSIONS			
Indicated in diarrhea, hyperurination, extreme loss of electrolyte, fluid imbalance			
RINTOSE	Wochardt	500 ml inj	(Dextrose 20g, NaCl 0.6g, KCl 0.04 g, $CaCl_2$ 0.027g, Na lactate 0.312 g)/100 ml
VITROSE	Vetindia	500 ml inj	(Dextrose 20g, NaCl 0.6g, KCl 0.04 g, $CaCl_2$ 0.027g, Na lactate 0.312 g)/100 ml
INTALYTE	Neovet Intas	500 ml FFS bottle	each 100 ml contains dextrose 20 gm, NaCl: 0.6 gm, KCl : 0.04 gm, $CaCl^2$: 0.027 gm, Na lactate 0.312 gm
MANNITOL			
Osmotic diuretic, reduces intracranial or intraocular pressure associated with cerebral oedema in conditions like polioencephalaomalacia, glaucoma, toxicity. Indicated in renal failure, hyponatremia, Cerebral oedema. C/I in pulmonary congestion, anuria, dehydration, intracranial bleeding, progressive renal damage.			
MANNITOL 5%	Krishan keshav	350 ml, 500 ml	mannitol 5%
MANNITOL 10%	Krishan keshav	350 ml, 500 ml	mannitol 10%
MANNITOL 20 %	Mount mettur	350 ml, 500 ml	mannitol 20%
MANNITOL 20 %	Albert david	350 ml, 500 ml	mannitol 20%
RINGER LACTATE			
Indicated in Extracellular fluid deficit, burns, peritoneal irrigation, metabolic acidosis, neonatal diarrhea, diabetic ketosis, during anaesthesia, metabolic acidosis. Electrolytes concentration in ringer lactate is almost the same as that of plasma. The lactate serves as bicarbonate precursor for treating mild to moderate metabolic acidosis. It is found useful in making good the extracellular and intravascular fluid loss during surgery. It restores normal fluid shift due to burn, fracture, cardiovascular emergencies or due to any other clinical conditions.			
Ringer lactate	Albert david	500 ml, 1000 ml	Lactic Acid 0.24 ml, NaOH: 114 mg, NaCl- 600 mg, KCl -40mg, CaCl2 Hydrated- 40 mg
Ringer lactate	Mount mettur	500 ml, 1000 ml	Lactic Acid 0.24 ml, NaOH, 114 mg, NaCl 600 mg, KCl 40mg, CaCl2 Hydrated 40 mg
SODIUM CHLORIDE: dehydration, shock, fluid loss, vomition, diarrhea			
Sodium chloride 0.45%	Mount mettur	540 ml	Sodium chloride 0.45%
Sodium chloride 0.9%	Albert david	500 ml	Sodium chloride 0.9%

AMINOACID INFUSION			
Indicated in hypoproteinemia, malnutrition, cachexia, parenteral nutrient supply when oral feeding is not possible.			
AMINODRIP	Wockhardt	200 ml Infusion	Amino acids 7.5gm (equivalent to 1.29 gms, Nitrogen) per 100 ml, L- Arginine 495.00 mg, L-Histidine 33.75 mg, L-Lysine 1229.25 mg, L-tyrosine 56.25 mg, L-Phenyl Alanine 253.05mg, L-Tryptophan 0.55mg, L-Cystcine 5.60mg, L-Methionine 316.80 mg, L-Glutamic Acid 450.00 mg, L-Hydroxyproline 315.00mg, L-Threomine 129.30mg, L-Leuclne 756.75 mg, L- Isoleucine 106.80 mg, L-valine 157.50 mg, L-Alamine 675.00 mg, L-Proline 345.00 mg, L-Serine 165.00mg, Glycine 1650.00 mg, L- Aspartic acid 360.00 mg Total Essential amino acids 3.54063gm/100ml. Bran ched chain aromatic amino acids 3.30, Sodium not more than 8.7 mEq/100ml Potassium not more than 1.5 mEq per 100 ml
HERMIN	Alembic	200ml Inf	L -Lysine HCl 19.2mg, l -Threonine 7mg, l-Methionine 6.8mg, l -Tryptophan 3mg, l -Leucine 10mg, I-Isoleucine 6.6mg, I-Phenylalanine 9.6mg, I -Valine 6.4mg, I -Arginine HCl 10.9mg, I -Histidine HCl 4.7mg, Glycine 6mg, Sorbitol 50mg/ml
HERMIN -T	Alembic	200ml Soln	Each 100ml contains L-Isoleucine 560mg, L-Leucine 1250mg, I -Threonine 650mg, I-Methionine 350mg, I -Tryptophan 130mg, I-Valine 955mg, L-Aspartic Acid 380mg, L-Cysteine HCl 145mg, L-Glutamic Acid 650mg, L -Histidine HCl 811mg, L-Proline 330mg, Glycine 1070mg, Xylitol 5g, Water for injection q.s
ASTYMIN-SN	Tablets India	200ml Inf	L-isoleucine 5.6mg, L-leucine methionine 3.5mg, L-phenylalanine 9.35mg, l-threonine 6.5mg, L-trypt-ophan 1.3mg, L-valine 4.5mg, L-alanine 6.2mg, L-arginine HCl 9.55 mg, L-aspartic acid 3.8mg, L-cysteine HCl 1.45mg, L-glutamic acid 6.5mg, L-histidine HCl 8.11mg, L-proline 3.3mg, L-serine 2.2mg, L-tyrosine 0.35mg, glycine 10.7mg, xylitol 50mg, per ml. Each 200ml contains : total amino acids 21.282g, total essential amino acids 10.85 g, total nonessential amino acids 10.432g, free amino acid content 10%, total branched chain amino acid 22.6%, total nitrogen content 3.04g

Chapter 15
Biologicals

BIOLOGICALS			
Name of product	**Company**	**Presentation/Dosage**	**Composition**
RUMINANTS' VACCINES			
Anthrax Spore Vaccine	Intervet	100 ml, Injection. 1 ml SC in endemic areas	Live spore of *B. anthracis* in glycerine saline
Black Quarter vaccine	Brilliant	100 ml, Injection. 2 ml SC at 6 month. Annual revaccination	Inactivated *Cl. chauvoei* antigens in Al $(OH)_3$ gel
Black Quarter vaccine	Intervet	100 ml, Injection. 2 ml SC at 6 month. Annual revaccination	Inactivated *Cl. chauvoei* antigens in Al $(OH)_3$ gel
Brucella vaccine	Intervet	25 ml, Injection 5 ml SC at 8th month of age in female calves	Live strain of B. abortus C-19 in sterile freeze dried form
Bruvax	Indian Immunologicals	5 dose freeze dried vaccine with 10 ml diluent. Seronegative female calves of 4-8 month age group are vaccinated with 2 ml reconstituted vaccine by s/c route.	Brucella abortus Strain 19 vaccine Live vaccine
Clovax (FMD)	Intervet	30 ml, 90 ml, Injection 3 ml SC or IM (Cattle/Buffalo) 3 ml IM (pig)	Tetravalent oil adjuvant vaccine containing FMD virus O, A, C and Asia-1

Enterotoxemia vaccine	Biomed	100 ml, Injection 1 ml SC at 4-6 weeks age (vaccinated dam) or 1 week age (unvaccinated dam); Booster after 3-6 weeks of first vaccination. Revaccination at every 6 month	*Cl. welchii* (Type D) toxoid
Enterotoxemia vaccine	Intervet	100 ml, Injection 5 ml SC at 4-6 weeks age (vaccinated dam) or 1 week age (unvaccinated dam); Booster after 3-6 weeks of first vaccination. Revaccination at every 6 month	*Cl. welchii* (Type C & D) toxoid in Al $(OH)_3$ gel
Enterotoxemia vaccine	Intervet	100 ml, Injection 2.5 ml SC at 4-6 weeks age (vaccinated dam) or 1 week age (unvaccinated dam); Booster after 3-6 weeks of first vaccination. Revaccination at every 6 month	*Cl. welchii* (Type D) toxoid in Al $(OH)_3$ gel
Foot & Mouth Disease vaccine	Intervet	50 ml, Injection 5 ml SC (Cattle/Buffalo) Primary Vaccination at 8 weeks, 3 months, 6 months of age. Booster dose after 1 month of Primary vaccination. Revaccination at every 6 months.	Super concentrated Tetravalent vaccine containing FMD virus O, A_{22}, C and Asia-1
F.D. CELL CULTURE SHEEP POX vaccine	IVRI	100 doses	freeze dried cell culture of sheep pox virus standard strain
Haemorrhagic septicaemia vaccine	Brilliant	100 ml, Injection 2 ml SC (Ruminants) Primary Vaccination at 6 month of age. Annual revaccination	Inactivated *Pasteurella multocida* absorbed in Aluminium hydroxide as adjuvant

Haemorrhagic septicaemia vaccine	Intervet	100 ml, Injection 2 ml SC (Ruminants) Primary Vaccination at 6 month of age. Annual revaccination	Inactivated *Pasteurella multocida* absorbed in Aluminium hydroxide as adjuvant
IBRIVAX (Infectious Bovine Rhinotracheitis)	Intervet	20 ml Injection 2 ml SC/IM Primary at 6 weeks of age, Booster after 3 months. Annual revaccination.	Inactivated Bovine herpes virus cell culture.
PPR vaccine	IVRI	100 doses	Live attenuated virus on vero cell and freeze dried
Raksha Anthrax	Indian Immunologicals	50 ml vial. 1 ml (10 million viable spores) I/M or S/C route one month before grazing season or as per advice.	Brucella anthracis spore vaccine (Live)
Raksha Biovac (HS and FMD)	Indian Immunologicals	30 ml, 90 ml, Injection 3 ml deep IM (cattle/buffalo) Primary vaccination at 4 month, booster after 9 months. Annual revaccination.	Oil adjuvant with inactivated FMD virus (O, A, C&Asia1) and *P. multocida*.
Raksha HS+BQ	Indian Immunologicals	90 ml, Injection. 3 ml SC Primary vaccination at 6 month. Annual revaccination.	Formalin inactivated culture of P. multocida and *Cl. chauvoei* with aluminium hydroxide.
Raksha Triovac (FMD, HS, BQ)	Indian Immunologicals	30 ml, 90 ml. Injection. 3 ml deep IM Primary at 4 month and booster after 9 months. Annual revaccination.	Oil adjuvant with inactivated FMD virus (O, A, C&Asia1), *Cl. chauvoei* and *P. multocida* culture.
Raksha-BQ	Indian Immunologicals	100 ml, Injection. 2 ml SC at 6 month. Annual revaccination	Inactivated *Cl. chauvoei* antigens in Al $(OH)_3$ gel
Raksha-ET (enterotoxemia)	Indian Immunologicals	100 ml, Injection 2.0 ml SC at 4 months age; Annual Revaccination.	*Cl. welchii* (Type D) toxoid in Al $(OH)_3$ gel

Raksha	Indian Immunologicals	30 ml. Injection 3 ml SC (Cattle, Buffalo) 1^0 Vaccination at 4 month followed by booster after 4 weeks. Revaccination at every 6 months.	Tissue culture inactivated FMD virus antigens O, A and Asia-1 on Aluminium Hydroxide and saponin adjuvant
Raksha-HS	Indian Immunologicals	100 ml, Injection 2 ml SC (Ruminants) Primary Vaccination at 6 month of age. Annual revaccination	Formalin Inactivated *Pasteurella multocida* absorbed in Aluminium hydroxide as adjuvant
Raksha-OVAC	Indian Immunologicals	10 ml, 30 ml, 50 ml, Injection 2 ml SC (Cattle, Buffalo) 1^0 Vaccination at 4 month of age. Revaccination at every 9 month.	Tissue culture inactivated FMD virus antigens O, A, C and Asia-1 adjuvanted into mineral oil.
Raksha-PPR	Indian Immunologicals	25 ml, 50 ml, 100 ml vial, injection 1 ml SC at 4 month of age (primary vaccination) before monsoon. Revaccination once in 3 years.	Live attenuated PPR virus grown on vero cell culture and freeze dried. Virus is composed of Sungri 96 strain.
Raksha-SP (Sheep pox)	Indian Immunologicals	25,50, 100 ml. Injection. 1 ml IM Primary vaccination at 3 month age	Live attenuated sheep pox virus on lamb testicle cells
Rakshavac-T (Theileriosis)	Indian Immunologicals	50 dose vial+diluent, Injection 3 ml SC cattle Primary vaccination at 2 months of age. Revaccination at every 3 years.	Attenuated Live schizont in cell culture
Swine fever vaccine	Intervet	5 ml, injection 1 ml IM Primary vaccination at 8 weeks of age. Annual revaccination	Attenuated Swine fever virus in tissue culture

CANINE VACCINES			
Adenomune-7	Biocor	1 ml vial 1 ml SC/IM Primary at 9-14 wk. Booster after 4 weeks. Annual revaccination.	Live strain of CD, adeno virus type-II, ICH, canine parainfluenza, parvovirus and killed strain of Leptospira
Anigen-DHL+R (ICH, CD, Leptospirosis, Rabies)	Virbac	1 ml vial 1 ml SC/IM Primary at 7 wk. booster after 4 weeks. Annual revaccination.	Freeze dried vaccine with live viruses of CD, ICH ad inactivated Leptospiral somatic and rabies antigen
Candur-DHL+P (CD, ICH, Leptospira, CPV)	Intervet	1 ml vial single dose IM Primary at 7- 9 weeks. Booster at 12-14 wks. Annual revaccination.	Freeze dried attenuated live CD virus + inactivated Leptospira + Canine parvovirus + ICH virus with Aluminium hydroxide
Candur-R (rabies)	Intervet	1ml, 10 ml, Injection 1 ml SC/IM (All animals) Primary at 7 wk. Booster after 6 wks. Annual revaccination. Post exposure: on 0, 3, 7, 14, 28, 90 days.	Inactivated rabies virus (1 IU)
Commander 7L	Bayer	1 ml vial single dose IM Primary at 7- 9 weeks. Booster at 12-14 wks. Annual revaccination.	CD virus, Adenovirus type II, Parainfluenza virus, Parvo virus, Leptospira antigens
Defensor® 1	Pfizer	Single 1ml dose at 3 months of age or older to healthy dog and cats. Repeat dose 1 yr later.	Rabies Vaccine, Killed Virus
First Dose CV	Pfizer	50 X 1 ml vials. Healthy dogs 6 weeks of age or older should receive 3 doses, each administered 3 weeks apart. Annual revaccination with single dose is recommended.	Killed Coraona Virus Vaccine.

Megavac-6	Indian Immunologicals	1 ml single dose vial SC/IM. Primary at 8-9 wks. Booster at 12 wks. Annual revaccination.	Freeze dried attenuated live vaccine against CD, ICH(type II), CPV and inactivated antigens of ICH(type-I), L. *canicola* and L. *icterohemorrhagiae*
Megavac-CC (canine corona virus)	Indian Immunologicals	1 ml vial, Injection 1 ml SC/IM Primary vaccination at 8th weeks. Booster dose at 12 week. Annual revaccination.	Inactivated tissue culture canine corona virus antigen
Megavac-D (canine distemper)	Indian Immunologicals	1 ml vial, Injection 1 ml SC/IM Primary vaccination at 6th weeks. Annual revaccination.	Live freeze dried virus
Megavac-DHRL	Indian Immunologicals	1 ml single dose vial SC/IM. Primary at 8-9 wks. Booster at 12 wks. Annual revaccination.	Freeze dried attenuated live vaccine against CD, ICH(type II) and inactivated antigens of Rabies, L. *canicola* and L. *icterohemorrhagiae*
Megavac-P (inactivated Parvo virus)	Indian Immunologicals	1 ml vial, Injection 1 ml SC/IM Primary at 9 wk, annual revaccination	Aqueous inactivated virus
Megavac-P (live) (Parvo virus)	Indian Immunologicals	1 ml vial, Injection 1 ml SC/IM Primary at 6 wk, annual revaccination	Freeze dried live attenuated virus
Megavac-R	Indian Immunologicals	multidose vial of 10 ml. 1 ml s/c or I/M route at 3 month of age. Revaccination at 2 years.	
Nobivac-DHPPi	Intervet	Single dose vial 1 ml, IM. Primary at 9-12 wks. Annual revaccination.	Live attenuated CD virus, ICH virus, CPV and canine parainfluenza virus grown in cell line culture

Nobivac-L (Leptospirosis)	Intervet	1 ml vial 1 ml SC Primary at 9-12 wk, booster after 4 wks. Annual revaccination	Inactivated bivalent Leptospira
Rabigen (Rabies)	Virbac	1, 5, 10 ml. Injection. 1 ml SC/IM (All animals) Primary at 3 month. Annual revaccination. Post exposure: on 0, 3, 7, 14, 28, 90 days.	Fixed strain rabies virus BHK21 cell line, with Aluminium hydroxide
Raksharab (rabies)	Indian Immunologicals	1, 5, 10 ml. Injection. 1 ml SC/IM (All animals) Primary at 3 month. Annual revaccination. Post exposure: on 0, 3, 7, 14, 28, 90 days.	Inactivated tissue culture rabies virus, CVBS strain produced on BHK21 cell line, with Aluminium hydroxide
Vanguard-CPV	Pfizer	1 ml, 10 ml, Injection 1 ml SC Primary at 16 wks, annual revaccination	Killed Parvo virus vaccine
Vanguard Plus 5 Cv/L	Pfizer	Pack 25X 1 ml vials. Dosage Healthy dogs 6 weeks of age or older should receive 3 doses, each administered 3 weeks apart. Puppies are vaccinated for the first time at 10-12 weeks of age, only2 vaccinations 3-4 weeks apart need to be given at the veterinariarn's discretion Annual revaccination with a single dose is recommended	Composition High titer low passage polyvalent vaccine providing protection against Canine Distemper Virus Canine Parvovirus Virus Canine Parainfluenza Virus Canine Adenovirus Virus Canine Corona Virus L.canicola L.icterohaemorrhagiae
		SWINE VACCINE	
F.D. LAPINIZED SWINE FEVER VACCINE	IVRI	5 Doses	Lapinized swine fever virus strain

POULTRY VACCINES			
EDS-76 vaccine	Sarabhai zydus	500 ml vial 0.5 ml SC at point of lay	Inactivated water in oil emulsion of adeno virus 127 strain
Nobivac EDS 76	Intervet	500 ml vial 0.5 ml SC at point of lay	Inactivated water in oil emulsion of adeno virus BC14 strain
Cholerin Triple	Sarabhai zydus	500 ml vial 0.5 ml SC at 8-12 wks and 15-18 wks of age.	Inactivated P. multocida serotype 1, 3 and 4) oil adjuvant
FC vax	Indovax	500 ml vial 0.5 ml SC at 6-9 wks (primary) and 25 wks of age (booster).	Inactivated P. multocida indigenous strain in oil adjuvant
Fowl cholera killed vaccine	Ventri	400 doses, 1000 dose vial	Killed P. multocida bacterin
Fowl pox	Indovax	500 doses, 1000 doses. 0.2 ml IM at 6 wks (primary) and at 16-18 wks (booster)	Freeze dried fowl pox virus
Fowl pox vaccine	Ventri	200, 500 doses, 1000 doses. 0.2 ml IM at 6 wks (primary) and at 16-18 wks (booster)	Live fowl pox virus lyophilized
SG vaccine Nobilis (Fowl typhoid)	Intervet	500, 1000 doses. 0.2 ml SC at 6 wks (primary) and at 16-18 wks (revaccination)	Live vaccine with 9R William smith strain of S. gallinarum
H P Vax (Hydropericardium syndrome)	Indovax	500, 1000, 2500 doses vial. 0.2 ml SC at 7 day age	Inactivated suspension from chicken infected with HPS/Inclusion Body Hepatitis with oil based emulsion
Inclusion body hepatitis inactivated vaccine (HPS)	Ventri	500, 1000, 2500 doses vial. 0.2 ml SC at 7 day age	Inactivated suspension from chicken infected with HPS/Inclusion Body Hepatitis with oil based emulsion

Avian I.B. vaccine living (Mass)	Ventri	200, 500, 1000, 2000, 5000 doses. Oculonasal/drinking water method	Lyophilized IB (Massachusetts type) virus of chick embryo origin
Infectious Bronchitis killed vaccine	Ventri	400, 1000 doses vial	Killed I.B. virus vaccine
Burvax (IBD)	Indovax	500, 1000 doses 0.5 ml SC/IM at 18-22 wks (primary) and at 40-45 wks (revaccination)	Inactivated IBD virus strain oil emulsion
Infectious Bursal Disease Killed vaccine (Intermediate plus)	Ventri	200,400,1000 doses	Inactivated IBD virus in oil emulsion for booster vaccination
Infectious Bursal Disease live vaccine (Intermediate plus)	Ventri	200, 500, 1000, 2000 doses	Live virus vaccine with intermediate plus strain
Infectious Bursal Disease live vaccine (Lukert)	Ventri	200, 500, 1000, 2000,5000 doses	Live IBD virus vaccine with Lukert strain
IV 95 strain (IBD)	Indovax	200, 500, 1000, 2000 doses Oral @ 3 g/lit DW with skim milk powder at 10 days-14 wks of age	Freeze dried with intermediate strain
IBDV killed	Intervet	1000 doses vial Primary vaccination @ 0.3 ml SC/IM at 14 days age. Booster @ 0.5 ml SC/IM at 16-18 wks (layers) or 40th wks (breeders)	Inactivated killed IBD RNA virus

Haemovax (Infectious coryza)	Glaxo	1000 doses vial 0.3 ml SC/IM in layers or breeders at 6th wks (primary) and 14th wks (revaccination)	Adjuvanted inactivated bacterin of *Hemophilus gallinarum* vaccine
Infectious coryza killed vaccine	Ventri	400, 1000 doses vial 0.5 ml SC/IM at 8th wks (Primary) and Revaccination after 4 weeks.	Oil emulsion inactivated bacterin of *Hemophilus gallinarum* vaccine
Marek's disease vaccine	Indovax	500, 1000, 2000 doses. 0.2 ml SC at 1st day age at back of neck	Live freeze dried Turkey herpes virus (FC 126) vaccine
Marek's disease vaccine	Intervet	500, 1000 doses. 0.2 ml SC/IM at 1st day age at back of neck	Live freeze dried Turkey herpes virus (FC 126) vaccine
Marek's disease vaccine	Ventri	500, 1000, 2000, 2500 doses. 0.2 ml SC at 1st day age at back of neck	Live freeze dried Turkey herpes virus (FC 126) vaccine
Marek's disease vaccine	Ventri	500, 1000, 2000 doses.	Live cell associated Turkey herpes virus (SB-1) vaccine
Nobivac MG (Mycoplasma gallisepticum)	Intervet	1000 doses	Inactivated *Mycoplasma gallisepticum* antigen
ENCIVAX	Indovax	500, 1000 doses vial 0.5 ml SC/IM at point of lay (primary) and at middle of laying (revaccination)	Inactivated New Castle disease virus vaccine in oil emulsion
F-strain	Indovax	100, 200, 500, 1000, 2000 doses Intraocular/intranasal administration at 4-10 days of age	Freeze dried lentogenic F strain of NCD virus

Lasota strain	Indovax	100, 200, 500, 1000, 2000 doses Intraocular/intranasal/oral administration at 4-8 wks, 9-10 wks,11-20 wks as per directions	Freeze dried lentogenic Lasota strain of NCD virus
Mukteshwar strain (R_2B)	Indovax	100, 400, 1000 doses 0.5 ml SC/IM at 8th wks (Primary) and Revaccination at 16 weeks.	Live Freeze dried mesogenic Mukteshwar (R_2B) strain of NCD virus
NDV-F	Intervet	100, 500, 1000, 2000 doses 1 drop into nostril/eye at 4-7 days of age	Live Freeze dried lentogenic F strain of NCD virus
NDV-Killed	Intervet	100, 1000 doses 0.2 ml SC/IM at 4-7 day age. 0.5 ml SC/IM at 16-20 wks and at 40th wks of age	Inactivated killed virus
NDV-R_2B	Intervet	100, 500, 1000 doses 0.5 ml SC/IM at 10-12 wks (Primary) and Booster at 16-18 weeks.	Live Freeze dried mesogenic Mukteshwar (R_2B) strain of NCD virus
New castle disease vaccine (Lasota strain)	Ventri	100, 200, 500, 1000, 10,000 doses Intraocular/intranasal/oral administration at 4-10 days, 15-16 wks as per directions	Freeze dried lentogenic Lasota strain of NCD virus
New castle disease vaccine -R_2B	Ventri	200, 400, 1000 doses 0.5 ml SC/IM at 10-12 wks (Primary) and Booster at 16-18 weeks.	Live Freeze dried mesogenic Mukteshwar (R_2B) strain of NCD virus
Spirochaetosis Killed vaccine	Ventri	100 doses	Killed Spirochaetes bacterin
Tenosynovitis (Reo virus)	Intervet	1000 doses	Inactivated reo virus
Combined killed vaccine (ND+IBD)	Ventri	400, 1000 doses	Killed antigen of NCD and IBD virus

Combined Live vaccine (Lasota + IB)	Ventri	500, 1000 doses	Live freeze dried attenuated Lasota strain of NCD and Infectious bronchitis virus
EDS+ND vaccine	Sarabhai Zydus	500, 1000 doses 0.5 ml IM/SC at 18-20 wks of age	Inactivated (EDS-76 adeno 127 strain virus and NCD virus)
Fowl cholera + Infectious coryza killed vaccine	Ventri	200,500 doses	Killed virus vaccine against Fowl cholera and Inf. Coryza
IB+ND+EDS vaccine	Sarabhai zydus	500 ml 0.5 ml SC/IM at 18-20 wks	Inactivated IB virus, ND virus and EDS-76 adeno virus127 strain
Nobivac IB+ND+EDS vaccine	Intervet	1000 doses	Inactivated IB virus, ND virus and EDS-76 adeno virus127 strain
Nobivac Reo+IB+G+ ND vaccine	Intervet	1000 doses	Inactivated reo virus, Gumboro virus, IB virus, ND virus strain

Chapter 16
Diagnostics

DIAGNOSTICS			
ABORTUS BANG RING ANTIGEN	IVRI	20 ml vial	Stained suspension of Brucella abortus strain 99
BRUCELLA ABORTUS POSITIVE SERUM	IVRI	10 ML	antibodies against Brucella abortus
BRUCELLA ABORTUS SERUM AGGLUTINATION TEST ANTIGEN	IVRI	250 ml	Stained suspension of Brucella abortus strain 99
JOHNIN PPD	IVRI	10 doses	--
MALLEIN PPD	IVRI	10 doses	--
MASTECT	Indian Immunolo gical	paper strips	Bromothymo blue impregnated paper strip
ROSE BENGAL PLATE TEST ANTIGEN	IVRI	20 ml vial	Stained suspension of Brucella abortus strain 99 (coloured antigen)
SALMONELLA 'O' sera	IVRI	01 ml	---
SALMONELLA ABORTUS EQUI H antigen	IVRI	250 ml	---
SALMONELLA PULLORUM COLOURED ANTIGEN	IVRI	20 ml	---
SALMONELLA PULLORUM PLAIN ANTIGEN	IVRI	250 ml	---
SALMONELLA PULLORUM POSITIVE SERUM	IVRI	01 ml	----
SALMONELLA PULLORUM STAINED ANTIGEN	Solvay	10 ml vial	inactivated stained suspension of S. pullorum
TUBERCULIN BOVINE PPD	IVRI	10 doses	----

Chapter 17

Immune System

MISCELLANEOUS IMMUNOLOGICAL PRODUCTS

- ➢ TETANUS ANTITOXIN
- ➢ TETANUS IMMUNOGLOBULIN
- ➢ TETANUS TOXOID
- ➢ EQUIMUNE
- ➢ RABIES IMMUNOGLOBULIN
- ➢ ANTISNAKE VENOM

MISCELLANEOUS IMMUNOLOGICAL PRODUCTS

TETANUS ANTITOXIN:

It is obtained from horse; is inferior to human antitoxin and should be used in non-immunized persons who have received a contaminated wound and who are at high risk of developing tetanus only when tetanus immunoglobulin is not available.

Indications : Prophylaxis after injury in high risk patients.

Dosage (Prophylactic)

Cattle, Horse: 1500-3000 IU S/C; Calf, sheep, pig: 500 – 1500 IU S/C; Dog: 250-500 IU S/C

Therapeutic dose is administered I/V or I/M in above stated dosage.

Special precautions : Test dose of tetanus antitoxin should always be given prior to injection. Tetanus antitoxin should not be injected into the same site as TT inj. and should not be mixed in the same syringe as tetanus toxoid.

TETANUS IMMUNOGLOBULIN

It is a sterile solution of Immunoglobulin obtained from the plasma of healthy volunteers specifically immunised against tetanus.

Indications : It is indicated for prophylaxis in non-immunized cases receiving a contaminated wound who are at high risk of developing tetanus e.g. extensive soft tissue and bony injury. May be given in treatement of tetanus also.

Dosage: Prophylaxis : 250-500 i.u. I.M. Inj. Therapeutic : 3000-6000 I.M. Inj. and/or 250-500 i.u. intrathecal.

Special precautions : I.V. injection to be avoided.

Adverse drug rections : Low grade fever, chills, malaise. Local tenderness, muscle soreness or stiffness may occur occasionally at the injection site.

TETANUS TOXOID:
It is a formalin treated exotoxin of tetanus bacilli. Two types of preparations – fluid and adsorbed (on almunium phosphate) are available. The adsorbed toxoid is superior – induces higher antibody titers and more prolonged immunity.
Indications : Active immunisation against tetanus.
Dosage :
Large animals: 5 ml S/C; Small animals: 3 ml S/C.
Contraindications : Acute febrile illness of unknown origin. Known hypersensitivity, outbreaks of poliomyelitis.
Special precautions : Delay dose during outbreak of poliomyelitis. In Cases, receiving corticosteroid or other immunosuppressive drugs.
Adverse drug reactions : Local erythema, pain and induration is not uncommen. Axillary lymph nodes may enlarge. Fever, chills, malaise, aches and pains occur occasionally. Paresis and other neurological complications are rare.

TETANUS ANTI-TOXIN	Bengal Immunity	Inj	1500 IU/ vial; 10,000 IU / vial; 20, 000 IU/vial
TETANUS ANTI-TOXIN	B.E.	Inj	1500 IU/ vial
TETANUS ANTI-TOXIN	HBPCL	Inj	1500 IU/ vial; 10,000 IU / vial; 20, 000 IU/vial
TETANUS TOXOID (Adsorbed)	B.E.	Inj	0.5 ml toxoid per ampoule; 5 ml vial
TETANUS TOXOID (Adsorbed)	HBPCL	Inj	0.5 ml toxoid per ampoule; 5 ml vial
TETANUS TOXOID (Adsorbed)	Glaxo	Inj	0.5 ml toxoid per ampoule; 5 ml vial
TETANUS TOXOID (Adsorbed)	Serum Institute	Inj	0.5 ml toxoid per ampoule; 5 ml vial

EQUIMUNE (Vetripharm Inc): Mycobacterial cell wall fraction immunostimulant. Indicated in Equine Upper Respiratory Disease Complex (caused by Herpes virus), Influenza A Equine 1 and Influenza A Equine 2. Dose: 1.5 ml I.V weekly interval for three times.

RABIES IMMUNOGLOBULIN
It is of two types :
a) Antirabies serum (ARS) Also called 'equine rabies immunoglobulin' (ERIG) is refined, concentrated and lyophilized serum from horses' hyperimmunized by repeated injections of liver rabies virus.
b) Rabies immunoglobulin human (HRIG) it is used in the same manner as ARS and is superior to it.
Indications : It is indicated promptly after suspected exposure and is given simultaneously with rabies vaccine to nonimmunized individuals.
Dosage : ARS : 40 IU/kg. Infiltrate in and around the wound.

HRIG : 20 IU/kg infiltrated around the wound (part dose may be given I.M. at a separate site).			
ERig	Cadila Newgen	5 ml vial	Anti-rabies serum 1000 IU per ml
PARS	Cadila Newgen	5 ml vial	Fragments of Equine rabies Immunoglobulin >1000 IU per ml

ANTI-SNAKE VENOM

It is available as purified, enzyme refined and concentrated equine globulins in lyophilized vials with 10ml ampoule of distilled water. After reconstitution, each ml neutralizes :

- 0.6mg of standard Cobra (Naja Naja) venom.
- 0.6mg of standard Russel's viper (vipera russelli) venom.
- 0.45mg of standard Sawscaled viper (Echis carinatus) venom.
- 0.45mg of standard Krait (Bungarus caeruleus) venom.

Indications : Treatment of snake bite along with appropriate medical management.

Dosage : Mix 10 ml water in a vial and shake

Dog : 20 ml slow i/v (1 ml per minute) repeat 2nd dose after 2 hr.

Exclude hypresensitivity by intradermal injection of 0.02ml of 1:10 diluted antivenin.

Special precautions : If time permits sensitivity tests should be done before injection. Emergency resuscitation drugs should be available. Antihistaminic and steroids injections may be given prophylactically.

Adverse drug reaction: Allergic reactions with anaphylaxis.

ANTISNAKE VENOM POLYVALENT	Serum Institute	Injection	serum neutralized standard venom of Cobra, Viper, Krait.
SNAKE ANTIVENIN	HBPCL	Injection	serum neutralized standard venom of Cobra, Viper, Krait.

Chapter 18

Drugs for Respiratory System

- ❖ **BRONCHODILATORS**
  - ➢ AMINOPHYLLINE
  - ➢ ATROPINE SULPHATE
  - ➢ TERBUTALINE
  - ➢ THEOPHYLLINE
- ❖ **EXPECTORANTS & MUCOLYTICS**
- ❖ **RESPIRATORY STIMULANTS**
  - ➢ DOXAPRAM

BRONCHODILATORS **AMINOPHYLLINE:** potent inhibitor of phosphodiesterase enzyme leading to increase in intracellular cAMP, stimulates endogenous catecholamine, inhibits cGMP. Relaxes bronchial smooth muscle. Indicated in bronchial asthma, supportive to treatmetn of CHF. Dogs: 6-11 mg/kg BW TID IM, IV, Oral; cats: 4 mg/kg BW BID IM, IV, Oral.			
Product	**Company**	**Presentation**	**Composition**
Aminophylline	Burrough Wellcome	pack of 100 tabs, inj of 10 ml vial	tab has 100 mg; inj has 250 mg/2 ml
ATROPINE SULPHATE is indicated in respiratory distress, bronchospasm in dogs @ 0.04 mg/kg BW TID IM, IV, SC.			
TERBUTALINE: beta adrenoceptor agonist with selective action on Beta-1 receptors effecting bronchodilation @ 0.05 mg/kg BW TID in dogs and cats. C/I in pregnancy and lactation.			
BRICANYL DURULES tabs	Astra IDL	strip of 10 tabs	each tab has 5 mg, 7.5 mg
THEOPHYLLINE: inhibit Phosphodiesterase enzyme leading to accumulation of cAMP. Relaxes bronchial smooth muscle. Indicated in bronchial asthma, supportive to treatmetn of CHF. Dogs: 6-11 mg/kg BW TID IM, IV, Oral; cats: 4 mg/kg BW BID IM, IV, Oral. May induce hypocalcemia.			
DERIPHYLLIN inj	German remedies	2 ml ampoule	Each 2 ml contains Theophylline 50.6 mg, Etophylline 169.4 mg
DERIPHYLLIN	German	strip of 10 tabs	Each tab contains

tab	remedies		Theophylline 23 mg, Etophylline 77 mg
EXPECTORANTS & MUCOLYTICS			
GLYCODIN	Alembic	50 ml, 100 ml bottle	each 5 ml contains Terpene 10 mg, Dexamethorphan 10 mg, Menthol 3.75 mg.
V-COFEX	Varsha labs	500 ml pack	Diphenhydramine HCl 8 mg, Bromhexine HCl 4 mg, NH_4Cl 100 mg, Na citrate 50 mg, Menthol 1 mg/5 ml
CAFLON powder	Natural Remedies	100 gm, 1 kg bag	herbal
CATCOUGH electuary	Cattle Remedies	100 gm, 250 gm, 1 Kg	Herbal
Breather syrup	Cipla	Bottle of 100ml	Herbal expectorant& respiratory stimulant
CLENBUTEROL: It is beta adrenergic receptor agonist drug and indicated in Rx of chronic obstructive pulmonary disease (COPD) in horses. It is a repartitioning agent and redirects nutrients away from adipose tissue and towards muscle. **Dose rate:** Horses: 0.8-3.2 mg mcg/kg, PO, BID or 0.8 mcg/kg IV BID.			
Respeze Powder	Cipla	500gm, 1kg	Clenbuterol HCl 16mcg/gm
Respeze Oral Paste	Cipla	500 ml, 10ml	Clenbuterol hydrochloride 40mcg/ml
SALBUTAMOL(Albuterol): It is beta adrenergic receptor agonist drug and indicated in bronchoconstriction. Contraindicated in glaucoma, renal and cardiac disease. **Dose rate:** ➢ Dogs: 0.05 mg/kg, PO, tid; ➢ Horses: 8 mcg/kg, PO, bid			
Salbutamol Eq-Haler	Cipla	Each containing 200 metered Doses	Salbutamol 120 mcg /actuation
RESPIRATORY STIMULANTS			
DOXAPRAM: Acts directly upon chemoreceptors of carotid and aortic regions, stimulates medullary respiratory centre, leading to increase in tidal volume. **Indications** : Apnoea in premature neonates, respiratoty depression following drug poisoning, drowning, post operative respiratory depression and acute respiratory failure, barbiturate induced depression. **Dosage** ➢ Dogs : 5-10 mg/kg BW IV, SC, Sublingual; ➢ Horse: 0.5 mg/kg BW IV, SC, Sublingual.			

<table>
<tr><td colspan="4">➢ Foal: 0.02-0.05 mg/kg/min, I/V.
Drug induced CNS depression : 2mg/kg. repeat in 5 min. and then every 1-2 hours untill patients recovers. Max dose 3gm.
Contraindications : Cardiovascular diseases like ischaemic heart disease, hypertension, CNS diseases like, cerebral edema, convulsive disorders, epilepsy, cerebro vascular diseases, pheochromocytoma, hyperthyroidism.
Special precautions : Monitoring of cardio respiratory status is essential. To be used with caution in liver disease, and COPD.
Adverse drug reactions : Hypotension, cerebral irritation, excitation, muscle fasciculation, spascity, convulsions, hyperpyrexia. Nausea, diarrhoea.
Status in
1. Pregancy : Use with caution.
2. Lacation : Use with caution.
3. Old age : Use with extreme caution.</td></tr>
<tr><td>CAROPRAM inj</td><td>Khandelval</td><td>5 ml vial</td><td>20 mg/ml</td></tr>
</table>

BECLOMETHASONE DIPROPIOANTE			
Beclate-200 Eq-Haler	Cipla	Each containing 200 metered Doses	Beclomethasone dipropioante 200mcg/actuation

Chapter 19

Surgery and Anaesthesia Products

GENERAL ANAESTHETIC			
KETAMINE: potent inhibitor of GABA which enhance CNS inhibitory maechanisms. It inhibits GABA reuptake at synapses where it is normally liberated. Indicated in immobilisation and surgery. C/I in head injuries, status epilepticus. Dogs: 10 mg/kg BW IM; Pig: 15-20 mg/kgBW IM, SC; Horse: 2.2 mg/kgBW IV; Goat: 22-44 mg/kgBW IM, SC.			
Product	**Company**	**Presentation**	**Composition**
KETALAR	Parke Davis	injection 10 ml, 2 ml; 20ml Inj	10 mg/ml in 20 ml vial, 50 mg/ml in 2 ml and 10 ml vial
KETMIN	Themis	injection 2ml 10 ml, 20 ml	10 mg/ml in 10 ml, 20 ml Inj vial; 50 mg/ml in 2 ml, 10 ml vials.
THIOPENTONE SODIUM			
INTRAVAL SODIUM	RhonePoulenc	50 Amp	500mg/amp; 1g/amp
PENTOTHAL	Abbott	Injection Vial	500mg/vial; 1g/vial
THIOSOL	Neon Labs	Injection Vial	500mg/vial; 1g/vial
LOCAL ANAESTHETIC			
BUPIVACAINE & combination			
SENSORCAINE 0.5% with ADRENALINE	Astra Zeneca	20ml Inj.	(Bupivacaine HCl 5mg, Adrenaline (as bitart) 0.005mg, Sod. Chl. 8mg, Sod. Metabisulph 0.5mg, Methylparaben 1mg/ml)
SENSORCAINE	Astra Zeneca	20ml Vial	0.25% w/v, 0.5% w/v
SENSORCAINE HEAVY	Astra Zeneca	10x4ml Inj.	Bupivacaine HCl 5mg, Dextrose monohydrate 80mg/ml
SENSORCAINE SPINAL	Astra Zeneca	5x4ml Inj. 0.5%	Bupivacaine HCl 8mg, Sodium Chloride 8mg/ml
LIGNOCAINE & combination			
XYLOCAINE 5% HEAVY	Astra Zeneca	25x2ml Inj.	Lignocaine HCl 53.3mg, Dextrose 75mg/ml

XYLO	Drakt Pharma	30ml Inj.	Lignocaine HCl 2%
Xylocard 2%	Astra Zeneca	50ml Vial	Lignocaine HCI 21.3mg, Sodium chloride 6mg water for inj to make 1 ml
XYLOCAINE	Astra Zeneca	30ml Vial: 1%; 30ml: 2%; 5x2ml Amp: 2%; 5x5ml: 2%; 5x10ml:2%	
LIDOCAINE preparation			
Lidocaine inj	Cipla	50 ml vial	**Lidocaine hydrochloride 20mg/ml**

PREANAESTHETIC **ATROPINE SULPHATE**			
Product	**Company**	**Presentation**	**Composition**
ATROPINE SULPHATE	Samarth Pharma	10ml, 50ml Inj.	6mg/ml in 1 ml amp; 30mg/ml in 50 ml vial
ATROPINE INJ	Life Pharma	1ml/1Amp	Atropine Sulphate 0.6mg/ml
CHLORPROMAZINE: Phenothiazine derivative. Blocks alfa adrenoceptors. Indicated for nervous and aggressive animals, as pre anaesthetic. Dogs: 1-2 mg/kg BW IV, IM, 3 mg/kg oral; Swine: 1.1 mg/kg BW IV; 2-4mg/Kg BW IM; Cattle: 1 mg/kg BW IM. C/I in equines. Do not use with adrenalin. Avoid in o-p poisoning and very weak animals.			
CHLORPROMA ZINE	Rhone poulenc	Strip of 10 tabs, injection of 2ml amp.	each tab contains 10 mg; 25mg, 50 mg, 100 mg; Injection has 2.5 %
MEGATIL	Intas	Strip of 10 tabs, injection of 2ml amp.	each tab contains 25mg, 50 mg, 100 mg, 200 mg; Injection has 50mg/2ml.
TRIFLUPROMAZINE: neuroleptic agent. Antagonise central dopamine D2 receptors. Prominent antiemetic activity. Dog: 2-4 mg/kg BW IM, 1-2 mg/kg BW IV. Administration with epinephrine is contraindicated.			
Siquil injection	Sarabhai zydus	5 ml vial	Each ml has Triflupromazine HCl: 20 mg
Siquil tab	Sarabhai zydus	Strip Of 10 Tabs	Each tab has Triflupromazine HCl: 10 mg
ANICALM	**Intas**	Strip Of 10 Tabs, inj of 5 ml vial	Each tab has Triflupromazine HCl: 5 mg, 10 mg; injection has 20 mg/ml
SUGIL	**Biomedica**	inj of 5 ml vial	injection has 20 mg/ml

XYLAZINE:
activates alfa-2 adrenoceptors with potent antinociceptive/analgesic action. Indicated for sedation, analgesia, muscle relaxation, immobilisation of animals. Horse/dog/cat: 1-2mg/kgBW IM, 0.5-1.1 mg/Kg BW IV; Cattle: 0.1-0.2 mg/kg BW IM, 0.05 mg/kg BW IV. C/I in GIT obstruction, stomach torsion, hernia, later stage of pregnancy. Antidote : Yohimbine HCl, 4-aminopyridine.

Xylodac injection	Sarabhai zydus	2 ml & 10 ml vials	Each ml has Xylazine HCl: 23.32 mg
XYLAXIN	Indian Immunologicals	2 ml & 10 ml, 30 ml vials	Each ml has Xylazine HCl: 23.32 mg
XYLOCAD INJ	Cadila Pharmaceuticals Limited	5 ml vial	Each ml has Xylazine HCl: 23.32 mg
PENTAZOCINE			
PENTAZOCINE	Biochem	10x1ml Inj	30mg/ml

MISCELLANEOUS PRODUCTS FOR SURGEON'S PERUSAL

SERRATIOPEPTIDASE:
Proteolytic enzyme, releives inflammation associated with infection, trauma and chronic venous insufficiency.

Dose rate: Dog, cat: 10 mg BID total dose, orally.

Indications : Releif of edema associated with trauma, infection or venous insufficiency.

Contraindications : Bleeding disorders.

Special precautions : Hepatic or renal disorders.

Adverse drug reactions : GI disturbance, epistaxis.

SUCCINYL CHOLINE:
It is an ultrashort acting depolarizing agent. It induces rapid, complete and predictable paralysis within 1 minute and has spontaneus recovery in 5 mins. It is rapidly hydrolysed by plasma pseudocholinesterases.

Dosage: Dogs: 0.3 mg/KgBW IV; Cattle/goat: 0.01 – 0.02 mg/KgBW IV; Pig: 02 mg/KgBW IV; **Horse**: 0.08 mg/KgBW IV

Indications : Most commonly used adjuvant in surgical anaesthesia for endotracheal intubation and skeletal muscle relaxation in various surgeries. It is also used during brief surgical procedures like laryngoscopy, bronchoscopya, esophagoscopy and reduction of fractures.

Special precautions : Renal, hepatic and CVS disorders, myasthenia gravis, electrolyte disorders and neonates.

Status in

1. Pregnancy : Use with caution, (category C drug). In labour succinylcholine is commonly used to provide muscle relaxation during delivery by cesarean section.
2. Lactation : Use with caution.

3. Old age : Use with caution. 4. Neonates : Use with caution. Interactions: Beta blockers, lithium, chloroquine, magnesium salts, Calcium channel blockers (verapamil) : Potentiate neuromuscular block; Opioid analgesics : Increase incidence of bradycardia and cardiac arrest; Digitalis, potassium sparing diuretics: Can cause life threatening hyperkalemia; Halothane : May cause malignant hyperthermia in predisposed patients; Thiopentone : Should not be mixed in the same syringe.			
TOLPA	Micro Labs	10 Tab	Serratiopeptidase 10mg
MIDARINE	Burr. Wellcome	2ml Inj.	Succinyl Choline 50mg/ml
SCOLINE	GSK	2ml Inj.	Succinyl Choline 50mg/ml
SUXOMIN	VHB Life Sciences	10ml Inj.	Succinyl Choline 50mg/ml

ABSORBABLE SUTURE MATERIALS

- CATGUT
- CATGUT PLAIN
- POLYDIOXANONE
- POLYGALACTIN 910

SUTURES NON-ABSORBABLE

- POLYAMIDE – MONOFILAMENT
- POLYPROPYLENE MONOFILAMENT
- SILK – BLACK BRAIDED

SURGICAL STAPLES

TISSUE ADHESIVE

- N-BUTYL 2 CYANOACRYLATE

MISCELLANEOUS PRODUCTS

ABSORBABLE SUTURE MATERIALS		
CATGUT: absorbable suture, from intestinal sub mucosa of sheep and goat. Indicated in visceral surgery, ophthalmic surgery. Starts loosing tensile strength within 15-21 days.		
SUTURE MATERIAL	COMPANY	Suture Length - Needle Type-Needle Length

ETHICON STERILIZED SURGICAL GUT CHROMIC (3-0)	ETHICON	152 cm long
ETHICON STERILIZED SURGICAL GUT CHROMIC (2-0)	ETHICON	152 cm long
ETHICON STERILIZED SURGICAL GUT CHROMIC (1-0)	ETHICON	152 cm long
ETHICON STERILIZED SURGICAL GUT CHROMIC (1)	ETHICON	152 cm long
ETHICON STERILIZED SURGICAL GUT CHROMIC (2)	ETHICON	152 cm long
MERSUTURES-CHROMIC (5-0)	ETHICON	76 cm - 3/8 RC-12 mm
MERSUTURES-CHROMIC (4-0)	ETHICON	76 cm - 3/8 C-16 mm 76 cm - 3/8 RB-16 mm
MERSUTURES-CHROMIC (3-0)	ETHICON	76 cm - 3/8 C- 22 mm 76 cm - 1/2 RB- 20 mm 76 cm - 3/8 RC visiblack-12 mm 76 cm - 3/8 C-16 mm
MERSUTURES-CHROMIC (2-0)	ETHICON	76 cm - 3/8 RB - 30 mm 76 cm - 3/8 RB - 40 mm 76 cm - 1/2 RB- 30 mm 76 cm - 1/2 RB visiblack-12 mm 76 cm - 1/2 RB - 40 mm 76 cm - 1/2 C- 30 mmH 152 cmDN-1/2 RB, ½ RC- 36 mm
MERSUTURES-CHROMIC (1-0)	ETHICON	76 cm - SRB - 45 mm 76 cm - 3/8 RB - 30 mm 76 cm - 3/8 RB - 40 mm 76 cm - 3/8 RB - 45 mm 100 cm - 1/2 RB- 45 mmH 76 cm - 1/2 RB - 30 mm 76 cm - 1/2 RB - 40 mm 76 cm - 1/2 RB- 30 mmH 76 cm - 1/2 RB - 40 mmH 100 cm - 1/2 TP - 40 mm
MERSUTURES-CHROMIC (1)	ETHICON	76 cm – 3/8RB - 45 mm 76 cm - 3/8 RB visiblack- 45 mm

		100 cm - 1/2 RB - 45 mmH 100 cm - 1/2 TP - 40 mm 100 cm - 1/2 RB- 50 mmH 76 cm - 1/2 RB - 40 mmH 76 cm - 1/2 RB visiblack - 40 mm
MERSUTURES-CHROMIC (2)	ETHICON	100 cm - 1/2 RB - 45 mmH 100 cm - 1/2 TP - 40 mmH
PROGUT-CHROMIC (5-0)	FUTURA	30 cm – 5/8 TP - 10 mm 76 cm - 3/8 RC - 12 mm 76 cm - 3/8 RB - 16 mm
PROGUT-CHROMIC (4-0)	FUTURA	38 cm – 3/8 RC - 12 mm 76 cm - 3/8 RB - 16 mm 76 cm - 3/8 C - 16 mm
CATGUT PLAIN		
ETHICON STERILIZED SURGICAL GUT PLAIN (3-0)	ETHICON	152 cm long, 76 cm (Precut half length), 50.7 cm (precut third length)
ETHICON STERILIZED SURGICAL GUT PLAIN (2-0)	ETHICON	152 cm long, 76 cm (Precut half length), 50.7 cm (precut third length)
ETHICON STERILIZED SURGICAL GUT PLAIN (1-0)	ETHICON	152 cm long, 76 cm (Precut half length), 50.7 cm (precut third length)
ETHICON STERILIZED SURGICAL GUT PLAIN (1)	ETHICON	152 cm long, 76 cm (Precut half length), 50.7 cm (precut third length)
ETHICON STERILIZED SURGICAL GUT PLAIN (2)	ETHICON	152 cm long, 76 cm (Precut half length), 50.7 cm (precut third length)
MERSUTURES-PLAIN (3-0)	ETHICON	76 cm - 3/8 C- 16 mm 76 cm - 3/8 C -22 mm 76 cm - 3/8 C- 26 mm
PROGUT- PLAIN (4-0)	FUTURA	76 cm - 3/8 C - 16 mm
PROGUT- PLAIN (5-0)	FUTURA	76 cm - 3/8 C - 12 mm
PROGUT- PLAIN (1-0)	FUTURA	152 cm (Precut)
POLYDIOXANONE synthetic absorbable monofilament suture. Complete absorption takes place in 180 days.		
PDS II (1-0)	ETHICON	90 cm – ½ RB – 40 mmH
POLYGALACTIN 910 synthetic absorbable suture material made from glycolic lactic acid polymer and C calcium stearate. Complete absorption occurs in 90 days. Stable in contaminated		

wound. Rapid absorption in alkaline medium.		
VICRYL (8-0)	ETHICON	30 cm DN-3/8 MPS- 6 mm
VICRYL (7-0)	ETHICON	30 cm -3/8 MPS- 6 mm
VICRYL (6-0)	ETHICON	45 cm DN-1/4 MPS- 8 mm
VICRYL (5-0)	ETHICON	45 cm -1/2 RB - 16 mm 45 cm -3/8 C - 16 mm 45 cm - 3/8 RC - 12 mm
VICRYL (4-0)	ETHICON	70 cm -1/2 RB - 16 mm 70 cm -1/2 RB - 20 mm 70 cm - 3/8 C – 16 mm 45 cm - 5/8 C – 16 mm 45 cm – 3/8 RC – 12 mm
VICRYL (1)	ETHICON	70 cm - 3/8 RB - 45 mm 90 cm - 1/2 RB - 40 mmH 70 cm - 1/2 RB – 40 mmH 70 cm – ½ TP – 40 mmH 90 cm – ½ TP – 40 mmH 100 cm- ½ RB – 50 mmH 90 cm - ½ RC – 50 mmH
SUTURES NON-ABSORBABLE **POLYAMIDE – MONOFILAMENT:** non-absorbable inert material, excellent for general closure, skin and plastic surgery. Excellent knot security, smooth texture, does not support infection.		
ETHICON (10-0)	ETHICON	25 cm - 3/8 RB - 4 mm 20 cmDN - 3/8 AMPS - 6 mm 38 cmDN - 3/8 MPS - 6 mm 38 cm - 3/8 MPS - 6 mm 30 cmDN - 3/8 MPS - 6 mm 38 cmDN - 1/2 - 6 mm
ETHICON (9-0)	ETHICON	38 cmDN - 3/8 MPS - 6 mm 38 cm - 3/8 MPS - 6 mm
LINEX (6-0)	FUTURA	70 cm – 3/8 C – 26 mm
LINEX (1)	FUTURA	100 cm – 1/2 RB – 45 mmH 100 cm – 1/2 RC – 45 mmH 100 cm – 1/2 RC – 50 mmH 150 cm – 1/2 RB – 50 mmH 70 cm – 3/8 C – 90 mm
POLYESTER: non absorbable suture braided and coated with silicone. excellent for general closure, cardiovascular, orthopedic, skin and plastic surgery.		
ETHI BOND (4-0)	ETHICON	76 cm – 1/4 MPS – 8 mm
MERSILENE (5-0)	ETHICON	38 cm – 1/4 MPS – 8 mm
PROCARE (1)	FUTURA	100 cm – ½ RC – 50 mm

PROCARE (2)	FUTURA	100 cm – ½ TCP – 45 mmH
PROCARE (5)	FUTURA	100 cm – ½ TCP – 55 mmH 75 cm – ½ TCP – 55 mmH
POLYPROPYLENE MONOFILAMENT: non absorbable suture. Excellent knot security, smooth texture, do not support infection. excellent for general closure, cardiovascular, orthopaedic, skin and plastic surgery.		
DURACARE (6-0)	Futura	45 cm – 3/8 RC – 12 mm 70 cmDN – 3/8 RB – 13 mm 70 cm – 3/8 SBC – 15 mm
DURACARE (6-0)	Futura	70 cmDN – 3/8 RB – 12 mm 70 cm – 3/8 RC – 12 mm 70 cm – 3/8 SBC – 15 mm 70 cm – 3/8 RB – 16 mm 70 cm DN – 3/8 RB – 16 mm
PROLENE (1)	ETHICON	70 cm – 1/2 TC – 30 mmH 70 cm – 1/2 RB – 40 mmH 100 cm – 1/2 RC – 45 mmH 100 cm – ½ TP – 30 mmH
SILK – BLACK BRAIDED: non absorbable suture treated with silicon or wax for strength. Moderate tissue reaction, Excellent knot security, smooth texture. Avoid to use in presence of infection and urinary tract and bile duct surgery. Used for general closure, cardiovascular, orthopedic, skin and plastic surgery and as ligature.		
ETHICON VIRGIN SILK BLACK (8-0)	ETHICON	38 cm – ½ RC-MP-8 mm 38 cmDN – 3/8 MPS-6 mm 38 cm – 3/8 MPS -6 mm
MERSILK (6-0)	ETHICON	38 cm – 3/8 RC-MP- 10 mm 38 cm – 3/8 RC-MP-8 mm
SUTURA (I)	FUTURA	76 cm – 3/8 C – 60 mm
SUTURA (1-0)	FUTURA	76 cm – 3/8 RB – 30 mm 76 cm – 1/2 RB – 30 mm
SURGICAL STAPLES: metallic staples for skin closure. Easy to apply, disposable in nature, no tissue reaction.		
ETHICON PROX-MULTI DIR 35 PIN	EHTICON	35 pins x 6 pieces
ETHICON PROX-MULTI DIR 55 PIN	EHTICON	55 pins x 6 pieces
TISSUE ADHESIVE: Synthetic bio-adhesive used for closure of wounds, micro ligature where ligation is not possible. **N-BUTYL 2 CYANOACRYLATE**		
ENDOCRYL	Samarth pharma	0.5 ml ampoule

NECCTACRYL	Dr. reddy's	0.25 ml ampoule, 0.5 ml ampoule, 1 ml ampoule
MISCELLANEOUS PRODUCTS		
JOHNSONPLAST	Johnson & Johnson	Tube pack having 2.5 cm x10m; 5 cm x10, 7/5 cm x10m; 10cm x10m
RAPIDUR	Beierdorf	Plaster of paris. 2.7 m x 15 cm
SURGIPAD	Johnson & Johnson	10 cm x 10 cm; 7.5 cm x 20 cm; 10 cm x 20 cm
Umbilical cotton tape	Ethicon	(75 cm x 3 mm) 12's

Chapter 20

Drugs for Urogenital System

➢ DIURETICS

DIURETICS			
ACETAZOLAMIDE: carbonic anhydrase inhibitor. Indicated in acidic urine, glaucoma. Dogs: 2-5 mg/kg BW TID Oral. Avoid during pregnancy, lactation			
Product	**Company**	**Presentation**	**Composition**
DIAMOX	Cyanamid	strip of 10 tabs	each tab contains 250 mg.
FRUSEMIDE: Loop diuretic. Reduces active absorption of sodium and chloride from luminal phase of loop cells. Indicated in acute pulmonary oedema, cerebral oedema, ascites, CHF, post parturient edema. Dogs/cat: 2-4 mg/kg BW BID IM, IV, Oral. Cattle: 1-2 mg/kg BW IM, IV, oral. Ototoxicity results due to concurrent administration with Aminoglycoside.			
LASIX	Hoechst	Tab, Inj 2 ml	each tab contains 40 mg, inj contains 20 mg/ml
LASIX high dose	Hoechst	Tab, Inj 2 ml	each tab contains 500 mg, inj contains 250 mg/2ml
RIDEMA	Merind	inj 10 ml vial	each inj contains 50mg/ml
SPIRONOLACTONE: aldosterone antagonist. Increases Na, Ca and chloride excretion while reduces K, H, Ammonium ions. Indicated in acute pulmonary oedema, CHF, cerebral oedema, ascites. Indicated in acute pulmonary oedema, cerebral oedema, ascites, CHF. Dogs/cat: 1-2 mg/kg BW Oral. Use with precaution in renal failure, metabolic acidosis, diabetes mellitus.			
ALDACTONE	Searle	tablets	each tab contains 25 mg, 100 mg.
INDIGENOUS PRODUCTS			
NEPHORCARE	Caretech	Powder 500 gm pack. (@ 1 kg/ton feed in poultry)	Herbal

ECBOLIC / UTERINE CLEANSER			
Ecbolic is drug, as ergot, which by exciting uterine contractions promotes the expulsion of the contents of the uterus. **Indication:** Retention of Placenta, Delayed involution of uterus, Uterine tonic.			
Exapar bolus	Ayurvet	4'S Large animals: 10 tablets BID PO	Herbal

		for 2-3 weeks Small animals: 2-3 tablets BID PO for 2-3 weeks	
Exapar liquid	Ayurvet	500 ml Cow & Buffalo: 2-4 boli PO BID Ewe & Doe: 1-2 boli PO BID	Herbal
Explanta powder	Sarabhai Zydus	40 g 200g packet (@ Cow, Buffalo & Mare : 20 g BID PO)	Herbal
HimRop	Himalya	500 ml pp pack	Herbal
Prolase-In	Cattle remedies	Box 5x6 tabs with 20 gm powder pack	Herbal
Repel-R	Unim pharma	100 tab pack, 500 ml, 1 lt, 5 ltr plastic jar (10 tab bid PO in cow; 100 ml bid PO in cow)	Ayurvedic prepn.
Replanta	Indian Herbs	Carton of 100 gm. Poly bag of 500 gm and 1 kg. (Large animal :50-60 gm)	Herbal
Uterotone capsuls	Cattle remedies	Box 6 x8 capsules	Herbal
Uterotone liquid	Cattle remedies	225 ml, 450 ml, 900 ml (Cow & Buffalo : 100-125 ml)	Herbal
U-tone liq	Triveni herbal	500 ml, 1 ltr pack (Cow & Buffalo : 100-125 ml)	Herbal

ESTRUS INDUCING PREPARATIONs

Anoestrus due to non functional ovary. Delayed maturity due to non specific reasons in heifers. Non specific anestrus, silent estrus, non-ovulatory estrus, For inducing timely postpartum estrus and regulating ovarian function.

Product	compositio n	indication	Dosage	present ation	Compa ny
Agrimin-I bolus	Multivitami n-mineral bolus	Anoestrus due to mineral, vitamin deficiency	1 bolus per day PO per cow for 7-14 days	Pack of 14 boli	Virbac
Aloes Compoun d	Herbal	Infertility associated with ovarian dysfunctions like anoestrus, silent heat, delayed puberty and	Large animals : 5-10 tabs BID for 3-6 weeks Small animals : 2-3 tabs BID for 1 month	100'S	Alarsin

		infective conditions like metritis, endometritis, cervicitis and vaginitis			
Alona bolus	Herbal	Oestrus induction	1-2 boli BID	10'S	Theodor
Alona capsule	Herbal	As above	2 caps BID	10'S	Theodor
Clofert-Vet	Clomiphene : 300 mg/ tab	Anovulatory heat, repeat breeding, delayed puberty and oestrogen induced tumors	Cattle, Horse, Sheep, Goat, Pig: 1-1.5 mg/ kg body weight for 5 days PO Dog ; 25 mg/ kg body weight PO	5'S	Sigma
Cofecu tab	Each caplet contains Cu, Fe, Co	Anoestrus due to mineral deficiencey	1 caplet per animal daily	20 caplet pack	Indian Herbs
Estrona	Herbal	As above	2 caps daily	Vial containing 10 caps	Rakesh
Estrona forte	Herbal	As above	1-2 boli daily	10'S	Rakesh
Heat Up	Herbal	As above	Cattle, Buffalo & Mare: 3 caps daily for 2 days PO Ewe, Doe, Sow, Bitch: 2 caps OD PO	6'S	Century
Himfertin	Ayurvedic	Anoestrus	3 caps daily for 2-3 days PO per cow	6's strip	HImalaya
Janova	Herbal	Non specific anestrus , silent estrus, non ovulantory estrus , for inducing timely postpartum estrus and regulating ovarian function.	Cows, buffaloes,heifers & mares : 3 capsule per day. Ewes,bitches and sows :2 cap/day orally for 2 consecutive days.	Strip of 6 capsules	Dabur Ayurvet Limited

			Repeat after 10 days in case no estrus is observed .		
Mintrus caplet	Each caplet contains Cu, Fe, Co	Anoestrus due to mineral deficiencey	1 caplet per animal daily	20 caplet pack	Indian Herbs
Ovifertin Powder	Herbal	As above	Large animals: 10 g PO OD for 2 days Repeat the dose schedule after 10 days if required	10 g packet	Indian Herbs
Prajana	Herbal	Anoestrus due to non functional ovary. Delayed maturity due to non specific reasons in heifers.	Large animal :3 capsules Ewes & Does : 2 capsules orally with gur or feed on the first day followed by another dose on the second days.	Carton contain ing 20 pouche s of 6 capsule s; each vial of 6 capsule s.	Indian Herbs
Sajani	Herbal	As above	Large animals: 3 caps/ day for 3 days PO Small animals: 2 caps/ day for 2 days PO Repeat on 11th & 12th day in case of no oestrus	6'S	Sarbhai Zydus
TICO infertility kit	Each kit contains clomiphene 300 mg tab and two boli of CuSO4 750 mg each	Anoestrus due to non functional ovary. Delayed maturity	Each kit per day for five days	Kit contain ing 5 strip of white and blue tabs	Marc

HORMONES USED IN ANIMAL REPRODUCTION

- GONADOTROPIN RELEASING HORMONES
- PITUITARY GONADOTROPINS: (FOLLICLE STIMULATING HORMONE/ LUTEINIZING HORMONE)
- NON PITUITARY GONADOTROPINS: HUMAN CHORIONIC GONADOTROPIN, PREGNANT MARES SERUM GONADOTROPHIN
- OVARIAN STEROIDS: HYDROXY PROGESTERONE CAPROATE; MEDROXYPROGESTERONE ACETATE (MPA), NORGESTOMET
- OESTROGENS: OESTRADIOL VALERATE PROSTAGLANDINS CLOPROSTENOL, DINOPROST, LUPRASTIOL, TIAPROST
- OXYTOCIN
- VALETHAMATE

DRUGS FOR MALE GENITAL SYSTEM PROBLEMS:

- HUMAN CHORIONIC GONADOTROPIN,
- PREGNANT MARES SERUM GONADOTROPHIN,
- OESTROGENS,
- TESTOSTERONE PREPARATIONS,
- INDIGENOUS PREPARATIONS

GONADOTROPIN RELEASING HORMONES

BUSERELIN:

GnRH analogue. Stimulates follicular growth, estrus and ovulation by release of FSH and LH. Indicated in Anestrum, Silent heat, Anovulation, Delayed Ovulation, Follicular cyst, Improvement of conception rate. ***Contraindicated in swine.***

DOSAGE: Anovulation & Delayed Ovulation

Cattle/ Buffaloes- 2.5 ml i/m or i/v

True anestrum

Cattle/ Buffaloes 5ml i/m or i/v

Horse - 5 ml i/m or i/v

Sheep and Goat – 1 ml i/m or i/v

Follicular Cyst

Cattle/ Buffaloes 5ml i/m or i/v

Horse - 10 ml i/m or i/v

Receptal	Intervet	10 ml Vial	Buserelin acetate- 0.0042 mg/ml

GONADORELIN:

GnRH analogue. Stimulates follicular growth, estrus and ovulation by release of FSH and LH. Indicated in cystic ovarian disease (@ 100 mcg IM, IV in large animals), Delayed Ovulation, repeat breeder, Improvement of fertility rate post partum (@ 250 mcg IM, IV in Large animals). ***Contraindicated in swine.***

Fertagyl inj	Intervet	1 ml amp	Gonadorelin- 0.1 mg/ ml
Cystorelin inj	BCAHP	2ml & 10 ml vial	Gonadorelin- 50 μg/ ml

PITUITARY GONADOTROPINS

FOLLICLE STIMULATING HORMONE:

Pituitary Gonadotropin. Stimulates folliculogenesis in mature female ovaries. **Indicated** in True anestrum, Superovulation in embryo transfer donor cows.

Dose is 400 mg in 8 divided doses of 50 mg each at 12 hours interval for superovulation in cattle. ***(Contraindicated in swine).***

LUTEINIZING HORMONE:

Pituitary Gonadotropin. Stimulates maturation, estrogen production and finally ovulation and also growth of CL **Indicated** in Anovulation, Delayed Ovulation, Cystic Ovaries, Repeat breeding.

Dose : Cattle, buffalo& horse- 25 mg IV; Swine – 5 mg IV; Sheep & Goat – 2.5 mg IV. ***(Anaphylactic reaction may be seen in some cases. Epinephrine may be used in such cases)***

Folltropin- V	Vetrepharm Inc	Vial of 400 mg with diluent of 20 ml	FSH NIH (porcine) – 400 mg/ vial
Lutropin-V	Vetrepharm Inc	25 mg vial with 5 ml diluent	LH 25 mg/ vial

NON PITUITARY GONADOTROPINS

1. HUMAN CHORIONIC GONADOTROPIN: It is derived from urine of pregnant women. HCG mimics the effects of Pituitary LH causing Ovulation. It promotes formation and maintenance of LH. Indicated in Delayed Ovulation, Cystic Ovaries, Repeat breeding, Early embryonic death.

Dose rate:

Repeat breeding

Canines- 100-500 IU i/m on the day of service

Cattle & buffaloes- 1500-3000 IU, i/m on the day of service

Sheep & Goat-200-500 IU i/m on the day of service

Cystic Ovaries

Cattle & buffaloes- 1500-3000 IU; i/m, i/v

Mare- 1500-3000 IU i/m

Indications : Female infertility, to trigger ovulation and maintain luteal support. Also used in recurrent abortions. In males it is given for hypogonadotropic hypogonadism and cryptorchidism.

Contraindications : Known hypersensitivity, androgen dependant neoplasm, undiagnosed vaginal bleeding. Risk should be weighed in patients with bleeding disorders.

Specical Precautions : Avoid HCG injection if there are more than 3 follicles of 16mm on ultrasound after stimulation, cardiac disease, renal disease, epilepsy, migraine. Discontinue injection if signs of precautious property appear.

Adverse drug reactions: Allergic reactions like rash, pruritis and rarely anaphylaxis can occur.

Status in

1. Pregnancy : Use only if benefits outweigh risks.
2. Lactation : Not indicated.
3. Old age : Not indicated.

2. PREGNANT MARES SERUM GONADOTROPHIN:

PMSG affects FSH like action inducing follicular growth in inactive ovaries of mature animals. Indicated in Superovulation in embryo donors, True Anestrus with inactive ovaries, Bitch: Anoestrus –True subnormal oestrus with non acceptance, Bull &Stallion: Impaired spermatogenesis, Dog : Impaired spermatogenesis. ***(In cows mating at first estrus may cause superfetation. Repeated administration may cause anaphylactic shock)***

DOSE RATE:

Cow & Buffalo: 1500-3000 IU i/m or i/v. Oestrus normally results in 2-5 days. Repeat after 10-14 days if required.

Mare: 3000-6000 IU as i/m or subcut inj Oestrus results in 7 days.

Sheep and Goat: 1000 IU i/m or subcut. Oestrus results in 24 hours and lasts for 3 days. Reinject 750IU 24 hours after the first injection.

Bitch: 50-200 IU subcut Estrus symptoms appears in 8-10 days.

Chorulon	Intervet	1500 IU Vial	Human Chorionic Gonadotropin 1500 IU
Folligon	Intervet	1000 IU Vial & solvent	Pregnant mare serum Gonadotropin -1000 I.U/ vial
Syncro-Part PMSG 400	BCAHP	400 IU Vial and solvent	Pregnant mare serum Gonadotropin - 400 I.U/ vial
Syncro-Part PMSG 500	BCAHP	500 IU Vial and solvent	Pregnant mare serum Gonadotropin - 500 I.U/ vial
Syncro-Part PMSG 600	BCAHP	600 IU Vial and solvent	Pregnant mare serum Gonadotropin - 600 I.U/ vial
Syncro-Part PMSG 700	BCAHP	700 IU Vial and solvent	Pregnant mare serum Gonadotropin - 700 I.U/ vial
Syncro-Part	BCAHP	6000 IU Vial and	Pregnant mare serum

PMSG 6000		solvent	Gonadotropin - 6000 I.U/ vial
Trophovet	Indian Immunological	1000 IU Vial and solvent	Pregnant mare serum Gonadotropin - 1000 I.U/ vial

OVARIAN STEROIDS

HYDROXY PROGESTERONE CAPROATE: Stimulates luteal action and causes quieting of myometrium. Enhance endometrial glandular secretions and hence responsible for maintenance of pregnancy. At lower doses it also induce ovulation by indirect effect on LH release. Indicated in Repeat breeder, anoestrus, antipartem prolapse of vagina, habitual abortion. ***(Prolonged Progesterone administration may cause uterine glandular hypoplasia, accumulation of fluids in the uterus and endometritis)***

DOSE RATE:

Habitual Abortion in early pregnancy: 750 mg I/M.

after 1.5 month of pregnancy. Repeat 4 or 5 times at 10 days interval.

Repeat breeder with weak corpus Iuteum :500 -750 mg i/m followed per week for 3 weeks.

Prolapse of uterus: 750 mg i/m for two days.

Induction of estrus: 500 mg i/m if no response, repeat after 10 days.

Duraprogen inj	Vetcare	2ml amp	Each ml contains : Hydroxy progesterone caproate-250 mg in oil base
Pulp depot inj.	Morvel	2ml and 3 ml amp	Each ml contains : Hydroxy progesterone caproate-250 mg in oil base
P-Depot inj	Vetcare	2ml amp	Each ml contains : Hydroxy progesterone caproate-250 mg in oil base
Uniprogestin inj	Neu foreva	1 ml amp	Each ml contains : Hydroxy progesterone caproate-50 mg in oil base
Uniprogestin Depot inj	Neu foreva	1 ml, 2 ml amp	Each ml contains : Hydroxy progesterone caproate-250 mg in oil base, 500 mg in oil base.
Vetaprogen inj	Prima Vetcare	2 ml amp	Each ml contains : Hydroxy progesterone caproate-250 mg in oil base

MEDROXYPROGESTERONE ACETATE (MPA): Synthetic Progestagen. Stimulates luteal action, suppresses uterine motility and enhances glandular secretion. They also control ovulation and suppress estrus. Indicated in Postponement/ suppression of estrus, pseudo- pregnancy, mammary tumors,

<table>
<tr><td colspan="4">Habitual abortions. (Cystic endometrial hypoplasia may occur by use of this group of hormone)
DOSE RATE:
➢ Prevent abortion: Cat : 1-2 mg sub cut once weekly (Stop 7-10 days before parturition)
➢ Postpone/ suppress Estrus:
Dog (>25 Kg BW) : 5 mg daily PO
(<25 Kg BW) : 10 mg daily PO
50 mg sub cut at anestrus stage, repeat every 6 months
Cat : 2.5 mg daily PO</td></tr>
<tr><td>Depo-Provera inj</td><td>Max</td><td>1 ml vial</td><td>Each ml contains 150 mg MPA</td></tr>
<tr><td>Prestine inj</td><td>Novitech</td><td>2 ml and 3 ml vials</td><td>Each 2 ml vial contains 500 mg MPA and Each 2 ml vial contains 750 mg MPA.</td></tr>
<tr><td>Promone-E</td><td>BCAHP</td><td>5 ml vial</td><td>Each ml contains 50 mg MPA</td></tr>
<tr><td>Provera</td><td>Max</td><td>Tabs</td><td>Each tablet contains 10 mg MPA</td></tr>
<tr><td colspan="4">NORGESTOMET: Used for estrus synchronization. Progestagen in conjunction with Oestradiol exert a negative feedback on hypothalamic hypophysial system preventing final growth and maturation of follicles. Sudden withdrawl of Progerstagen-releasing implant lead to an increase of LH pulse frequency resulting in Oestrum and ovulation within 2-3 days. Indicated in Oestrus/ Ovulation synchronization.
Cattle and Buffaloes: Norgestomet 3 mg sub cut ear implant to be kept for 9 days 2 ml injection of Oestradiol valerate 5 mg and Norgestomet 3 mg/ ml to be injected at the time of implant application. (to be used in healthy animals only)</td></tr>
<tr><td>Crestar</td><td>Intervet</td><td>One implant + 2 ml injection</td><td>Implant contains Norgestomet 3 mg along with injection containing Oestradiol valerate 5 mg and Norgestomet 3 mg/ ml</td></tr>
<tr><td>Syncromate-B</td><td>BCAHP</td><td>One implant + 2 ml injection (Cattle and Buffaloes: Norgestomet 6 mg sub cut ear implant to be kept for 9 days 2 ml injection of Oestradiol valerate 5 mg and Norgestomet 3 mg/ ml to be injected at the</td><td>Implant contains Norgestomet 6 mg along with injection containing Oestradiol valerate 5 mg and Norgestomet 3 mg/ ml</td></tr>
</table>

		time of implant application.)	
OESTROGENS			
OESTRADIOL VALERATE: Natural steroidal estrogens are Oestradiol, Oestrone & Oestriols. They have low oral activity and so simple esters of Oestrogens such as benzoates or valerates are used in therapeutics which release the parent molecule on hydrolysis. Potency of estrogens is enhanced by adding ethinyl group to the molecule. **Indicated** in Misalliance, Urinary incontinence in old spayed bitches, Uterine infections, anal adenoma. **Dose rate**: Dogs : 1-3 mg daily, orally, 0.5-1.0 mg I/M (For Estrus induction in bitches)			
Progynon Depot	German Remedies	1 ml amp	Oestradiol Valerate 10 mg/ml
Progynon-C	German Remedies	tabs	Ethynyl estradiol 0.02 mg/ tablet
Evalon	Organon	tabs	Oestriol 1 mg/ tablet Oestriol 2 mg/ tablet
Premarin tablet	Wyeth lederle	20'S	Conjugated Oestrogen 0.625 mg
Premarin injection	Wyeth lederle	1 ml vial	Conjugated Oestrogen 25 mg/ml
PROSTAGLANDINS			
CLOPROSTENOL: Prostaglandin F 2 α analogue. Potent luteolytic action which brings about regression of CL and induces fertile heat. **Indicated** in Sub oestrum Luteal cyst, Estrus synchronization, Mummified fetus, Chronic endometritis & Pyometra, Induction of parturition. **Dose**: Cattle and Buffalo: 2 ml I/M. C/I in pregnancy; except if interested to terminate pregnancy.			
Synchromate	Prima Vetcare	4 ml vial	Cloprostenol sodium 263 μg/ ml
Vetmate	Vetcare	20 ml vial	Cloprostenol sodium 263 μg/ ml
DINOPROST: Prostaglandin F 2 α analogue. Potent luteolytic action, by constriction of Utero-ovarian vessels. Enhances cervical dilatation enhances cervical dilatation and also has selective spasmogenic action. **Indicated** in Sub oestrum Luteal cyst, Estrus synchronization. **Dose rate**: Bovine : 25 mg I/M, Equine : 5 mg I/M. C/I in pregnancy; except if interested to terminate pregnancy.			
Lutalyse inj	Novartis	10 ml Vial	Dinoprost : 5 mg/ ml
Hormo P_2 Alpha	BCAHP	5 ml Vial	Dinoprost : 5 mg/ ml

<table>
<tr><td colspan="4">LUPRASTIOL:
Causes regression of CL followed by follicular growth, estrus and ovulation in suboestrus, Pseudoestrus & anestrus.
Indicated in Sub-estrus, Pseudoestrus, Anestrus, Luteal Cyst, Persistent CL, Estrus synchronization.
Dose(I/M): Cow : 15 mg; Heifer, Horse : 7.5 mg. C/I in pregnancy; except if interested to terminate pregnancy.</td></tr>
<tr><td>Prosolvin</td><td>Intervet</td><td>2 ml, 10 ml, 20 ml Vial</td><td>Luprastiol 7.5 mg/ ml</td></tr>
<tr><td colspan="4">TIAPROST: Potent luteolytic activity by constriction of Utero-ovarian vessels. Enhances cervical dilatation and also has selective spasmogenic action. Indicated in Sub-estrus, Pseudoestrus, Anestrus, Luteal Cyst, Persistent CL, Estrus synchronization.</td></tr>
<tr><td>Iliren</td><td>Intervet</td><td>10 ml Vial (Cattle & Buffalo : 3.5 ml I/V; 5 ml I/M or subcut; Equine : 3 ml I/V; Caprine: 1-1.5 ml subcut)</td><td>Tiaprost : 0.196 mg/ ml</td></tr>
<tr><td colspan="4">OXYTOCIN: Nano peptide hormone. Acts on uterine smooth muscles and myoepithelial cells of mammary glands. Oxytocin binds to specific receptors present in the mammary gland and myometrium. This binding stimulates smooth muscle contractions promoting uterine motility and milk let down. Indicated in Induction of parturition (only when the cervix is completely dilated), Caesarian section as local infiltration to speed up involution and control bleeding after removal of fetus. For expulsion of placenta, placental debris. Uterine inertia/ Uterine prolapse.
DOSE
Cow & Buffaloes: 75-100 IU I/M, I/V
Mare : 75-100 IU I/M, I/V
Sow : 30-50 IU I/M, I/V
Ewe & Doe : 30-50 IU I/M, I/V
Bitch : 5-25 IU I/M, I/V
Queen : 5-10 IU I/M, I/V</td></tr>
<tr><td>Pitocin</td><td>Parke-Davis</td><td>0.5 ml amp</td><td>Oxytocin 5 IU / 0.5 ml</td></tr>
<tr><td>Syntocinon</td><td>Novartis</td><td>1 ml amp</td><td>Oxytocin 5 IU / ml</td></tr>
<tr><td colspan="4">VALETHAMATE: Anticholinergic. It ia quartenary ammonium compound, with peripheral actions similar to those of Atropin enabling cervical dilatation. Indicated for cervical dilatation. Dose: Cattle, Buffalo, Mare: 40-50 mg I/M; Sheep, Goat, Pig : 10-20 mg I/M; Dog, Cat : 5-10 mg I/M. Precaution should be taken while administering during gestation period.</td></tr>
<tr><td>Epidosin inj</td><td>TTK</td><td>1 ml vial</td><td>Valethamate 8 mg/ ml</td></tr>
<tr><td>Epidosin Vet inj</td><td>TTK</td><td>5 ml vial</td><td>Valethamate 10 mg/ ml</td></tr>
</table>

DRUGS FOR MALE GENITAL SYSTEM PROBLEMS

HUMAN CHORIONIC GONADOTROPIN: Mimics effect of pituitary Luteinizing hormone causing leydig cell stimulation and enhances androgen production.

Indicated in cryptorchidism, lack of sex drive, genital hypoplasia.

Dose: Bull/stallion: 1500-5000 IU twice weekly for 6 weeks. Dogs: 100-500 IU twice weekly for 6 weeks.

PREGNANT MARES SERUM GONADOTROPHIN:

PMSG affects FSH like action inducing follicular growth in inactive ovaries of mature animals.

Indicated in Superovulation in embryo donors, True Anestrus with inactive ovaries, Bitch: Anoestrus –True subnormal oestrus with non acceptance, Bull &Stallion: Impaired spermatogenesis, Dog : Impaired spermatogenesis. *(In cows mating at first estrus may cause superfetation. Repeated administration may cause anaphylactic shock)*

DOSE RATE: (repeat twice weekly for 6 weeks)

BULL: 1500-3000 IU I/M, I/V.

STALLION: 3000-6000 IU, I/M.

RAM/BUCK/BOAR: 1000 IU I/M.

DOG: 50-200 IU, I/M

Chorulon	Intervet	1500 IU Vial	Human Chorionic Gonadotropin 1500 IU
Folligon	Intervet	1000 IU Vial & solvent	Pregnant mare serum Gonadotropin -1000 I.U/ vial
Syncro-Part PMSG 400	BCAHP	400 IU Vial and solvent	Pregnant mare serum Gonadotropin - 400 I.U/ vial
Syncro-Part PMSG 500	BCAHP	500 IU Vial and solvent	Pregnant mare serum Gonadotropin - 500 I.U/ vial

OESTROGENS

Natural steroidal estrogens are Oestradiol, Oestrone & Oestriols. They have low oral activity and so simple esters of Oestrogens such as benzoates or valerates are used in therapeutics which release the parent molecule on hydrolysis. Potency of estrogens is enhanced by adding ethinyl group to the molecule.

Indicated in prostatic hypertrophy, excessive libido, anal adenoma.

Dose rate: Dogs : 1-3 mg daily, orally, 0.5-1.0 mg I/M. Chronic use may lead to feminization of male.

Progynon Depot	German Remedies	1 ml amp	Oestradiol Valerate 10 mg/ml
Progynon-C	German Remedies	Tabs	Ethynyl estradiol 0.02 mg/ tablet
Evalon	Organon	Tabs	Oestriol 1 mg/tablet

			Oestriol 2 mg/ tablet
TESTOSTERONE PREPARATIONS: **Indicated** in hypogonadism, oligospermia, cryptorchidism, premature senility, androgen deficiency. C/I in prostatic hyperplasia. **Dose Rate:** Bull/stallion: 100-300 mg I/M, S/C; Dog: 5-20 mg I/M, S/C.			
AQUAVIRON	Nicholas piramal	1 ml ampoule	each ml contains Testosterone 25 mg + Thiomersal 0.01 % w/v)
TESTOVIRON DEPOT	German Remedies	1 ml ampoule (100 mg; 250 mg)	Total Testosterone 100 mg/ml Total Testosterone 180 mg/ml
INDIGENOUS PREPARATIONS indicated in oligozoospermia, suboptimal sperm motility, low semen viscosity/sperm count, prostatic enlargement.			
Fortege Vet	Alarsin	pack of 100 tabs @ 10 tabs BID/Bull	Herbal
RATRAJ	BBB	10 gm, 1 kg pack Bull: 25-45 gm daily	Herbal
SEXONA	Universal Remedies	125 gm, 250 gm, 1 kg. 5 gm/cock/day oral	Herbal
SPEMAN VET powder	Himalaya	50 gm sachet Bull: 10 gm BID orally x 10 days	Herbal
TENTEX FORTE VET	Himalaya	10 gm sachet Bull: 5 gm BID orally x 10 days	Herbal

INTRAUTERINE PREPARATIONS					
Brand name	**Composition**	**Indications**	**Dosage**	**Presentation**	**Manufacturer**
Alincomycin Vet	Lincomycin 300 mg/ml	Metritis, Pyometra, Cervicitis, vaginitis, Retention of Placenta	1-2 ml diluted with water for injection i/Ut	5 ml vial	Vetnex
Anarobin	Each ml contains: Metronidazo	Pyometra,Metritis	4-15 ml/kg at 12 hr interval intravenously; 20-50	50 ml vial.	Unichem

	le 5 mg		ml I.U. on alternate days.		Laboratories
Ceflax Powder	Cephalexin 7.5 % w/w	Metritis, Pyometra, Vaginitis, retention of placenta	20 g/ 50 ml Distilled water	20 g sachet	Neospark
C-Flox I.U.	Ciprofloxacin Hydrochloride: 125 mg/ 5 ml Tinidazole : 150 mg/ 5 ml	Endometritis, Metritis, repeat Breeder	60 ml as intrauterine for 3-5 days for Endometritis & metritis Repeat breeders: 60 ml intrauterine 1 hr Post AI	60 ml	Intas
Chortetracycline bolus	Chortetracycline 500 mg/ bolus	As above	Large animals: 2-4 boli I/U Small animals: 1-2 boli I/U	12'S	AHP
Enuria bolus	Nitrofurazone 60 mg Urea 6 g	As above	Large animals: 2-4 boli I/U	4'S	Theodor
Furea bolus	As above	As above	2-4 boli/ infected horn	6'S	Pfizer
Gentamor –Vet	Inj. of gentamicine 40 mg/ml	Gram negative and Gram positive organism, repeat breeders.	Intrauterine: 2 ml diluted with 20-30 ml of distilled water in repeat breeders.	2 ml vial. 6 ml vial. 30 ml vial.	Morvel laboratories (p) ltd.
Intrim Forte bolus	Sulfa Methoxazole 2 g Timethoprim 0.4 g	As above	2-4 boli/ infected horn	5 X4'S	Intas
Lixen Dry Susp	Cephalexin 1.5 g & 4.5 g	As above	Reconstitute in 60 ml sterile water and infuse in uterus	1.5 g and 4.5 g pkt	Virbac
Lenovo I.U.	Each ml contains Levofloxacin 20mg +	Retention of placenta, metritis	30 ml Intrauterine infusion once	30ml, 60 ml pack I.U.	Intas

	alpha tocopherol 5 mg				
Lixen IU	Cephalexin 750 mg Urea 2.5 g	As above	2 boli / infected horn	2'S	Virbac
Marcogenta	Each ml contains : Gentamicin sulphate 40 mg	Metritis ,repeat breeders ,	5-10 ml in 20-40 ml of DW for intrauterine .	Vials of 2 ml ,5 ml ,10 ml, 30 ml.	Marc Laboratories Pvt Ltd
Metrijet solution	Oxytetracycline hydrochloride 500 mg, Furazolidone 500 mg, Cliquinol 500 mg, Ethinylestradiol 0.5 mg)/ 19 g	As above	Mild endometritis Cows & Buffaloes: 1 syringe during oestrus Severe endometritis Cows & Buffaloes: 1 syringe daily for 3- 5 days, Repeat if neccessary	19 g syringe	Intervet
Metron bolus	As above	As above	As above	4"S	Vetindia
Nefrea bolus	As above	As above	As above	5X4'S	Jeps
Pesuria Pessary	Nitrofurazone 60 mg, Urea 5 g & Metronidazole 1 g	As above	As above	10X4'S	Indian Immunologicals
Povidone Iodine Solution	Povidone iodine 10% equal to 1% w/v of available iodine	Post partum endometritis and infertility associated with mild endometritis.	Post partum endometritis Cattle, Buffalo: Dilute 1:5 in water and infuse 100 ml I.U. at 1-3 weeks of calving and 50 ml 3 weeks onward.	100 ml and 500 ml bottle	Ethicare ltd.
Steclin bolus	Tetracycline Hydrochloride 500 mg	Metritis, ROP, pyometra, repeat	Large animals: 1-2 bolus I/U Small animals: 0.5-1	500 mg and 1g bolus	Sarbhai Zydus

	and 1 g bolus	breeding	bolus per infected horn I/U	4'S	
Terramycin animal formula Tablets	Each tab contains oxytetracycline 500 mg	Pyometra, retention of placenta	Cows & mares 2-4 tab in uterus. Ewe,Sow bitch ½ -1 tab. In uterus.	In strips of 4	Pfizer Limited
Terramycin liquid	Each ml contains :Oxytetracyline HCL 50 mg	Mixed infection	10 -20 ml diluted with equal quantity of sterile water I/U.	Bottles of 30 ml & 100 ml.	Pfizer Limited
Uromet bolus	Nitrofurazone 50 mg Urea 6 g	ROP, pyometra	As above	6X4'S	Neospark
Uterofit bolus	Nitrofurazone 60 mg, Urea 5 g & Metronidazole 1 g	ROP, pyometra	2 boli/ infected horn	4'S	Alembic
Wokadine	Povidone-iodine 5% w/v with 0.5% w/v available active ingredient.	Metritis, ROP, pyometra	10-40 ml. intrauterine	100 ml in glassbottle & 500 ml in polyethylene container	Wockhardt

MISCELLANEOUS PRO-UROGENITAL PREPARATIONS			
UNISPAS	Walter Bushnell	Hyperspasticity, urinary incontinence	strip of 8 tabs Flavoxate 200 mg/tab
UROTONE	VHB	Neurogenic bladder atony, non-obstructive urinary retention (post operative, post partum)	100 tabs pack Bethanocol 25 mg/tab

URO-GENITAL ANTISPASMODIC PREPARATIONS:

- DICYCLOMINE
- DICYCLOMINE combination

URO-GENITAL ANTISPASMODIC PREPARATIONS			
DICYCLOMINE antispasmodic. Produces nonspcific direct relaxant action on smooth muscles. Indicated in renal, ureteric colic, spasmodic pain. **Dose** rate is 0.5 mg/KgBW IM in ruminants, horses; 0.1 mg/kg BW TID IM in dogs. • Avoid use in neonates, old age animals, frank urinary retention and GIT obstruction cases.			
Spasmo-Proxyvon	Wockhardt	injection 2ml, 30 ml	each ml contains 10 mg/ml
Spasmovet	Wockhardt	injection 30 ml	each ml contains 10 mg/ml
DICYCLOMINE combination:			
PECOREX	Pranav	strip of 4 boli	Each bolus contains Dicyclomine HCl 100 mg+Diclofenac Na + Paracetamol 1500 mg

ANTI-UROLITHIASIS PRODUCTS:

- ALLOPURINOL
- INDIGENOUS HERBAL PRODUCTS

ANTI-UROLITHIASIS PRODUCTS			
ALLOPURINOL: Xanthine Oxidase inhibitor. This enzyme converts hypoxanthine to xanthine and uric acid. **Dogs/cat**: 10 mg/kg BW TID x 3 days orally. Doses should be tapered gradually before withdrawl of drug.			
ALLGORIC	Kameron	strip of 10 tabs	100 mg/tab
ZYLORIC	Burroghs-Wellcome	strip of 100 mg tabs	100 mg/tab
INDIGENOUS HERBAL PRODUCTS			
CYSTONE	Himalaya	pack of 100 tabs @1-3 tabs TID oral	Herbal
CYSTONE powder	Himalaya	50 gm pack 2-4 gm TID oral	Herbal
Nefrotec	Himalaya	pack of 60 tabs Dog: 1-3 tabs BID	Herbal

Chapter 21

Veterinary Homeopathic Drugs

REPUTED VETERINARY HOMEO PRODUCTS OF INDIA

Product	Company	Presentation	Indication
ACTIVIT	Kathya Homeo Labs	5 ltr,1 ltr, 500 ml	General Break down of overall health, diminished appetite, milk reduction, slow growth rate with disturbance in reproductive process.
ANOSIS	Kathya Homeo Labs	225 ml , 450 ml	IBD / Gumboro
BITARIN	Kathya Homeo Labs	225 ml , 450 ml	Blue tongue
CANASULE G	Goel Vet Pharma	tablets in blister form / powder in dibby	For growth in pups & dog
CANASULE T	Goel Vet Pharma	Tabs Blister Form	A first aid for dogs
Canasule T	Goel vet Pharma	Presentation: Tablets in Blister Packing	Indication: A 24-hour first aid, A supplementary treatment of all ailments, Saves liver& enhance body metabolism, A digestive stimulant, tonic& disease resistant factor. Category: Canine(Pups& Dogs)
CIDONIL	Kathya Homeo Labs	225 ml , 450 ml	Caecal and intestinal Coccidiosis.

CONCEPTAL	Kathya Homeo Labs	10 ml	Late Heat, Irregular Oestrous of any form, Repeat Breeders, Early Abortion, Metritis in any form, Post Partum Prolapse etc.
CRYZA	Kathya Homeo Labs	225 ml , 450 ml	Infectious Coryza in fowls
DERONIL	Kathya Homeo Labs	30 ml 5 ml	Rinderpest / PPR / Parvovirus/ Specific or Non-specific Diarrhoea.
DIASULE	Goel Vet Pharma	BOLUS Blister Form	A treatment for diahrroea due to variety
EQUASULE	Goel Vet Pharma	BOLUS Blister Form	For indigestion and liver disorders in donkey & horses
FERTISULE	Goel Vet Pharma	5gm +100Tab	For treatment of repeat breeders & infertility
FOMOCIDE	Kathya Homeo Labs	30 ml	FMD
FOOMASULE	Goel Vet Pharma	BOLUS Blister Form	For foot & mouth disease -
HEMISEPT	Goel Vet Pharma	Liquid 105 ML in Bottle	For treatment of H.S. & bronchitis
HENJAI	Goel Vet Pharma	Liquid 450 ML in Bottle	A one for all formula for chicks & birds -
HIT-O-GEN	Goel Vet Pharma	Two Bolus in one Blister Form Packing	To induce heat in physiological anoestrus
MANDGOLE	Goel Vet Pharma	Liquid 105 ML in Bottle	For treatment of meningitis & brain fever
MILKFLO	Kathya Homeo Labs	100 ml	Agalactia / diminished milk.
MILKOGEN	Goel Vet Pharma	100 Tablets form in Dibby / 450 gm. granules in Pouch Packing	An excellent milk increaser in natural way

NECADE	Kathya Homeo Labs	225 ml , 450 ml	New castle disease / R.D.
Pet Safe (Pet Shampoo)	Goel vet Pharma	Bottle: 135 ml Sachet: 15 ml	Pet shampoo with arnica calendula & aloe vera-a special blend of nutritive herbal ingredients, keeps hair clean, soft, manageable and healthy Key ingredients: Arnica, calendula, and aloe vera etc.
PLOX	Kathya Homeo Labs	225 ml , 450 ml	Fowl pox - cutaneous / diphtheritic (wet)
POXONIL	Kathya Homeo Labs	30 ml	Pox in Sheep / Goats & Large animals.
PYROSULE	Goel Vet Pharma	BOLUS Blister Form	For all types of pyrexia
R.BLOATASULE	Goel Vet Pharma	BOLUS Blister Form	For treatment of indigestion anorexia & liver disorders
REFROMATE	Kathya Homeo Labs	50 tabs	Acute and sub acute mastitis
REFROMATE PLUS	Kathya Homeo Labs	50 tabs	Chronic mastitis.
RESPINORM	Kathya Homeo Labs	225 ml , 450 ml	Chronic Respiratory Disease (C. R. D.) with E. coli.
RHEUMASULE	Goel Vet Pharma	BOLUS Blister Form	For treatment of rheumatism & arthritis
TEATASULE	Goel Vet Pharma	BOLUS Blister Form	For treatment of acute, sub acute & chronic mastitis
UTEROGEN	Goel Vet Pharma	Liquid 105 ML in Bottle	A multipurpose uterine remedy

Vet Safe (Antiseptic Soap)	Goel vet Pharma	Sachet 15 ml	Antiseptic liquid soap with anti bacterial and antifungal action moisturizes your skin without drying.

Apppendix

LIST OF VETERINARY COMPANIES OF INDIA

- Dosch Pharmaceuticals Pvt Ltd
  15-C, LAXMI IND ESTATE, NEW LINK ROAD, ANDHERI (WEST)
  MUMBAI- 400 053, Phone number : +022 26321315
- Alved Pharma & Foods Pvt Ltd, 549, 14TH STREET, IV SECTOR, K K NAGAR, 600078,CHENNAI, India +91-44-24834885
- Vetindia Pharmaceuticals Limited, A-6/1, Electronic Complex, Kushaiguda- 500062, Hyderabad, Andhra Pradesh. India. +91-40-27127184
- Alembic Limited
  Address: Veterinary Division : Alembic Road,, Vadodara, Gujarat, India - 390 003
  Phone: +91 - 265 - 228 0550 (3 Lines) Fax: +91 - 265 - 228 1508 / 228 2934
- Alved Pharma & Foods
  Address: Plot No549, 14 th Street, IV Sector, KKNagar, Chennai, Tamil Nadu, India - 600078
  Phone: +91- 44-24836279 / 24834885 / 24723542 / 24816874 Fax: +91- 44-24838344
- Amak Homoeo Pharmaceuticals
  Address: DNo: 9-4-77/A/4, Nizam Colony, Toli Chowki,, Hyderabad, Andhra Pradesh, India - 500008
  Phone: +91 - 40 - 23561626 Fax: +91 - 40 - 23560186
- Ayurvet Limited
  Address: 6 th Floor, Sagar Plaza, Disttt Centre, Laxmi Nagar, Delhi, Delhi, India - 110092
  Phone: +91-11- 22455992-94 Fax: +91-11-22455991
- B & T Pharmaceuticals
  Address: Animal Healthcare Phase - 1, Shed# 33, I DA, Cherlapally, Ranga Reddy, Andhra Pradesh, India - 500762
  Phone: +91-40-55766647
- Bio-Med Private Limited
  Address: C-96, Site No:1, Bulandshahr Road Industrial Area, Ghaziabad, Uttar Pradesh, India - 201001

Phone: 0091-120-2700881,2753255, 2702333, 2701765, 3948358 Fax: 0091-120-2700825

- Brilliant Industries Limited
  Address: TGV Mansion, 6-2-1012, 3rd Floor, Khairatabad , Hyderabad, Andhra Pradesh, India - 500004
  Phone: +91-40-55667464 Fax: +91-40-55104915
- Cadila Pharmaceuticals Limited
  Address: Veterinary Division: Sarkhej - Dholka Road, Bhat, Ahmedabad, Gujarat, India - 382210
  Phone: 91-2718-225001 (15 Lines) Fax: 91-2718-225039
- Concept Group of Companies
  Address: Animal Health Division, 167,CST Road, Kalinga Santacruz(E), Mumbai, Maharashtra, India - 400098
  Phone: +91-22-26528888 Fax: +91-22-26525800
- Deccan Homoeo Pharmacy
  Address: Opp: Sagar Talkies, Abid Road,, Hyderabad, Andhra Pradesh, India - 500001
  Phone: +91 - 40 - 24603911
- Daffodills Pharmaceuticals Ltd., Meerut.U.P.
- GLAXO SMITH KLINE PHARMACEUTICALS LIMITED
  Address: Agrivet Farm Care,252, Dr Annie Besant Road, Worli,, Mumbai, Maharashtra, India - 400025
  Phone: +91 22 2495 9595 Fax: +91 22 2495 9494
- Goel Vet Pharma
  102 Agarwal Complex Sharda road, meerut, Uttar Pradesh, India
- GROTEK PHARMA LTD
  Address: 20, Ganesh Park, Dhabasa,,, Vadodara, Gujarat, India - 391440
- Hindustan Therapeutics (P) Ltd
  Address: 5-5-35/40, Prashanthi Nagar, IE, Kukatpally, Ranga Reddy, Andhra Pradesh, India - 500072
  Phone: +91 - 40 - 23076823
- ICON BIOLOGICAL PVT LTD
  Address: #23-8-1/A, SESHADRI STREET, SATYANARAYANA PURAM, Vijayawada, Andhra Pradesh, India - 520 011
  Phone: +91-866-2539657 Fax: +91- 866 - 2442157
- Indian Pet Products
  Address: 2069, East End "B" Main Road, 9th Block Jayanagar, Bangalore,

Karnataka, India - 560069
Phone: +91 - 80 - 6657841 / 6580394 Fax: +91 - 80 - 6911254

- Indian Herbs Research & Supply Co Ltd
  Address: Post Box No 5, Sharda Nagar , Saharanpur, Uttar Pradesh, India - 247 001
  Phone: +91-132-725 044, 725 045, 725 046, 725 459 Fax: +91 (132) 726288

- Indian Immunologicals
  Address: A Wholly Owned Subsidary of the National Dairy Development Board Road No: 44, Jubilee Hills, Hyderabad, Andhra Pradesh, India - 500033
  Phone: +91 - 40 - 23544585 / 23544593 Fax: +91 - 40 - 23544007

- Indus Healthcare
  Address: 219, Heena Arcade , S V Road, Jogeshwari(W), Mumbai, Maharashtra, India - 400102
  Phone: +91-22-56960903 Fax: +91-22-56960903

- Intas Pharmaceuticals Ltd
  Address: Neovet Division Chinubhai Centre, Ashram Road,, Ahmedabad, Gujarat, India - 380009
  Phone: +91 79 26576655 Fax: +91 79 26576616

- Intervet India Pvt Ltd
  Address: 'Intervet House' 33, Pune-Nagar Road, (Behind Eden Gardens), , Pune, Maharashtra, India - 411 014
  Phone: +91-20-4050400 / 4050401 Fax: +91-20-4050410

- Karnataka Antibiotics
  Address: Animal Health Division KARNATAKA ANTIBIOTICS & PHARMACEUTICALS LIMITED -A Govt of India Enterprise Nirman Bhavan, Dr Rajkumar Road, 1st Block, Rajajinagar, Bangalore, Karnataka, India - 560010
  Phone: +91 - 80 - 3323301 - 4, 3322123 , 3322555 Fax: +91 - 80 - 3321350

- Lyka Exports Limited
  Address: Lyka Animal Healthcare Division, 77, Nehru road, Vile Parle (E),, Mumbai, Maharashtra, India - 400099
  Phone: +91 - 22 - 2610 5900/ 5030/ 6754/ 26183033 Fax: +91 - 22 - 2611 1024

- Natural Remedies Pvt Ltd
  Address: "Ashwathalakshmi Mansion" # 364, 16th Main, 4th 'T' Block Jayanagar, Bangalore, Karnataka, India - 560082
  Phone: + 91-80-26535891(5 lines) Fax: + 91-80-26656652, 26535889

- Neospark Drugs and Chemicals Private Limited
  Address: Corporate Center, 241, BL Bagh, Panjagutta,, Hyderabad, Andhra Pradesh, India - 500082
  Phone: +91 - 40 - 23416725 / 23408234 Fax: + 91 - 40 - 234118706
- Novartis India Limited
  Address: Animal Health Sector 14, J Tata Road, Churchgate, Mumbai, Maharashtra, India - 400020
  Phone: +91 - 22 - 22823434 Fax: +91 - 22 - 22822246
- Parvy Pharma Pvt Limited
  Address: Plot no: 117, Samathapuri, New Nagole, Hyderabad, Andhra Pradesh, India - 500035
  Phone: +91 - 40 - 24042068 Fax: +91 - 40 - 24040224
- Pedigree
  Address: Effem India Private Limited 1st Floor, Ashoka Hitech Chambers, Banjara Hills, Road No3, Hyderabad, Andhra Pradesh, India - 500034
  Phone: +91- 040 - 23555900 Toll Free No: 1600-112121 Fax: +91 - 040 - 23551528
- Pet Care
  Address: Divn of TETRAGON CHEMIE PVT LTD IS-40, KHB Ind Area, Yelahanka New Town,, Bangalore, Karnataka, India - 560064
  Phone: +91 - 80 - 28461241 / 28462055 / 56 Fax: +91 - 80 - 28461240
- Pfizer Limited
  Address: Pfizer Centre, Patel Estate, SV Raod, Jogeshwari(w),, Mumbai, Maharashtra, India - 400102
  Phone: +91 - 22 - 5693 2000 Fax: +91- 22 - 5693 2444
- Pranav Agrl Industries Ltd
  Address: Nav Maharashtra House, 43, Shaniwar Peth,, Pune, Maharashtra, India - 411030
  Phone: +91 - 20 - 4461021 / 22 / 23 Fax: +91 - 20 - 4493578
- Sarabhai Zydus Animal Health Limited
  Address: Administration Building Gorwa Road,, Vadodara, Gujarat, India - 390023
  Phone: +91 - 265 - 2282110 Fax: +91 - 265 - 228479
- Stallen
  Address: STALLEN South Asia Pvt Ltd 101, Shyam Kamal "D" Bldg Vile Parle (East),, Mumbai, Maharashtra, India - 400057
  Phone: +91 - 22 - 26105147 / 26111577 Fax: +91 - 22 - 26161590

- Stanmax Pharma Pvt Ltd
Address: 2-16-115/A, Street No3, Prashanthnagar, Uppal, Hyderabad, Andhra Pradesh, India - 500039
Phone: +91 - 40 - 27201376 Fax: +91 - 40 - 27203014
- The Himalaya Drug Company
Address: Animal Health Division, Makali, Bangalore, Karnataka, India - 562 123
Phone: +91 - 80 - 23714444 Fax: +91 - 80 - 23714484
- TTK Pharma
Address: Animal Welfare Division, 8, Old Trunk Road,, Chennai, Tamil Nadu, India - 600043
- Unichem Laboratories Limited
Address: Unichem Bhavan, Off S V Road, Jogeshwari (West),, Mumbai, Maharashtra, India - 400 102
Phone: +91 - 22 - 2678 0643 / 2678 2644 Fax: +91 - 22 - 26576616
- Venky's (India) Limited
Address: Animal Health Products Division Venkateshwara House, SNo 114/A/2,Sinhagad Road, , Pune, Maharashtra, India - 411030
Phone: +91 - 20 - 24251530 to 41 Fax: +91 - 20 - 24251077 / 24251060
- Venky's Pet
Address: Venky's (India) Limited Venkateshwara House, S No 114/A/2, Pune - Sinhagad Road, , Pune, Maharashtra, India - 411030
Phone: +91 - 20 - 24251530 to 41 Fax: +91 - 20 - 24251077 / 24251060
- Ventri Biologicals
Address: VENKATESHWARA HATCHERIES LTD (VENTRI BIOLOGICALS, VACCINE DIVISION) 17/6, Milestone, Girinagar, Pune Panshet Road,, Pune, Maharashtra, India - 411025
Phone: +91 - 20 - 4389471 / 4389474 Fax: +91 - 20 - 4389471
- Vesper Pharmaceuticals
Address: Village Singapura, Vidyaranyapura post, Bangalore, Karnataka, India - 560097
Phone: +91 -80 - 28388942 / 23453192 Fax: +91 - 80 - 28388571
- Vetcare
Address: Vet Care, Divn of TETRAGON CHEMIE LTD IS-40, KHB Ind Area, Yelahanka New Town,, Bangalore, Karnataka, India - 560064
Phone: +91 - 80 - 8460060 / 8461241 / 42 / 8462055 / 56 Fax: +91 - 80 - 8461240

- Vetindia Pharmaceuticals Limited
  Address: 1-7-187/D-16, Kamalanagar, ECIL "X" Road, Hyderabad, Andhra Pradesh, India - 500 062
  Phone: +91 - 40 - 27127184 / 27143103 / 27137716 Fax: +91 - 40 - 27123563
- Wockhardt Limited
  Address: Wockhardt Towers, Bandra Kurla Complex, Bandra (East), Mumbai, Maharashtra, India - 400 051
  Phone: +91 - 22 - 26534444 Fax: +91 - 22 - 2653 424

LIST OF IMPORTANT HOMEOCOMPANIES OF INDIA

1. Hahnemann Publishing Co., 165, Bipin Bihari, Ganguly Street, Calcutta.
2. M/s. SBL Ltd., A-3, Site IV, Sahibabad, Ghaziabad-201010.
3. Bhandari Homoeopathic Laboratories, 14th Mile Stone, DLF Indl.Estate No.1, Delhi- Mathura Road, Faridabad-121003.
4. Dr. Willmar Schwabe India Pvt. Ltd., A-36, Sector-60, Phase – III, NOIDA-201 307(U.P.)
5. M/s. Bakson Drugs & Pharmaceuticals Pvt. Ltd., F-64, Okhla Industrial Area, Phase I, New Delhi-110020
6. Sree Krishna Homoeo Pharmacy, Chinchward Industrial Area, Poona.
7. Sintex International Limited, Near Seven Garnala, Kalol (N. Gujarat), 382721
8. Dr. Prakashan Homoeopathic Pharmacy Pvt. Ltd., 11/640 A, Chelannur, Palusssery Road, Calicut-673616.
9. State Cooperative Homoeopathic Pharmacy, Alapuzha, Kerala.
10 M/S Hahnemann Laboratory, 285, Bipin Behari Ganguly Street, Calcutta, 700012.
11. M.Bhattacharya & Co (P) Ltd., 73, Netaji Subhash Road, Calcutta, 700001.
12. National Homoeo Laboratory, 110, Acharya Jagadish Bose Road, Calcutta, 700014.
13. Sunder Homoeo Sadan, 113, Netaji Subash Road, Calcutta, 700001.
14. Hahnemann Laboratory, 13, Majudendra Dutta Road, Calcutta, 700001.
15. Economic Homoeo Pharmacy, 89, Netaji Subash Road, Calcutta, 700001.
16. M/S. S. Chaudhary & Co., 43/1, Stand Road, Calcutta, 700001.
17. M/S Everest Homoeo Laboratory, Bagha Jatin Road, Balasore.

18. M/S International; Homoeo Research, 1, Ram Mohan Mullick Garder Lane, Calcutta. 700010.
19. M/S N.P.Dutta & Sons, 26, Stand Road, Calcutta, 700001.
20. M/S Duke Pharmaceuticals, 404, Stand Road, Calcutta, 700001.
21. Boerick Homoeo Pharmacy, 85, Netaji Subash Road, Calcutta, 700001.
22. Powell Homoe Research Laboratory, Sushil Jyoti Avenue, Ravindra Pally, P.O. Profulla Kanan, Calcutta, 700059.
23. Homoeopathic Research Institute, Garden Beach Road, Calcutta., 700023.
24. Lord Hahnemann laboratory, 7, Moor Mohamad lane, Clacutta, 700009.
25. M/S P.Banerjee, Mehijam, Santhal Parganas, Bihar.
26. M/S P.Banerjee, 109, D.Shyama prasad Mukherjee Road, Calcutta,700028.
27. M/S Hahnemann Pharmaceutical laboratory, P-4, Beliaghata Road, Calcutta, 700015.
28. M/S Himani Limited, 13, B.T Road, P.O, Belghoria, Calcutta, 700087.
29. M/S King & Company, 90/6-A, Mahatma Gandhi Road, Calcutta. 700007.
30. M/S Reliable Homoeo Pharmacy, Sabji Bagh, Patna-4.
31. M/S Roy Choudhary & Co., 135, Bipin Behari Ganguly Street, Calcutta 12.
32. M/S Srivastava Homoeo Pharmacy, MIDCD- 2, No. 67-D, Pimpri, Ghonohwad, POONA.
33. M/S Beck & Koll, Plot No 37 A, Government Industrial Estate, Kandivali (West) Mumbai-400067.
34. M/S New Era Homoeopathic Pharmacy (P) Ltd., Noor Building, Opp. Western Railway station, dadar, Mumbai.400028.
35. M/S Champak lal magan Lal Homoeo Pharmacy, 41/43, Vithalvadi Industrial Area, Bhava Nagar. 364001.
36. M/S Holistic Remedies Pvt Ltd., 10, Mohtar House, 36, Pandit Rama Bai Road, Chowpaathy, Mumbai, 400007.
37. M/S Roy & Co., 176, Princes Street, Mumbai. Mumbai-2.
38. M/s Bharat Homoeo Pharmacy Ltd., Post Box 85, 20/60, Ashok Marg, Lucknow-l.
39. M/s R.S. Bhargava Pharmacy, P.O. Bhargava Pharmacy, Anupshahar, Bhulandshahar U.P.
40. M/s Harjeet Enterprises, ` 22 E/A, Industrial Area, Panipat, Haryana.
41. M/s Bhartiya Pharmaceuticals, 8A, Central Market, Lajpat Nagar, New Delhi.

42. M/s Hahnemann Pharmaceuticals, Phase I, Naraina Industrial Area, New Delhi-110028.
43. M/s Wheezal Laboratories, 157, Rajpur Road, Dehradun U.P.
44. M/s Suresh Laboratory (Homoeopaths), Varanasi U.P.
45. M/s Homoeo Research Institute, 138, V.N. Marg, Allahabad U.P.
46. M/s Hahnemann Scientific Laboratory, 2, Subash Marg, Lucknow U.P.
47. M/s Hahnemann Pure Drug Co., Azamgarh U.P.
48. Dr. Wellman's Homoeopathic Laboratory, AM-4, Dilkhush Industrial Estate, G.T. Karnal Road, Delhi-110033.
49. M/s Lord Homoeopathic Pharmacy, B-49, Naraina Industrial Estate, New Delhi-110028.
50. M/s Benzers & Taffels, L/56, Narankaari Colony, Delhi-110009.
51. M/s Meerut Homoeo Pharmacy, 773-D, Sotiganj, Meerut.
52. M/s United Globules, Dujana House, Matia Mahal, Delhi.
53. M/s Ram Krishna Pharmaceuticals, L-231, Katedon Industrial Complex, Hyderabad.
54. M/s Bohala Pharmaceuticals, Homoeopathic Pharmacist, 21, Gandhi Nagar, Kumbakonam Distt. Thanivur, Tamilnadu.
55. M/s St. George Homoeo Clinic Pharmacy, K-6-139, A. Balamatta, Kanakanady, P.O. Box 505, Mangalore-2.
56. M/s Sudha Homoeo Pharmaceuticals, 10-22, Ram Nathpur, Hyderabad.
57. M/s Father Mullori Homoeopathic Poor Dispensary, Post Box 501, Kankandy, Mangalore.
58. Dr. De Chane's Homoeo Division, Hyderabad.
59. M/s K.M.P. Oil Industries Ltd., KMP Nagar, Cochin-682 006.
60. M/s Chemmanur Clinic & Laboratory, Chorghat, Kerala.
61. M/s American Homoeo Pharmacy, Trichur.
62. M/s Trans Pharmaceuticals, A-9, Co-op Industrial Estate P.B. No. 96, Jalgaon 425 003.
63. M/s Allen Pharmaceuticals Pvt. Ltd., 1/5, Sanvid Nagar, Sakat Side Road, Indore-452 001.
64. M/s Anand Homoeopathic Medical College & Research Institute, Anand, Opp. Town Hall, Anand (Gujarat)
65. M/s Sareen Homoeo Laboratories, Court Road, Jagadhari-135 003 (Haryana).

66. Doliosis Homoeo Pharma Pvt.Ltd "Pushkar"
269/1,E-5, Varsha Park,
Near Green Park Hotel, Baner Road,
Baner, Pune,
Maharashtra, India 411045.
Landline +91 020 40788380, 020 40788381 , 020 32949860
Telefax +91 020 27292015 , 020 40788383
Email info@doliosis.com

67. Kathya Homeo Labs
(A unit of Kathya Drugs Private Limited)
Plot No. 398, Hariharapuram,
Vanasthalipuram, HYDERABAD – 500 070
Tele-Fax : +91+40+24241978 ;
Mobile : +91+9440057669

STANDARD VACCINATION SCHEDULE

VACCINATION SCHEDULE FOR PIGS					
Sr. No.	**Name of disease**	**Type of vaccine**	**Time of vaccination**	**Duration of immunity period**	**Remarks**
1	Anthrax	Spore vaccine	Once in a year, premonsoon vaccination	One season	
2	Hog Cholera	Crystal Violet vaccine	After weaning	One year	
3	Foot and mouth disease	Polyvalent tissue culture vaccine	At about six months of age with booster done after 4 months	One season	After vaccine repeat Vaccination every year in October/November
4	Swine Erysipelas	Alum treated vaccine	After weaning with a booster dose after 3-4 weeks	About one year	
5	Tuberculo sis	B.C.G vaccine	At about six months of age	One to two years	To be repeated every 2 or 3 years

DOGS

Diseases	Primary Vaccination	Secondary Vaccination	Re-Vaccination
Canine Distemper Canine Hepatitis (CanineAdenovirus 2) Corona Viral Enteritis Canine Parainfluenza Parvo Virus Infection Leptospirosis (Canicola) (icterohaemorrhagiae)	6 weeks of age	2-3 weeks later upto 16 weeks of age	Annual
Rabies	3 months of age	After 3 months	Annual

VACCINATION OF FARM ANIMALS					
Sr. No.	**Name of disease**	**Type of vaccine**	**Type of vaccination**	**Duration of immunity**	**Remarks**
1	**2**	**3**	**4**	**5**	**6**
1	Anthrax (Gorhi)	Spore vaccine	Once in an year premonsoon vaccination	One season	-
2	Black Quarter (Sujab)	Killed vaccine	- do -	- do -	-
3	Haemorrhagic Septicaemia (Galghotu)	Ocladjuvant vaccine	- do -	- do -	-
4	Brucellosis (Contagious abortion)	Cotton strain 19 (live bacteria)	At about 6 months of age	3 or 4 calvings	To be done only in infected herds
5	Foot and Mouth disease (Muhkhar)	Polyvalent tissue culture vaccine	At about 6 months of age with booster dose 4 months later	One season	After vaccination repeat vaccination every year in Oct./Nov.

6	Rinderpest (Mata)	Lapinised avianised vaccine for exotic and crossbred catte, caprinised vaccine for zebu cattle.	At about 6 months of age	Life long	It is better to repeat after 3 to 4 years

Vaccination Schedule for Broilers				
Name of disease	**Name of Vaccination**	**Days/weeks of vaccination**	**Route of inoculation**	**Remarks**
Marek's disease	Herpes virus turkey vaccination	1 day old	Sub cutaneous	Life long immunity
Ranikhet disease	RD vaccine (Lasota 'F` strain)	4-7 days old	Intra-nasal Intra-ocular	Immunity is up to 10 weeks old
Fowl pox	Chick embryo adopted fowl	6-8 weeks of age	Wing web method	If the disease is prevalent in the area. Once vaccinated gives life long immunity.
During chick rearing the disease most likely to occur is coccidiosis. Its organisms thrive on wet litter and so keep the litter dry. The feed mixed with coccidiosis should be used. In case of an outbreak, the Coccidiocidal drug in drinking water should be used at recommended level.				

VACCINATION CALENDER FOR POULTRY LAYER FARMING The vaccination schedule is a general guide. Each farm and area will require some changes in the schedule. Following table can be used as a geneal guideline.		
Name of Vaccine	**Route**	**Age of birds**
La Sota or F vaccine Ranikhet	Intranasal drop	3 to 7 days
Marek's vaccine (in Hatchery)	Intramuscular	1 day
Infectious Bronchitis (1st dose)	Eye drops	2 - 3 weeks
La Sota Ranikhet	Drinking water	5 - 6 weeks
Fowl Pox (1st dose)	Wing Web	7 - 8 weeks
R2B Ranikhet	Sub cut or Intramuscular	9 - 10 weeks
Infectious Bronchitis	Eye drop or drinking water	16 weeks
Fowl Pox (2nd dose)	Skin Scarification	18 weeks
La Sota (if necessary) Ranikhet	Drinking Water	20 weeks

La Sota (if necessary) Ranikhet	Drinking Water	40 weeks
IBD :		
Mildly invasive vaccine	Drinking Water	0 - 3 day
Intermediately invasive vaccine	Drinking Water	15th day
Intermediately invasive vaccine	Drinking Water	28-30th day

LIST OF ICAR INSTITUTIONS OF INDIA

- Central Agricultural Research Institute, Port Blair
- Central Arid Zone Research Institute, Jodhpur, Rajasthan
- Central Avian Research Institute, Izatnagar, Uttar Pradesh
- Central Inland Fishries Research Institute, Barrackpore, West Bengal
- Central Institute for Cotton Research, Nagpur, Maharashtra
- Central Institute for Research on Goats, Farah, Uttar Pradesh
- Central Institute for Research on Cotton Technology, Mumbai, Maharashtra
- Central Institute of Agricultural Engineering, Bhopal, Madhya Pradesh.
- Central Institute for Arid Horticulture, Bikaner, Rajasthan
- Central Institute for Research on Buffaloes, Hissar, Haryana
- Central Institute of Brakishwater Aquaculture, Chennai, Tamilnadu
- Central Institute of Freshwater Aquaculture, Bhubaneswar, Orissa
- Central Institute of Fisheries Education, Mumbai, Maharashtra
- Central Institute of Post Harvest Engineering & Technology, Ludhiana, Punjab
- Central Marine Fisheries Research Institute, Kochin, Kerala
- Central Plantation Crops Research Institute, Kasaragod, Kerala
- Central Potato Research Institute, Shimla, Himachal Pradesh
- Central Research Institute for Dryland Agriculture, Hyderabad, Andhra Pradesh
- Central Research Institute for Jute and Allied Fiber, Barrackpore, West Bengal
- Central Rice Research Institute, Cuttack, Orissa

- Central Sheep & Wool Research Institute, Avikanagar, Rajasthan
- Central Soil Salinity Research Institute, Karnal, Haryana
- Central Tuber Crops Research Institute, Thiruvananthapuram, Kerala
- Indian Agricultural Research Institute, New Delhi
- Indian Agricultural Statistics Research Institute New Delhi
- ICAR Research Complex For Goa, Ela Old, Goa
- Indian Grassland and Fodder Research Institute, Gwalior, Jhansi
- Indian Institute of Horticultural Research, Bangalore, Karnataka
- Indian Institute of Pulses Research, Kanpur, Uttar Pradesh
- Indian Instritute of Soil Science , Bhopal, Madhya Pradesh
- Indian Institute of Spices Research, Calicut, Kerala
- Indian Institute of Sugarcane Research, Lucknow, Uttar Pradesh
- Indian Institute of Vegetable Research, Varanasi, Uttar Pradesh
- Indian Lac Research Institute, Namkum, Ranchi
- National Academy of Agricultural Research Management, Hyderabad, Andhra Pradesh
- National Dairy Research Institute, Karnal, Haryana
- National Institute of Animal Nutrition and Physiology, Bangalore, Karnataka
- National Institute for Research on Jute & Allied Fibres Technology, West Bengal (formerly JTRL)
- Sugarcane Breeding Institute, Coimbatore, Tamilnadu
- Vivekanand Parvatiya Krishi Anusandhan Sansthan, Almora, Uttaranchal

Bureaus

- National Bureaue of Animal Genetic Resources, Karnal, Haryana
- National Bureaue of Fish Genetic Resources, Lucknow, Uttar Pradesh
- National Bureaue of Plant Genetic Resources, New Delhi.
- National Bureaue of Soil Survey & Land Use Planning, Nagpur, Maharashtra
- National Bureaue of Agriculturally Important Microorganisms, Distt. Mau, Uttar Pradesh

National Research Centres

- National Centre for Agril Economics & Policy Research, New Delhi
- National Research Centre for Agroforestry, Jhansi, Uttar Pradesh
- National Research Centre for Cachew, Puttur, Karnataka
- National Research Centre on Camel, Bikaner, Rajasthan
- National Research Centre for Coldwater Fisheries, Bhimtal, Uttaranchal
- National Research Centre on Equines, Hissar, Haryana
- National Research Centre for Grapes, Pune, Maharashtra
- National Research Centre for Groundnut, Junagadh, Gujarat
- National Research Centre for Integrated Pest Management, New Delhi
- National Research Centre for Medicinal & Aromatic Plants, Boriavi, Gujarat
- National Research Centre for Mithun, Nagaland
- National Research Centre for Mushroom, Solan, Himachal Pradesh
- National Research Centre for Onion and Garlic, Rajgurunagar, Pune, Maharashtra
- National Research Centre for Oilpalm, Pedavegi, Andhra Pradesh
- National Research Centre for Orchid, Pakyong, Sikkim
- National Research Centre for Weed Science, Madhya Pradesh
- National Research Centre for Yak, Dirang, Arunachal Pradesh

Project Directorates

- Project Directorate of Biological Control, Bangalore
- Project Directorate on Cattle, Meerut, Uttar Pradesh
- Project Directorate of Cropping System Research, Modipuram, Uttar Pradesh
- Project Directorate of Oilseed Research, Rajendranagar, Hyderabad
- Project Directorate of Poultry, Rajendranagar, Hyderabad,
- Project Directorate of Rice Research, Hyderabad
- Water Technology Centre for Eastern Region, Bhubaneswar, Orissa

List of related Important CSIR institutions

1. Centre for Cellular & Molecular Biology, Hyderabad
2. Central Drug Research Institute, Lucknow
3. Central Food Technological Research Institute, Mysore
4. Central Institute of Medicinal & Aromatic Plants, Lucknow
5. Central Scientific Instruments Organisation, Chandigarh
6. Institute of Genomics and Integrative Biology, Delhi
7. Institute of Himalayan Bioresource Technology, Palampur
8. Indian Institute of Chemical Biology, Kolkata
9. Indian Institute of Chemical Technology, Hyderabad
10. Indian Institute of Integrative Medicine(IIIM), Jammu
11. Industrial Toxicology Research Centre, Lucknow
12. Institute of Microbial Technology, Chandigarh
13. National Institute of Science Communication And Information Resources, New Delhi
14. National Institute of Science, Technology And Development Studies, New Delhi

Related Autonomous S&T Institutions of India

- Agharkar Research Institute, Pune
- Jawaharlal Nehru Centre for Advanced Scientific Research, Bangalore
- Sreechitra Tirunal Institute for Medical Sciences & Technology, Thiruvananthapuram
- Technology Information, Forecasting & Assessment Council (TIFAC), New Delhi
- Vigyan Prasar, New Delhi
- Centre For DNA Fingerprinting And Diagnostics (CDFD), Hyderabad (http://www.cdfd.org.in)
- Institute of Bioresources and Sustainable Development (IBSD), Imphal, Manipur (http://www.ibsd-imphal.nic.in)
- Institute of Life Sciences, Bhuvaneswar (http://www.ilsc.org)

- National Institute Of Immunology, New Delhi (http://www.nii.res.in)
- National Centre For Plant Genome Research (NCPGR), JNU, New Delhi (http://www.ncpgr.nic.in)
- National Brain Research Centre (NBRC), Gurgaon (http://www.nbrc.ac.in)
- National Centre for Cell Sciences, Pune (http://www.nccs.res.in)
- Bharat Immunologicals & Biologicals Corporation Limited, Bulandshahar
- Indian Vaccines Corporation Limited, Gurgaon

VETERINARY FORMULARY

Definition of pharmacological preparations:

Aquae- It is solution of volatile substances in water, e.g. aquae chloroformi. It is used as vehicle for mixture.

Powders- Powders are prepared by reducing the drugs by trituration to a state of fine division.

Mixture / Mistura- Mixtures are the preparation for internal use consisting of one or more drugs dissolved/ suspended in water.

Vinegars/ Aceta- Drug dissolved in acetic acid are called Vinegars/ Aceta, e.g. vinegar of squill.

Glycerines- Glycerines are the solution of a drug in glycerine, e.g. Boro glycerine.

Mellita/ honey - Drug mixed with honey or sometimes glycerine ae called Mellita/ honey, e.g. honey of borax.

Oxymels/ Oxymellita- Oxymels are the mixture of a drug in with honey and acetic acid, e.g. oxymel of squill.

Elixir- It consists of syrup, alcohol and an aromatic drug, e.g. elixir paregoric.

Unguentum/ Ontment- It is a semisolid soft preparation in Vaseline or paraffin bases for topical application.

Liniment- Liniments are the liquid preparations in oil, alcohol or soap for external use. It is applied by rubbing in the form of massage.

Lotion/ Lotio - Lotions are aqueous preparations of soluble as well as insoluble drugs for external application.

Tinctura/ Tincture- Tinctura/ Tincture are alcoholic or hydro alcoholic solutions of non volatile drugs. They can b classified as Simple (contaning onbly one ingredient) and compound (containing more than one ingredient).

Liquor- Preparation of non volatile substances generally in distilled water. Alcohol, oils and other solvents are also sometimes used in exceptional cases.

Spirit- Solution of volatile substance in alcohol e.g. Aromatic spirit of ammonia.

Syrups/ Syrupus- Consists of sugar, water and a water soluble drugs.

Electuary- It is medicinal paste in semi solid form prepared in vehicles like honey, glycerine etc. It is meant for internal us and is applied to the base of the tongue. It is used when he animal cannot take powder or liquid medicine due to difficulty in swallowing.

Emulsion- These are the aqueous preparation where resinous or fatty substances are suspended by means of other viscid materials. Gum acacia, gelatin, egg yolk are frequently used for this purpose. This also helps to reduce irritability of highly irritant drugs.

Collodions/ Collodia- These are the compound containing solutions of pyrexylin with ether and alcohol.

Bolus- Bolus literally means a lump. It can be defined as a large pill or a cylindrical mass with rounded ends. The length may be 2″ to 2.5″ and may weigh 1.5 to 2 ounce.

SELECTED PHARMACEUTICAL PREPARATIONS IN VETERINARY PRACTICE

1. Tinctura Iodi Fortis

Iodum	2.5 g
Pot iodide	1.5 g
Aqua add.	2.5 ml
Alcohol 90 % ad.	25 ml

Sig: to be applied externally

2. Tinctura Iodi Mitis

Iodum	2.5 g
Pot iodide	1.5 g
Aqua add.	2.5 ml
Alcohol 90 % ad.	100 ml

Sig: to be applied externally

3. Lugols Solution

Iodum	0.4 g
Pot iodide	0.8 g
Aqua add.	20 ml

Sig: to be applied i/v intermmitantly or used as intrauterine preparation after dilution

4. Dressing oil

Pulv camphore	2 g
Oil terebinth	2 ml
Oil eucalyptus	2 ml
Oil lini ad.	20 ml

Sig: to be applied externally

5. Dusting powder

Boric acid	10 g
Zinc oxide	10 g
Amylum	10 g

Sig: to be applied externally

6. Expectorant mixture for small animal

Sodi-bi-carb	1 g
Pot iodide	0.2 g
Spt-amon arom	1 ml
Syrup vasak	4 ml
Tr. ginger	1 ml
Tr. card co.	1 ml
Aqua ad	1 ml

Sig: 30 ml T.I.D.

7. Expectorant mixture for a dog

Ammon carb	0.5 g
Tr. scilli	3.5 g
Spt. chlyreformi	3.5 g
Aqua ad.	6 ml

Sig: to be given orally 2 teaspoonful every 4 hours

8. Influenza mixture for common cold, cough etc.

Sodi-bi-carb	0.6 g
Sodi salicylus	0.6 g
Spt. ammon arom	1.2 ml
Tr. Carb Co	0.6 ml
Aqua ad	30 ml

Sig: to be given T.I.D.

9. Electuary for Chronic cough in bovines

Ext. Bellad liq.	1 ml
Pot iodide	1.5 g
Liq. Arsenicalis	8 ml
Glycerine	4 ml
Syrup simplex	15 ml

Mft. Elect (1) Send such (6)

Sig: to be given 1 tablespoonful B.I.D.

10. Analgesic and antipyretic mixture for dog

Sodi salicylas	0.5 g
Sodi- benzoas	0.5 g
Sodi-bi-carb	0.5 G
Spt. Ammon arom	7 ml
Tr. urginea	0.5 ml
Aqua ad	30 ml

Sig: 30 ml T.I.D.

11. Triple carb for dog (Gastric antacid or gastric sedative)

Sodi bi carb	0.6 g
Mag carb levis	0.6 g
Bismuth carb	0.6 g
Water ad.	3.0 ml

Sig: to be given orally in gastritis and hyperacidity in dog

12. Carminative mixture

Sodi-bi-carb	1.5 g
Tr. carb co.	2 ml
Spt. amon arom	1 ml
Spt. Chloroformi	1 ml
Tr. ginger	1 ml
Aqua menth pipp	30 ml

Sig: 1 dose T.I.D.

13. Carminative mixture for small animals

Sodi-bi-carb	1.5 g
Spt. amon arom	1 ml
Spt. Chloroformi	1 ml
Tr. card co.	2 ml
Aqua month pip	30 ml

Sig: one dose T.I.D.

14. Stomachic, gastric stimulant, tonic for horse and cattle

Pulv nuxvom	4 g
Sodi chlor	16 g
Sodi bi carb	16 g

Sig: to administered orally B.I.D.

15. Alkaline stomachic powder for bovine

Sodi bi carb	8 g
Ammon carb	2 g
Pulv nuxvom	1 g
Pulv gentian	8 g

Sig: to be administered orally B.I.D. in anorexia or inappetance

16. Astringent Powder

Tannic acid	2 g
Pulv catechu	4 g
Creta preparata	30 g

Sig: to be given B.I.D. one dose should be given with 300ml of rice gruel

17 . Emetic for dog

Sodi chlor	4 g
Mustard flour	2 g
Luke warm water	120 ml

Sig: administered orally immediately to induce vomiting in case ingestion of poison

18. Mistura alba for dog

Mag carb levis	2 g
Mag sulph	4 g
Aqua ad	60 ml

Sig: to be administered B.I.D. one teaspoonful at a time

19. Cleansing Draught for a cow

Extergot liq.	8 ml
Mag sulph	210 g
Pot nitrous	8 g
Tr. ginger	30 ml
Aqua ad.	500 ml
Aqua menth pip	8 ml

Sig: to be given B.I.D.

20. Hematinic tonic for acow

Ferri sulph	4 g
Cupri sulph	1 g
Pulv gentian	4 g
Pulv chirreta	4 g
Pulv nuxvom	2 g

Sig: to be administered orally as directed

21. Mandle's Paint or throat paint

Iodine	360 mg
Pot iodide	720 mg
Oil pipermint	0.25 ml
Distilled water add	0.8 ml
Glycerine ad.	3 ml

Sig: to be used as throat paint in tonsillitis or pharyngitis

22. Mel Boracts

Borax	10 g
Glycerine	5 ml
Honey	85 ml

Sig: to be used Q.I.D. as mouth wash

23. Iodine ointment

Iodum	1 g
Pot iodide	1 g
Glycerine ad	3 ml
Vaseline	25 g

Sig: for external application

24. Salisylic acid ointment

Salisylic acid 0.5 g
Vaseline 25 g
Sig: to be applied externally

25. Sulpher ointment

Sulpher sublimatum 2.5 g
Vaseline ad 25 g
Sig: to be applied externally

26. Turpentine ointment

Oil turpentine 2.5 g
Vaseline ad 25 g
Sig: to be applied externally

27. Iodoform ointment

Iodoform 2.5 g
Vaseline ad 25 g
Sig: to be applied externally

28. Red ointment

Hydragyri iodium rubrum 5 g
Vaseline ad 50 g
Sig: to be applied externally

29. Yellow ointment

Hydragyri iodium flavum 0.125 g
White Vaseline ad 25 g
Sig: to be applied in eye

30. Boric acid ointment

Boric acid 0.5 g
Vaseline ad 25 g
Sig: to be applied externally

31. Zinc oxide ointment

Zinc oxide 3.7 g
Vaseline ad 25 g
Sig: to be applied externally

32. Boro zinc ointment

Boric acid 2.5 g
Zinc oxide 2.5 g
Vaseline ad 25 g
Sig: to be applied externally

33. Zinc Iodoform Paraffin Paste (Z.I.P.P.)

Zinc oxide 1 g
Iodoform 2 g
Liquid paraffin q.s.
Sig: to be applid in deep seated wounds/ sinuses/ fistula

34. Bismuth Iodoform Paraffin Paste (B.I.P.P.)

Bismuth sub-nitrate 1 g
Iodoform 2 g
Liquid paraffin q.s.
Sig: to be applied externally in sinus/ fistula

34. Zinc Sulph Paste

Zinc sulph 1 g
Copper sulph 1 g
Ferri sulph 1 g
Liquid paraffin q.s.
Sig: to be applied externally

35. White Lotion

Plumbi acetas 1 g
Zinc sulphate 0.75 g
Aqua ad 20 g
Sig: to be applied externally

36. Calamina Lotion

Calamina preparata 3 g
Zinc oxide 1 g
Glycerine 1 ml
Aqua ad 20 ml
Sig: to be applied externally

37. Refrigerent Lotion

Pot nitrus 1 g
Sodi chlor 1 g
Ammon Chlor 1 g
Aqua ad. 20 ml
Sig: for external application

38. Boric acid Lotion

Boric acid	0.25 g
Aqua ad.	50 ml

Sig: to be used as collyrium

39. Zinc sulph Lotion

Zinc sulphate	0.25 g
Aqua ad.	50 ml

Sig: to be used as collyrium

40. Boro Zinc Lotion

Boric acid	0.25 g
Zinc sulphate	0.25 g
Aqua ad.	50 ml

41. Silver nitrate Lotion

Argenti nitrus	25 g
Aqua dist ad.	50 ml

Sig: to applied in eye diseases like corneal opacity, conjunctivitis, ulcer etc.

42. Boroglycerine Lotion

Borax	12 g
Glycerine	100 ml

Sig: to be aqpplied externally in stomatitis

43. Ammonia Liniment

Liq Ammon fort	2 ml
Pulv camphore	2 g
Oil turpentine	2 ml
Oil lini ad.	20 ml

Sig: to be applied externally

44. Turpentine Liniment

Oil turpentine	16.25 ml
Oil lini ad.	25 ml

Sig: to be applied externally

45. Camphore Liniment

Pulv camphore	4 g
Oil lini ad.	20 ml

Sig: to be applied externally

46. A.B.C. Liniment

Pulv Aconite	2 g
Bellad radix	2 g
Liq Chloroforme	2 ml

Sig: to be applied externally

47. Sodium salicylate injectable

Sodi salicylas	4 g
Tripple glass distilled water	30 ml

Sig: to be injected sub cut every alternate day for 5-6 days for treatment of rheumatism, fever, rheumatic arthritis, mild inflammation

48. Karpin lotion

Sodi thio sulph	20 g
Sodi hydroxide	50 mg
Sodi benzoas	500 mg
Water ad.	100 ml

Sig: to be applied externally

49. Caron oil

Lime water	1 part
Coconut oil	1 part

Sig: to be applied externally in cases of fresh burn

50. Anthelmintic Emulsion for dog

Oil chenopodium	0.3 ml
Oil turpentine	0.3 ml
Spt. chloroformi	0.6 ml
Castor oil	30 ml
Gum acacia	q.s.

Sig: to be administered in empty stomach in hookworm infection

51. Antidot of poisoning in large animals

Egg yolk	5 nos
Gum acacia	30 g
Milk	500 ml
Syrup simplex	60 ml

Sig: to be given immidately after ingestion of poison to prevent further absorption.

52. Sheep dip for Ectoparasites

Arsenic tri oxide	900 g
Pot carbonate	900 g
Sulphur sublime	900 g
Soft soap	2 kg
Boiling water	10 gallon

Mft (1) This amount is to be mixed with 100 gallon of cold water

Sig: to be applied externally

53. Saline Purgative for cattle

Mag sulph	120 g
Sodi sulph	120 g
Sodi chlor	120 g

Sig: to be given as directed

54. Drug for actinobacillosis and actinomycosis

Pot iodide	8 g
Aqua ad.	500 ml

Sig: to be given orally B.I.D. for 8-10 day

55. Drug for dandruff

Cetrimide solution	1 ml
Water ad.	10000 ml

Sig: 1 cup in a bucket of water

Model Bankable Project: DAIRY FARMING

1. GENERAL

i) Name of the sponsoring bank

ii) Address of the controlling ofice sponsoring the scheme

iii) Nature and objectives of the proposed scheme

iv) Details of proposed investments

S.No	Investment	No. Of units
(a)		
(b)		
(c)		

v) Specification of the scheme area (Name of District & Block/s)

S.No.	District	Block

vi) Names of the financing bank's branches:

S.No.	Name of the Branch/District

Appendix

(a)	
(b)	
(c)	

vii) Status of beneficiary/ies:

(indidivual/Partnership/Company/Corporation/Co-operative Society / Others)

viii) In case of area based schemes, coverage of borrowers in weaker sections (landless labourers, small, medium & large farmers as per NABARD's norms, SC/ST, etc.)

ix) Details of borrowers profile (Not applicable to area based schemes)

(a) Capability

(b) Experience

(c) Financial Soundness

(d) Technical/Other special Qualificaitons

(e) Technical/Managerial Staff and adequacy thereof

2. TECHNICAL ASPECTS :

a) Location, Land and Land Development :

i) Location details of the project

ii) Total Area of land and its cost

iii) Site map

iv) Particulars of land development, fencing, gates, etc.

b) Civil Structures :

Detailed cost estimates along with measurements of vaious civil structure

- Sheds

- Store room

- Milk room

- Quarters, etc.

c) Equipment/Plant and Machinery :

i) Chaff cutter

ii) Silo pit

iii) Milking machine

iv) Feed grinder and mixer

v) Milking pails/milk cans

vi) Biogas plant

vii) Bulk coolers

viii)Equipment for manufacture of products

ix) Truck/van (price quotations for the above equipments)

d) Housing :

i) Type of housing

ii) Area requirement

- Adults

- Heifers (1-3 years)

- Calves (less than 1 year)

e) Animals :
i) Proposed species
ii) Proposed breed
iii) Source of purchase
iv) Place of purchase
v) Distance (kms.)
vi) Cost of animal (Rs.)
f) Production parameters :
i) Order of lactation
ii) Milk yield (ltrs. per day)
iii) Lactation days
iv) Dry days
v) Conception rate
vi) Mortality(%)
- Adults
- Young stock
g) Herd projection (with all assumptions) :
h) Feeding :
i) Source of fodder and feed - Green fodder
- Dry fodder
- Concentrates
ii) Fodder crop rotations
- Kharif
- Rabi
- Summer
iii) Fodder cultivation expenses
iv) Requirement and costs :
Quantity required (kg./day)

	Cost(Rs. / Kg)	Lactation	Dry Period	Young Stock
Green Fodder				
Dry Fodder				
Concentrates				

i) Breeding Facilities :
i) Source :
ii) Location :
iii) Distance (km.) :
iv) Availability of semen :
v) Availability of staff :
vi) Expenditure per animal/year
j) Veterinary Aid :
i) Source
ii) Location

iii) Distance (km.)
iv) Availability of staff
v) Types of facilities available
vi) If own arrangements are made -
a) Employed a veterinary doctor/stockman/consultant
b) Periodicity of visit
c) Amount paid/visit (Rs.)
vii)Expenditure per animal per year (Rs.)
k) Electricity :
i) Source
ii) Approval from SEB
iii) Connected load
iv) Problems of power failure
v) Arrangements for generator
l) Water :
i) Source
ii) Quality of water
iii) Abvailability of sufficient quantity for drinking, cleaning nad fodder production
iv) If investment has to be made, type of strucutre, design and cost
m) Marketing of milk :
i) Source of sales
ii) Place of disposal
iii) Distance (km.)
iv) Price realised - (Rs. per liter of milk)
v) Basis of payment
vi) Periodicity of paymen
n) Marketing of other products :
i) Animal - age
- place of sale
- price expected
ii) Manure - Qty./animal
Price/unit (Rs.)
iii) Empty gunny bags
- Number
- Cost/bag (Rs.)
o) Beneficiary's experience :
p) Comments on technical feasibility :
q) Government restrictions, if any :

3. FINANCIAL ASPECTS :
i) Unit Cost :

Sr.No	Name of the Investment	Physical units and specification	Unit cost with component wise break-up (Rs.)	Whether approved by state level unit cost committee
	Total			

Ii) Down payment/margin/subsidy(Indicate source & extent of subsidy):
iii) Year-wise physical & financial programme :

Year 1	Invest-Ment 2	Physical Units 3	Unit Cost (Rs.) 4	Total Outlay (Rs.) 5	Margin/ Subsidy (Rs.) 6	Bank loan (Rs.) 7	Refinance Assistance (Rs.) 8
Total							

Iv) Financial viability (comment on the cash flow projection on a farm model/unit and enclose the same.)
Particulars :
a) Internal Rate of Return (IRR) :
b) Benefit Cost Ratio (BCR) :
c) Net Present Worth (NPW) :
v) Financial position of the borrowers (to be furnished in case of corporate bodies/partnership firms)
a) Profitability Ratio :
i) GP Ratio
ii) NP Ratio
b) Debt Equity Ratio :
c) Whether Income Tax & other tax obligations are paid upto date :
d) Whether audit is upto date (enclose copies of audited financial statements for the last three years)
vi) Lending Terms :
i) Rate of Interest :
ii) Grace Period :
iii) Repayment Period :
iv) Nature of Security :
v) Availability of Government guarantee wherever necessary :
4. INFRASTRUCTURAL FACILITIES :
a) Availability of technical staff with bank/implementing authority for monitoring
b) Details of -
i) technical guidance
ii) training facilities

iii) Govt support/extention support
c) Tie-up arrangements with marketing agencies for loan recovery
d) Insurance -
- Type of policy
- Periodicity
- Rate of premium
e) Whether any subsidy is available, if so amount per unit
f) Arrangements for supply of green fodder and cattle feed

Cattle and Buffalo Breeds Important Characteristics/Description

Sr. No.	Name Breed	Habitat/Main State	Breeding Tract Districts	Assembling Centres	Areas of demand	Remarks
1	2	3	4	5	6	7
A)	CATTLE	(INDIGENOUS)				
1	Amrith mahal	Erstwhile Mysore State now part of Karnataka	Tumkur and Chitradurg	Erstwhile Mysore State	Karnataka and adjoining area	Draught breed
2	Dangi	Maharashtra and Gujarat	Ahmednagar, Khandesh, Raigad, Nasik, Thane, Surat	Weekly markets in Ahmednagar, Nasik, Thane and West Khandesh district	Rocky ghat areas with heavy rainfall	Draught breed
3	Denoi	Andhra Pradesh Karnataka and Maharashtra	Medak, Nizambad, Mahboobnagar, Adilabad Gulbarga, Bidar, Osmanabad, Nanded	Weekly cattle markets, Jatras and fairs in Bidar and adjoining districts	Bidar and adjoining districts	Draught purposse breed
4	Gir	Gir Hills and forest of South Kathiawar	Junagarh, Also maintained by NDRI, Bangalore	_	Gujarat, Rajasthan, Maharashtra	Dairy purpose breed
5	Hallikar	Karnataka	Tumkur, Hassan & Mysore	Dodbalapur, Chickballapur , Harikar, Devargudda, Chikkuvalli, Karuvalli, Chittavadgi	Dharwar, North Kanara, Bellary (KT) Anantur & Chittur (A.P.),	Draught breed

				(T.N.) North Arcot (T.N.) Hindupur, Somaghatta, Anantpur (A.P.)	Coimbatore North Arcot, Salem (T.M.)	
6	Hariana	Haryana and Delhi, Punjab, Rajasthan	Rohtak, Hissar, Gurgaon, Karnal, Patiala, Sangrur, Jaipur, Jodhpur, Alwar, Bharatpur Western districts	Cattle fairs at Jehazgarh, Mahim and Bhadurgarh (Rohtak dist.) Hansi & Bhiwani (Hissar dist.)	Throughout the country	Dual purpose breed
7	Kangaya m	Tamil Nadu	Coimbatore	Avanashi, Tirppur, Kannauram, Madurai Athicombu	Southern Districts of Tamil Nadu	Draught breed
8	Kankrej	Gujarat	Ahmedabad, Banaskantha	Ahmedabad, Radhanpur	Rajasthan, Maharashtra	
9	Khillari	Maharashtra	Solapur, Kolhapur, Satara	Southern Districts of Maharashtra and adjoining districts of Andhra Pradesh and Karnataka		Draught breed
10	Krishna Valley	Maharashtra, Andhra Pradesh, Karnataka	Watersheds of Krishna and adjoining areas of A.P. and KT	Ichalkaranji. (Kolhapur), Chincahli (Gulbarga)		
11	Malvi	Madhya Pradesh	Guna, Vidisha, Raisen Sehora, Ujjain, Indore, Dewas, Gwalior, Shivpuri, Mandsaur, Jhabus & Dhar	Agar (Shajapur) Singaj (Nimar) Sehore & Ashta (Sehore)		Draught purpose
		Rajasthan	Jhalwar and Kotah	Karimnagar (A.P.)		
12	Nagori or Nagauri	Rajasthan	Jodhpur & Nagaur	Nagaur Parbatsar (Nagpur),	Rajasthan, Haryana, Uttar	Draught purpose

				Balotra (Barmer), Puskar (Ajmer), Hissar, Hansi (Haryana State)	Pradesh	
13	Ongole	Andhra Pradesh	Ongole, Guntur, Narasaraopet, Bapatla and Nellore	Available in Ongole tract of Andhra Pradesh	-	Dual Purpose
14	Rathi	Rajasthan	Alwar, Bharatpur, Jaipur	Alwar, Rewari (Gurgaon), Pushkar (Ajmer)	- -	- Dairy breed
15	Sahiwal	Punjab, Haryana, Delhi, U.P., Bihar, M.P., W.B.	Sahiwal (erstwhile Montgomery)	Jullundar, Gurdaspur, Amritsar, Kapurthala, Ferozepur (Punjab), NDRI, Karnal, Hissar, Anhora Durg (M.P), Lucknow, Meerut, Bihar, W.B.	-	Dairy breed
16	Red Sindhi	Pakisatan All parts of India	-	-	-	Dairy breed
17	Siri	Sikkim, Bhutan	Darjeeling Hill Tract	Darjeeling (Brought by dealers)	-	Dual purpose
18	Tharparka r	Pakisatn (sind)	Umarkot, Naukot, Dhoro Naro Chor	Balotra (Jodhpur), Puskar (Ajmer), Gujarat State	-	Dairy breed

B) CATTLE (EXOTIC)

B) CATTLE (EXOTIC)

1	Brown Swiss	Switzerland	-	India, Pakisatan & other Asian countries	-	Dairy breed
2	Holstein Friesian	Holland	Province of North Holland and West Friesland	Through out the country (crossbreds)	-	Dairy breed
3	Jersy	British Isles	Island of Jersey	Crossbreds available in all states/U.Ts	-	Dairy breed

B) BUFFALOES

Reproductive and Productive Parameters (Traits) in Indian Cattle and Buffaloes

Sr.No	Name of the breed	Age at first calving (months)	Calving interval (months)	Lactation yield (kg.)	Lactation length (days)	Dry period (days)	Milk yield kg/day during lactat-ion
1	2	3	4	5	6	7	8
i)	Cattle						
a)	Indian breeds						
1	Dangi	54	17	600	300	210	2.0
2	Deogir	48	15	1,500	300	150	5.0
3	Deoni	53	14	810	270	150	3.0
4	Gir	48	16	1,350	270	210	5.0
5	Gaolao	46	16	600	300	180	2.0
6	Hallikar	46	20	600	300	300	2.0
7	Hariana	58	13	1,200	240	150	5.0
8	Kangayam	44	16	600	240	240	2.5
9	Kankrej	48	17	1,800	360	150	5.0
10	Khilari	52	16	240	240	240	1.0
11	Ongole	40	19	630	210	360	3.0
12	Rathi	40	19	1,815	330	240	5.5
13	Red Sindhi	42	14	1,620	270	150	6.0
14	Sahiwal	40	14	1,620	270	150	6.0
15	Tharparkar	50	14	1,620	270	150	6.0
16	Umblachery	46	17	360	240	270	1.5
17	Non-descript	60	19	405	270	300	1.5

B) Crossbred Cattle (Bos indicus Fx Bostaurus M)

1	H x F	34	14	2,970	330	90	9.0
2	H x BS	29	15	2,805	330	120	8.5
3	H x J	33	13	2,850	300	90	9.5

4	G x J	25	13	2,640	330	60	8.0
5	G x F	25	13	2,160	270	120	8.0
6	RS x F	29	12	2,295	270	90	8.5
7	RS x RD	28	12	2,160	270	90	8.0
8	RS x J	29	12	1,500	300	90	5.0
9	R x J	32	12	2,700	300	60	9.0
10	T x F	33	13	2,550	300	90	8.5
11	S x F	33	14	2,400	300	120	8.0

C) Buffaloes

1	Bhadawari	50	15	1,080	270	180	4.0
2	Murrah	42	16	1,800	300	180	6.0
3	Nili-Ravi	54	16	1,950	300	180	6.5
4	Surti	44	16	1,765	330	150	5.5
5	Mehsani	50	14	1,620	270	150	6.0
6	Jaffarabadi	50	14	1,620	270	150	6.0
7	Pandharpuri	56	14	1,350	270	150	5.0
8	Marathwadi	50	14	1,015	270	150	3.5
9	Nagpuri	50	14	1,350	270	150	5.0
10	Dharwari	50	14	1,350	270	150	5.0
11	Non-descript	50	16	540	270	210	2.0

Key : H = Hariana S = Sahiwal RS = Red Sindhi
G = Gir T = Tharparkar L = Non-descript
R = Rathi F = Friesian BS = Brown Swiss
RD = Red dane J = Jersey

Annexure - IV

Unit cost of cows and buffaloes Approved by NABARD in some of the major States in India

Economics of two animal unit (buffaloes)

Project at a Glance

1	Unit Size	:	2 Animals
2	Breed	:	Graded Murrah
3	State	:	Karnataka
4	Unit Cost (Rs.)	:	18,223
5	Bank Loan (Rs.)	:	15,400
6	Margin Money (Rs.)	:	2,823
7	Repayment period	:	5
8	Interest rate (%)	:	12
9	BCR at 15% DF	:	1.50:1
10	NPW at 15% DF (Rs.)	:	29,187
11	IRR(%)	:	>50%

MODEL PROJECT FOR TWO ANIMAL UNIT(BUFFALOES)

A INVESTMENT COST

Sr. No .	Items	Specifications	Phy units	Unit Cost (Rs. /Unit)	Total Cost (Rs.)
1	Cost of animals		2	8,200	16,400
2	Insurance		2	689	1,378
3	Conc. Feed (4.5 kg/day/animal for 30 days)	135 Kg	1	3.3	446
4	Total cost				18,223
5	Margin money (15% of total cost)			Say Rs.	2,733 2723
6	Bank laon (85% of total cost)			Say Rs.	15490 15500

B TECHNO ECONOMIC PARAMETERS

i)	No.of milch animals	2
ii)	Cost of milch animals	8,200
iii)	Lactation period (days)	280
iv)	Dry period (days)	150
v)	Milk yield (lts./day)	7
vi)	Sale price of milk (Rs./lt)	7.75
vii)	Sale of manure/animal/year (Rs.)	300
viii)	Insurance premium for five years (%)	8.4
ix)	Veterinary aid/animal/year (Rs.)	150
x)	Labour (Rs.)	Family labour
xi)	Cost of electricity & water (Rs./animal)	100
xii)	Interest rate (%)	12
xiii	Repayment period (years)	5
xiv)	Income from sale of gunny bags 20 bags/tonne @ Rs. 5/bag	100
xv)	Feeding schedule	

S.No.	Type of fodder/feed	Price (Rs./kg)	(Quantity in kg/day) Lactation Dry Period Period
a)	Green fodder	0.2	25 25
b)	Dry fodder	0.5	5 5
c)	Concentrate	3.3	4.5 1

xvi) Animals will be purchased in two batches at an interval of 5 - 6 months

xvii) It is assumed that the expenditure on calf rearing will nullify the sale value of calf / hiefer.
xviii) Closing stock value (Rs. per animal) 4100
C LACTATION CHART

Sr.No	Particulars	Years				
		I	II	III	IV	V
i)	Lactation Days					
a)	First batch	250	280	250	210	210
b)	Second batch	180	210	210	210	210
	Total	430	490	460	420	420
ii)	Dry Days					
a)	First batch	110	80	110	150	150
b)	Second batch	-	150	150	150	150
	Total	110	230	260	300	300

D CASH FLOW ANALYSIS

Sr.No.	Particulars	Years				
		I	II	III	IV	V
I	Costs:					
1	Capital cost*	17,777				
2	Recurring cost					
a)	Feeding during lactation period					
	Green fodder	2,150	2,450	2,300	2,100	2,100
	Dry fodder	1,075	1,225	1,150	1,050	1,050
	Concentrate	6,386	7,277	6,831	6,237	6,237
	Total	9,611	10,952	10,281	9,387	9,387
b)	Feeding during dry period					
	Green fodder	550	1,150	1,300	1,500	1,500
	Dry fodder	275	575	575	750	750
	Concentrate	363	759	858	990	990
	Total	1,188	2,484	2,733	3,240	3,240
c)	Veterinary aid & breeding cover	225	300	300	300	300
d)	Cost of electricity & water	150	200	200	200	200

	Total	28,951	13,936	13,514	13,127	13,127	
II	BENEFITS						
a)	Sale of milk	23,328	26,583	24,955	22,785	22,785	
b)	Sale of Gunny bags	205	232	218	200	200	
c)	Sale of manure	450	600	600	600	600	
d)	Closing stock value					8,200	
	Total	23,982	27,414	25,773	23,585	31,785	
III	DF @15%	0.870	0.756	0.658	0.572	0.497	
IV	DISCOUNTED COSTS AT 15%	25,175	10,537	8,886	7,505	6,526	58,630
V	DISCOUNTED BENEFITS AT 15%	20,854	20,729	16,946	13,485	15,803	87,817
VI	NPW @ 15%	29,187					
VII	BCR @ 15%	1.50:1					
VIII	DF @ 50%	0.667	0.444	0.296	0.198	0.132	
IX	NET BENEFITS	-4,969	13,479	12,259	10,458	18,658	
X	DISCOUNTED NET BENEFITS AT 50%	-3,313	5,990	3,632	2,066	2,457	10,833
XI	IRR	>50%					

** excluding the capitalised expenditure on concentrated feed*

E REPAYMENT SCHEDULE

Bank Loan (Rs) - 15500
Interest Rate (%) - 12
Capital recovery factor - 0.277

Year	Income	Expenses	Gross surplus	Equated annual instalment	Net surplus
I	23,982	10,728	13,254	4,294	8,961
II	27,414	13,936	13,479	4,294	9,185
III	25,773	13,514	12,259	4,294	7,966
IV	23,585	13,127	10,458	4,294	6,165
V	23,585	13,127	10,458	4,294	6,165

ECONOMICS OF A MINI DAIRY UNIT
TEN ANIMAL UNIT (BUFFALOES)

PROJECT AT A GLANCE

1	Unit size	:	10 animals
2	Breed	:	Graded Murrah
3	State	:	Karnataka
4	Unit cost (Rs)	:	155,030
5	Bank loan (Rs)	:	131,700
6	Margin money (Rs)	:	23,330
7	Repayment period (yrs)	:	5
8	Interest rate (%)	:	13.5
9	BCR at 15% DF	:	1.53:1
10	NPW at 15% DF(Rs)	:	154,403
11	IRR (%)	:	>50

MODEL PROJECT FOR TEN ANIMAL UNIT (BUFFALOES)

A INVESTMENT COST

S.No.	Items	Specifications	Phy.units	Unit Cost (Rs./unit)	Total Cost (Rs.)
1	Cost of animals		10	8,200	8,200
2	Transportation cost of animals		10	300	3,000
3	Cost of construction of shed	Sq.ft.	650	55	35,750
4	Cost of Store cum office	Sq.ft.	200	100	20,000
5	Equipments (chaff cutter, milking pails, cans, technicians		10	500	5,000
6	Insurance		10	328	3,280
7	Fodder raising expenses @ Rs.3000/acre		2	3,000	6,000
8	Total cost				155,030
9	Margin money (15% of total cost)			Say	23255 23330
10	Bank loan (85% of total cost)			Say	131776 131700

ANNEXURE VI (contd)		
B TECHNO ECONOMIC PARAMETERS		
i	Animals will be purchased in two batches at an interval of 5-6 months	
ii	Second/Third lactation animals within 30 days of calving will be purchased in first year	
iii	No. of acres of irrigated land for fodder production considered in the project. Green fodder will be produced on the farm. Fodder production expenses is considered in the cash flow analysis. During first year only two seasons are considered.	2
iv	In the first year the fodder production expenses are capitalised for one season (Rs. per acre per season) and manure is utilised for fodder production	3,000
v	It is assumed that the expenditure on calf rearing will nullify the income realised from its sale. However, the heifer will be retained on the farm and the old animals will be sold out.	
vi	No. of milch animals	10
vii	Cost of milch animals	8,200
viii	Transportation cost (Rs. per milch animal including followers)	300
ix	Civil structures:	
	a) Shed (sft. per milch animal) b) Store and office (sft)	65 200
x	Cost of construction a) Shed (Rs. per sft) b) Store and office	55 100
xi	Cost of equipment (Rs per milch animals)	500
xii	Lactation period (days)	280
xiii	Dry period (days)	150
xiv	Milk yield (lts/day)	7
xv	Sale price of milk (Rs/lt)	7.75
xvi	Income from sale of gunny bags (20 bags/tonne @ Rs.5/bag)	100
xvii	Expenditure on dry fodder for dry and lactation period requirement (kg/day)	5 0.5

	Cost (Rs/kg)	
xviii	Expenditure on concentrates a) Requirement (kg/day) Lactation period Dry period b) Cost (Rs/kg)	4.5 1 3.3
xix	Veterinary aid/animal/year (Rs)	150
xx	Labour (Rs./month)	900
xxi	Insurance premium (%)	4
xxii	Cost of electricity, water & other overheads (Rs/animal)	200
xxiii	Depreciation(%) a) Sheds b) Equipment	5 10
xxiv	Value of closing stock	4,100
xxv	Interest rate(%)	13.5
xxvi	Repayment period (years)	5

C. Lactation Chart

S.No	Particulars		I	II	Years III	IV	V
I	Lactation Days						
a)	First batch		1,250	1,400	1,250	1,050	1,050
b)	Second batch		900	1,050	1,050	1,050	1,050
		Total	2,150	2,450	2,300	2,100	2,100
II	Dry days						
a)	First batch		550	400	550	750	750
	Second batch		-	750	750	750	750
		Total	550	1,150	1,300	1,500	1,500

D CASH FLOW ANALYSIS

Sr.No	Particulars	I	II	Year III	IV	IV
I	Costs					
1	Capital cost*	145,750				
2	Recurring cost					
a)	Green fodder raising	12,000	18,000	18,000	18,000	18,000

	expenses						
b)	Feeding during lactation period						
	Dry fodder	5,375	6,125	5,750	5,250	5,250	
	Concentrate	31,928	36,383	34,155	31,185	31,185	
	Total	37,303	42,508	39,905	36,435	36,435	
c)	Feeding during dry period						
	Dry Fodder	1,375	2,875	3,250	3,750	3,750	
	Concentrate	1,815	3,795	4,290	4,950	4,950	
	Total	3,190	6,670	7,540	8,700	8,700	
d)	Veterinary aid & breeding cover	1,125	1,500	1,500	1,500	1,500	
e)	Cost of electricity & water	1,500	2,000	2,000	2,000	2,000	
f)	Insurance	3,280	3,280	3,280	3,280	3,280	
g)	Labour cost	10,800	10,800	10,800	10,800	10,800	
	Total	188,868	52,678	50,945	49,503	48,635	
II	BENEFITS						
a)	Sale of milk	116,637	132,912	124,775	113,925	113,925	
b)	Sale of Gunny bags	1,023	1,218	1,165	1,095	1,095	
c)	Depreciated value of sheds	-				26,813	
d)	Depreciated value of equipments					2,500	
e)	Closing stock value					41,000	
	Total	117,660	134,130	125,940	115,020	185,333	
III	DF @ 15%	0.87	0.76	0.66	0.57	0.50	
IV	DISCOUNTED COSTS AT 15%	164,233	39,832	33,497	28,303	24,180	290,045
V	DISCOUNTED BENEFITS AT 15%	102,313	101,422	82,808	65,763	92,143	444,448
VI	NPW @ 15%	154,403					

VII	BCR @ 15%	1.53:1					
VIII	DF @ 50%	0.667	0.444	0.296	0.198	0.132	
IX	NET BENEFITS	-71,208	81,453	74,995	65,518	136,698	
X	DISCOUNTED NET BENEFITS AT 50%	47,472	36,201	22,221	12,942	18,001	41,893
XI	IRR	>50					

** excludes the capitalised cost for fodder raising for three months and insurance for one year*

E REPAYMENT SCHEDULE:

Bank Loan (Rs) - 131700

Interest rate(%) - 13.5

Capital recovery factor - 0.287

(in Rs.)

Year	Income	Expenses	Gross surplus	Equated annual installment	Net surplus
I	117,660	33,838	83,823	37,798	46,025
II	134,130	52,678	81,453	37,798	43,655
III	125,940	50,945	74,995	37,798	47,197
IV	115,020	49,503	65,518	37,798	27,720
V	115,020	48,635	66,385	37,798	28,587

Housing Space Requirements for Crossbred cattle

Age-group	Manger Space (mtr.)	Standing or covered area (sq.mtr.)	Open Space(sq.mtr.)
4-6 months	0.2-0.3	0.8-1.0	3.0-4.0
6-12 months	0.3-0.4	1.2-1.6	5.0-6.0
1-2 years	0.4-0.5	1.6-1.8	6.0-8.0
Cows	0.8-1.0	1.8-2.0	11.0-12.0
Pregnant cows	1.0-1.2	8.5-10.0	15.0-20.0
Bulls*	1.0-1.2	9.0-11.0	20.0-22.0

**To be housed individually*

Annexure - VIII

Feeding Schedules for Dairy Animals
(Quantity in Kgs.)

S.No.	Type of animal	Feeding during	Green Fodder	Dry Fodder	Concentrate
1	2	3	4	5	6
(A)	CROSSBRED COW				
a)	6 to 7 litres milk per day	Lactation days Dry days	20 to 25 15 to 20	5 to 6 6 to 7	3.0 to 3.5 0.5 to 1.0
b)	8 to 10 litres milk per day	Lactation days Dry days	25 to 30 20 to 25	4 to 5 6 to 7	4.0 to 4.5 0.5 to 1.0
(B)	BUFFALOES				
a)	Murrah (7 to 8 litres milk per day)	Lactation days Dry days	25 to 30 20 to 25	4 to 5 5 to 6	3.5 to 4.0 0.5 to 1.0
b)	Mehasana (6 to 7 litres milk per day)	Lactation days Dry days	15 to 20 10 to 15	4 to 5 5 to 6	3.0 to 3.5 0.5 to 1.0
c)	Surti (5 to 6 litrs milk per day)	Lactation days Dry days	10 to 15 5 to 10	4 to 5 5 to 6	2.5 to 3.0 0.5 to 1.0

Programme for vaccination of farm animals against contagious diseases

Sr. No.	Name of disease	Type of vaccine	Type of vaccination	Duration of immunity	Remarks
1	2	3	4	5	6
1	Anthrax (Gorhi)	Spore vaccine	Once in an year premonsoon vaccination	One season	-
2	Black Quarter (Sujab)	Killed vaccine	- do -	- do -	-
3	Haemorrhagic Septicaemia (Galghotu)	Ocladjuvant vaccine	- do -	- do -	-
4	Brucellosis (Contagious	Cotton strain 19 (live	At about 6 months of	3 or 4 calvings	To be done only in

	abortion)	bacteria)	age		infected herds
5	Foot and Mouth disease (Muhkhar)	Polyvalent tissue culture vaccine	At about 6 months of age with booster dose 4 months later	One season	After vaccination repeat vaccination every year in Oct./Nov.
6	Rinderpest (Mata)	Lapinised avianised vaccine for exotic and crossbred catte, caprinised vaccine for zebu cattle.	At about 6 months of age	Life long	It is better to repeat after 3 to 4 years

FORMAT FOR SUBMISSION

SCHEME: POULTRY - BROILER FARMING

1. General

i) Name of the sponsoring bank

ii) Address of the controlling office sponsoring the scheme

iii)Nature and objectives of the proposed scheme

iv)Details of proposed investments:

Sr.No.	Investment	No. of units
a)		
b)		
c)		

v)Specification of the scheme area (Name of District & Block/s)

Sr.No.	District	Block

vi) Names of the financing bank's branches:

vii) Status of beneficiary/ies' (Individual)/Partnership/Company/Corporation/Co-

operative/Others
viii) In case of area based schemes, coverage of borrowers
in weaker sections (landless labourers, small, medium & large farmers as per NABARD's norms, SC/ST, etc.)
ix) Details of borrowers profile (Not applicable to area based schemes)
(a) Capability
(b) Experience
(c) Financial soundness
(d) Technical/Other special Qualifications
(e) Technical/Managerial Staff and adequacy thereof

2. TECHNICAL ASPECTS:

a) Location, Land and Land Development:
i) Location details of the project
ii) Total Area of land and it's cost
iii) Site map
iv) Particulars of land development, fencing, gates etc.

b) Civil Structures:
Detailed cost estimates along with measurements of various civil structures
- Broiler Sheds
- Store room
- Dressing room
- Office room
- Quarters for staff
- Others

c) Equipment/Plant and machinery:
(i) Feeders
(ii) Waterers
(iii) Generator
(iv) Feed grinder and mixer
(v) Debeaker
(vi) Vaccinator
(vii) Fridge/Deep Freezer
(viii) Dressing equipment if necessary
(ix) Truck/van/Jeep
(Price quotations for the above equipments)

d) Housing:
i) Type of housing Deep Litter/Slat/Environment controlled
ii) Area required (sft./bird)

e) Birds:
i) Proposed strain
ii) No.of birds to be purchased
iii) Source of purchase
iv) Cost of birds (Rs. per bird)

v) Vaccination of purchased birds
vi) Proposed programmeof replacement
f) Production parameters:
i) Average body weight (kg.)
ii) Feed efficiency (kg. of feed/ kg.body weight gain)
iii) Mortality (%)
g) Flock Projection Chart:
h) Feeding:
i) Source of availability - Purchased or own feed manufacturing
ii) If purchased
a) Place of purchase
b) Brand
c) Cost (Rs./kg)
- Starter
- Finisher
iii) If manufactured on farm
a) Capacity of feed grinder and mixer
b) Source of raw materials
c) Feed formula
d) Cost of production (Rs./kg)
- Starter
- Finisher
iv) Requirement (kg/bird)
- Starter
- Finisher
i) Veterinary aid
i) Source
ii) Location
iii) Distance (km.)
iv) Availability of staff
v) Type of facilities available
vi) If own arrangements are made
a) Employed a verterinary doctor/stock man /consultant
b) Periodicity of visit
c) Amount paid (Rs.)
vii) Expenditure per bird per cycle (Rs.)
j) Electricity
i) Source SEB/Other
ii) Approval from electricity board
iii) Connected load
iv) Problems of power failure
v) Arrangements for generator
k) Water

i) Source
ii) Quality of water
iii) Availability of sufficient quantity for drinking and cleaning
iv) If investment has to be made type of strcture design and cost
l) Marketing of broilers
i) Source of sale
ii) Place of disposal
iii) Distance (km)
iv) Basis of payment (number or weight)
v) Price realised - (Rs. per kg live weight or live bird)
vi) Periodicity of payment

m) Marketing of other products
i) Manure - Qty./bird, price per unit (Rs./Ql)
ii) Empty gunny bags - Number and cost/bag
n) Beneficiary's experience
o) Comments on technical feasibility
p) Government restrictions, if any

3. FINANCIAL ASPECTS :

i) Unit Cost :

Sr.No.	Name of Investment	Physical unit and specification	Unit cost with component wise break-up (Rs.)	Whether approved by state level unit cost committee
			Total	

ii) Down payment/margin/subsidy (Indicate source & extent of subsidy)
iii) Year - wise physical & financial programme.

Year	Invest-ment	Physical units (Rs.)	Unit cost (Rs.)	Total outlay (Rs.)	Margin/ subsidy (Rs.)	Bank Loan (Rs.)	Refinance assistance (Rs.)
1	2	3	4	4	5	6	7
Total							

iv) Financial viability (comment on the cash flow projection on a farm model / unit and enclose the same) Particulars :
a) Internal Rate of Return (IRR):
b) Benefit Cost Ratio (BCR) :
c) Net Present Worth (NPW) :
v) Financial position of the borrowers (to be furnished in case of corporate

bodies/partnership firms)
a) Profitability ratio
i) Gross Profit ratio
ii) Net Profit ratio
b) Debt equity ratio
c)Whether Income tax & other tax obligations are paid upto date
d) Whether audit is upto date (enclose copies of audited financial statements for the last three years)
vi) Lending Terms :
i) Rate of interest
ii) Grace period
iii)Repayment period
iv) Nature of Security
v) Availability of Government guarantee wherever necessary

4. INFRASTRUCTURAL FACILITIES:

a) Availability of technical staff with bank/implementing authority for monitoring
b) Details of
i) technical guidance
ii) training facilities
iii) Govt support/ extention support
c) Tie-up arrangements with marketing agencies for loan recovery :
d) Insurance :
Type of policy
Periodicity
Rate of premium

Annexure IIa

Economics of Broiler Farming - at a Glance

1. Unit Size : 500 broiler birds per week
2. System of rearing : Deep litter system
3. State : Karnataka
4. Unit cost (Rs.) : 754926
5. Bank loan (Rs.) : 566195
6. Margin money (Rs.) :188732
7. Repayment period : 6 years with six months grace period
8. Interest rate (%) : 12
9. BCR at 15% DF : 1.823
10. NPW at 15% DF (Rs.) : 2616766
11. IRR (%) : × 40

Annexure - II b
ECONOMICS OF BROILER FARMING - INVESTMENT COST

Sr. No	Particulars	Specifications	Physical Units	Unit cost(Rs. / Unit)	Total cost (Rs.)
1	Sheds and other structures				
	a) Broiler sheds (8 sheds)	1 sft. per bird(DL)	4000 sft.	90	360,000
	b) Store room		200 sft	100	20,000
	c)Labour quarter		150 sft	100	15,000
	d) Slaughter room		100 sft	90	9,000
	e) Fencing	Barbed wire	750 rft	20	15000
2	Water supply system				
	a) Digging and construction of well	13'dia x33'depth	1 Ls	20000	20,000
	b) Water tank		5000 litres	2	10,000
	c) 3 HP electric motor/pumpset and other accessories and pipeline etc.		1 Ls	12000	12,000
	d) Electrical installation/equipment		4% of civil costs		16160
3	Equipments				
	a) Feeders and waterers		4000 birds	12	48000
	b) Dressing equipment		Ls		10,000
4	Capitalisation of recurring expenses for first 8 batches				
	a) Chick cost		4000 DOCs	13	52,000
	b) Feed cost for 4080 birds	3.2 kg/bird	13056 kg	11	143616
	c) Overheads such as cost of, Medicines, vaccine, insurance, litter	Rs.5.00/bird	4080 birds	5	20,400
	d) Labour cost	3 months	1250	3	3750
5	Total financial outlay (TFO)				754926

6	Margin money @ 25% of TFO			Say	188732
7	Bank loan @ 75% of TFO			Say	566195

Annexure - II c

ECONOMICS OF BROILER FARMING - TECHNO - ECONOMIC PARAMETERS

1	No. of birds (per week)	500
2	Rearing period (weeks)	
3	No. of batches per cycle	8
4	No. of batches introduced:	
	I year (on considering 3 months construction period)	40
	II year onwards	52
5	No. of batches sold:	
	I year (on considering construction period + rearing period)	33
	II year on wards	52
6	Space requirement per bird (s.ft.)	1
7	Cost of construction of shed (Rs./s.ft.)	90
8	Store room (s.ft.)	200
9	Cost of construction of store room (Rs./s.ft.)	100
10	Labour quarters (s.ft.)	150
11	Cost of construction of labour room (Rs./s.ft.)	100
12	Slaughter room (s.ft.)	100
13	Cost of construction of slaughter room (Rs. s.ft.)	100
14	Barbed wire fencing (Rs.rft.)	750
15	Cost of fencing (Rs./rft)	20
16	Cost of electrification (as % of civil costs)	4
17	Equipment cost (Rs./bird)	15
18	Mortality in 6-7 weeks (%)	4
19	Cost of DOCs (Rs./chick)	13
20	Supply of free chicks (%)	4
21	Feed requirement (kg./bird)	3.2
22	Feed cost (Rs./kg)	11
23	Expenditure on labour (Rs. per month) one labourer)	1250
24	Over heads cost (Cost of medicines, vaccine, insurance litter etc.) (Rs./bird)	8
25	Average body wt. of birds (Kg./bird)	1.5

26	Price of broilers (Rs./kg. body weight)	40
27	Sale price of bird (Rs./bird)	60
28	Income from manure (Rs. per bird)	1
29	No. of gunny bags (per ton of feed)	13.3
30	Income from gunny bags (Rs./bag)	10
31	Depreciation on sheds (%)	5
32	Depreciation on equipment (%)	10
33	Margin money (%)	25
34	Interest rate (%)	12
35	Repayment period (years)	6
36	Grace period (years)	0.5
37	Construction period ((months)	3
38	Rest period for broiler sheds (days)	7-10

Annexure - II d

ECONOMICS OF BROILER FARMING - FLOCK PROJECTION CHART

Year	No. of batches introduced	No. of batches sold
I	40	33
II	52	52
III	52	52
IV	52	52
V	52	52
VI	52	52

Note:

1) Initial period for three months, is considered as construction period and accordingly
only 40 batches will be introduced in first year.

2) Closing stock of 7 batches with an average age of 4 weeks will be there at the end of sixth year and the value of the same is taken into account for cash flow analysis.

3) The average value of the closing stock is considered at Rs. 35/- per bird.

Annexure - II e

ECONOMICS OF BROILER FARMING - CASH FLOW ANALYSIS

Sr. No	Particulars	I	II-V	VI	
I	Costs:				
1	Capital cost:*	535160	0	0	0

Appendix

2	Recurring costs:				
a)	Cost of chicks	260,000	3380000	3380000	
b)	Cost of feed	718080	933504	933504	
c)	Misc. expenses	95,110	132000	132,000	
d)	Labour cost	15000	15000	15000	
	Total Costs	1623350	1418504	1418504	
II	Benefits				
1	Sale of birds	990000	1560000	1560000	
2	Sale of manure	16500	26000	13,000	
3	Sale of gunny bags	8122	11286	11286	
4	Depreciated value of				
a)	Sheds	0	0	296977	
b)	Equipment (including water supply equipment)	0	0	59074	
5	Value of closing stock	0	0	122500	
6	Total Benefits	1014622	1597286	2075838	
	Net Benefits	-608728	178782	178782	
7	NPV				
a)	Cost	5546430.80			
b)	Benifits	5745128.16			
c)	NPW	198718			
8	BCR	01: 01.1			
9	IRR	>27%			

* Excluding the capitalised amount on chicks, feed, Misc. exp. and labour cost

Annexure - II f
ECONOMICS OF BROILER FARMING - REPAYMENT SCHEDULE
Bank loan (Rs.) : 566195
Interest rate :12 %
(Rupees)

Year	Income	Expenses	Gross surplus	Loan Balance	Interest	Repayment Int.	Repayment Pri.	Net surplus
I	1014622	868424 *	146198	566195	67944	67944	0	78255
II	1597286	1418504	178872	566195	67944	67944	66195	44642
III	1597286	1418504	178872	500000	60000	60000	75000	43782
IV	1597286	1418504	178872	425000	51000	51000	80000	47782
V	1597286	1418504	178872	345000	41400	41400	100000	37382
VI	1597286	1418504	178872	245000	29400	29400	125000	24382
VII	1597286	1418504	178872	120000	14400	14400	120000	44382

* During the first year it is the difference between the total costs and total project cost

Note : Average loan period in first year is considered as 10 months for working out interest amount.

Annexure - III
Floor space, Feeding space and watering space data for Broiler Chicks

Age weeks	Floor space Sq.ft./Chick	Feeding space inches/chick	Watering space inches/chick
1	0.2	1.5	0.5
2	0.2	2.0	0.7
3	0.3	2.0	0.7
4	0.4	2.5	0.8
5	0.6	2.5	0.8
6	0.8	3.0	1.0
7	0.9	3.0	1.0

Annexure - IV

Body weight, feed consumption and feed conversion of broiler chicks

Age		**Body weight & gain (kgs)**		**Feed consumption(kgs)**		**Feed conversion**	
Weeks	**Days**	**Average weight**	**Weekly gain**	**Weekly**	**Cummulative**	**Weekly**	**Cummulative**
1	7	0.17	-	0.1	0.1	0.81	0.81
2	14	0.28	0.15	0.23	0.34	1.53	1.21
3	21	0.48	0.2	0.34	0.67	1.64	1.4
4	28	0.73	0.25	0.47	1.14	1.93	1.50
5	35	1.00	0.29	0.63	1.77	2.16	1.77
6	42	1.32	0.33	0.74	2.51	2.26	1.89
7	49	1.66	0.33	0.82	3.32	2.47	2.01

Annexure V

Composition of Broiler diets

Ingredients	**Formulations**			
	1	2	3	4
Maize	51	58.5	47.5	53.25
Wheat bran	10	2.5	7.75	--
Groundnut cake	25.2	25	29.4	29.4
Fish Meal	10.8	11	12.6	12.6
Dicalcium Phosphate	1	1	1	1
Lime Stone	0.5	0.5	0.5	0.25
Salt	0.5	0.5	0.5	0.5
Premix*	1	1	1	1
	100	100	100	100
Crude protein %	22.1	22	24	24
ME. ICal/Kg.diet	2,800	3,000	2,800	3,000

* Premix added per 100 kg feed.

Vitamin (gm)		Vitabland (A1B2D3)	25
		Folic acid	0.1
		Vit.E	4
		Niacin	10
		Pyridoxine	1
		Choline Chloride	30
Mineral (gm)		Ferrous sulphate	20
		Zinc Sulphate	25
		Copper sulphate	25
		Manganese Sulphate	25
		Potassium iodate	0.1
Amino acid (gm)		L-lysine hydrochloride	220
		DL - Methionine	160

Annexure VI
Vaccination Schedule for Broilers

Name of disease	**Name of Vaccination**	**Days/weeks of vaccination**	**Route of inoculation**	**Remarks**
Marek's disease	Herpes virus turkey vaccination	1 day old	Sub cutaneous	Life long immunity
Ranikhet disease	RD vaccine (Lasota 'F` strain)	4-7 days old	Intra-nasal Intra-ocular	Immunity is up to 10 weeks old
Fowl pox	Chick embryo adopted fowl	6-8 weeks of age	Wing web method	If the disease is prevalent in the area. Once vaccinated gives life long immunity.

During chick rearing the disease most likely to occur is coccidiosis. Its organisms thrive on wet litter and so keep the litter dry. The feed mixed with coccidiosis should be used. In case of an outbreak, the Coccidiocidal drug in drinking water should be used at recommended level.

COMMON PHYSIOLOGICAL VALUES OF VARIOUS DOMESTICATED LIVESTOCK

Particulars	Cattle	Buffalo	Sheep	Goat	Pig	Horse	Dog	Cat	Camel	Elephant	Fowl
Rectal Temp^0 F	101.5	101.0	103.0	103.0	102.6	100.4	101-102	101	99.6	97.6	107
Normal pulse/ min	60-90	40-50	70-90	70-90	60-90	36-42	70-130	100-130	30-50	25-35	120-160
Normal Resp./ min	20-30	10-20	20-30	20-30	10-20	8-16	16-30	30-40	10-12	8-10	15-50
Duration of heat	6-30 hrs	6-48 hrs	1-2 d	2-3 d	3-4 d	6 day	11-18 d	7-10 d	5 d	–	
Age at first service (month)	15-18	24-27	8-12	8-12	8-10	16-18	6-12	6-15	–	–	
Gestation Period (days)	273-294 (283)	300–309 (304)	140–160 (150)	147–155 (150)	109–125 (115)	305–400 (340)	55–70 (63)	55–70 (56)	365-410 (370)	20 month	21 day hatching

SITES FOR PULSE RECORDING

Horse	Lower jaw, where the external maxillary artery is continued across the face as facial artery.
Cattle	Coccygeal artery on either sides of the under aspect of tail.
Sheep, Goat, Dog, Cat	Femoral artery inside the hind limb, more than half way between stifle & hip joint.
Fowl	Wing artery on the inner aspect of the wing

LIVESTOCK IDENTIFICATION

Sr	Method	Materials needed	Remarks
1.	Tattooing	Thin needles in the form of letters and numbers to form codes, Tattooing forceps, ink.	Applied on clear and light skin, like- inner aspect of pinna, under root of tail, escutcheon, gum. Applicable on white/ pink skin only (not in buffaloes). Good for calves, sheep & goat.
2.	Ear tagging	Metal Ear tags Plastic ear tags (Applicators, Pins)	

3.	Ear notching	Notching forceps	Requires skill and uniform coding system. Good for Pigs, sheep & goat.
4.	Branding (Hot & Cold	Long iron bars with protected handle having letters and numerals at tip.	It may be hot (red hot – furnace) and cold (liquid nitrogen: -196°C) branding. Not to be practiced in monsoon.

TEETH ERUPTION AND AGE DETERMINATION TABLE : HORSE

Age	Incisors	Canine	Cheek teeth
Up to 1 week	2. Temp. Centrals	-	-
2 – 4 weeks	2 Temp. Laterals	-	1st , 2nd ,3rd Temp.
7 – 9 months	2 Temp. Corners	-	4th Perm.
18-20 months	-	-	5 th Perm.
2.5 years	2 Perm. Centrals	-	1st, 2nd Perm.
3.5 years	2 Perm. Laterals	-	3rd Perm.
4.0 years	-	All 4	6th Perm.
4.5 years	2 Perm. Corners	-	-

ERUPTION TABLE FOR CATTLE

Age	Incisors	Cheek teeth
Up to 1 month	All Temp.	1st , 2nd , 3rd Temp.
6 months	-	4th Perm.
1.5 years	-	5th Perm.
2.0 years	Central Pair Perm.	1st, 2nd, 6th Perm.
2.5 years	-	3rd Perm.
3.0 years	Medial Pair Perm.	-
4.0 years	Lateral Pair Perm.	-
5.0 years	Corner pair Perm.	-

ERUPTION TABLE FOR BUFFALO

Age	Incisors	Cheek teeth
Up to 1 month	Central and medial Temp.	-
1.5 month	Lateral Temp.	1st , 2nd, 3rd Temp.
4.0 month	Corner Temp.	
6.0 month	-	4th Perm.
1.5 year	-	5th Perm.
2.0 year	-	1st, 2nd, 6th Perm.

3.0 year	Central Perm.	3rd Perm.
3.5 year	Medial Perm.	-
4.5 year	Lateral Perm.	-
5.5 year	Corner Perm.	-

ERUPTION TABLE FOR SHEEP & GOAT

Approx. age	Sheep	Goat
First year	One pair of central permanent incisors	Front teeth are small and sharp
Second yearing	Two pairs (central, medial) permanent incisors.	Central pair of incisors are replaced by permanent teeth
Third year	Three pairs (central, medial, lateral) central ones are replaced by permanent incisors.	One tooth on either side of the permanent teeth.
Fourth year	Four pairs (central, medial, lateral, corner) permanent incisors.	Six permanent incisors appear.
Fifth year	- do -	All permanent incisors appear.
Six year	Broken mouth condition may occur, that may later lead to Gummer condition.	onwards

BREEDS OF CAMEL

Name	Origin	Salient Features	Utility
Bikaneri	Bikaner	"STOP" and "Jheepras" present. Have > 50 % polulation	Riding & as Pack animal
Jaiselmeri	Jaiselmer	Streamlined body, shorter, lighter with no "STOP".	Riding
Mewari	Mewar	Short, stouter and have coarse body hair.	Pack animal in hilly areas.
Sindhi	Lower parts of Indus	Dark brown coat and can walk in marshy areas.	Pack animal
Tharparkar	Sindh	Well marked "STOP"	Riding
Kutchi	Kutch	Small	Riding and as pack

BREEDS OF HORSES

Sl.	Name	Origin	Salient features	Utility
1.	Kathiawari	Gujarat	*Sickle hocks, Ears inclined to meet at tips.*	Well known for pace (draft) and speed (race).
2.	Marwari	Rajasthan	*Handsome, Majestic, tough, sturdy with easy pace.*	Well known for riding skills.
3.	Spiti	Jammu and Kullu valley	*Well developed quarters. Legs covered with hair.*	Pack, Riding

4.	Bhutia	Himalayan ranges	*Surefooted, round quarters, coarse & hairy legs.*	Can walk long distances Known for their intelligence, used for polo, racing & as pack animal.
5.	Manipuri	Manipur	*Surefooted, well proportioned body.*	Known for elegance and speed. Military, Transport.
6.	Zanskari	Ladakh	*Well suited for snow bound areas.*	Well adapted in high altitudes as pack animal.

POULTRY BREEDS

Sl.	Name	Origin	Salient Features	Utility
I.	**American class:** Yellowish skin, clean shank, red ear lobe, brown shelled eggs.			
A.	Rhode Island Red	New England	Back flat and breast is carried well forward	Meat
B.	Plymouth Rock	America	Excellent Flesh, Single comb (whole white)	Dual
C.	Newhampshire	England	Chestnut red plumage, Single comb	Dual
II.	**Asiatic Class:** Yellow skin,red ear lobes,brown shelled eggs and feathered shank			
A.	Brahma	India	Massive, well feathered and pea comb	Dual
III.	**English Class:** Excellent flesh,white skin, red ear lobes, brown shelled eggs, clean shank			
A.	Sussex	England	Excellent flesh, single comb and coloured beak	Meat
B.	Australop	Australia	Single comb, black body and lustrous greenish black plumage	Dual
C.	Orpington	England	Well rounded and loose feathered	Dual
IV.	**Mediterranean Class:** Yellow/ white skin, white ear lobes, white shelled eggs and high egg production			
A.	Leg horn	Italy	World's No. 1 egg producer, small, active, neatest, single comb and stylish carriage	Egg
B.	Minorca	Spain	Largest and heaviest Mediterranean breed	Egg

WOOL FIBRE PARAMETERS

Indian wool fibre	Mean fibre diametre (mm)	% of India Production
North India Superior clothing white	0.032	4.9
North India clothing white	0.03 – 0.042	44.7
North India rug white	0.042 – 0.046	12.4
North India carpet white	0.046 and above	10.0
South India blanket type	0.042 – 0.046	23.5
South India Tannery type	0.046 above	4.5

ANIMAL UNITS OF LIVESTOCK

	Type of Livestock	Animal Units
Cattle:		
	□ Cow, with or without unweaned calf at side, or heifer 2 years old or older	1.0
	□ Bull, 2 years old or older	1.3
	□ Young cattle, 1 to 2 years	0.8
	□ Weaned calves to yearlings	0.6
Horses:		
	□ Horse, mature	1.3
	□ Horse, yearling	1.0
	□ Weaning colt or filly	0.75
Sheep:		
	□ 5 mature ewes, with or without unweaned lambs at side	1.0
	□ 5 rams, 2 years old or over	1.3
	□ 5 yearlings	0.8
	□ 5 weaned lambs to yearlings	0.6
Swine:		
	□ Sow	0.4
	□ Boar	0.5
	□ Pigs to 200 pounds	0.2
Chickens:		
	□ 75 layers or breeders	1.0
	□ 325 replacement pullets to 6 months of age	1.0
	□ 650 8–week–old broilers	1.0
Turkeys:		
	□ 35 breeders	1.0
	□ 40 turkeys raised to maturity	1.0
	□ 75 turkeys to 6 months of age	1.0

CARCASS CHARACTERISTICS

PARAMETERS	HORSE	OX
1. Side length	Unusual	Lesser
2. Muscular development of hind quarter	Great	Less
3. Thoracic cavity	Longer	Shorter
4. Ribs	18 pairs	13 pairs
5. Superior spinous process of first six vertebrae	Markedly developed	Less developed
6. Extension of ulna	Up to half the length of radius	Articulates with carpus
7. Articulation among last three lumbar vertebral	Articulates	Do not articulate
8. Flesh	Dark bluish red	Lacks blue tinge sweet taste, fibrous

CARCASS CHARACTERISTICS

FEATURE	SHEEP	GOAT
Back and withers	Round and well fleshed	Sharp, litter flesh
Thorax	Barrel shaped	Flattened laterally
Tail	Fairly broad	Thin
Radius	1 ¼ times length of metacarpus	Twice as long as metacarpus
Scapula	Short and broad	Long
Flesh	Pale red and fine	Dark red of coarse with goaty odour

IODINE VALUE OF MEAT

Animal species	Iodine value of meat
Horse	71 – 86 %
Ox	38-46 %
Sheep	35 – 46 %
Pig	50 -70 %
Good lard	66%

REFRACTIVE INDEX OF MEAT

Animal species	R. I. of meat fat
Horse	53.5
Ox	< 40
Pig	< 51.9

BIOLOGICAL VALUE OF LIVESTOCK PRODUCTS

Items	Biological Value
80	Whole milk
94	Whole egg
83	Egg white
67	Potato
67	Wheat
65	Oat

SITE OF THORACOCENTESIS

Animal	Right (ICS)	Left (ICS)
Horse	6th	7th
Cattle & Sheep	5th	6th
Dog & Cat	6th	7th

SITE OF PARACENTHESIS

	Heart Position	
Animal	**Base (ICS)**	**Apex (ICS)**
Horse, Cattle, Sheep, Pig	2nd	6th
Dog & Cat	3rd	6th
Animal	**Site for puncture**	
Horse	4th - 5th ICS	
Cattle	4th ICS	
Dog, Cat	4th - 5th ICS	

* ICS = Intercoastal space

LIVER BIOPSY

Animal	Site
Horse	Right Dorsal Half, 11th - 14th ICS
Cattle & Sheep	Upper third, righside, 11th ICS
Dog, Cat, Pig	Last 2 ICS close to costal arch

QUARANTINE PERIOD

Disease	Species	Period (OIE guidelines)
Infectious Bronchitis	Fowl	28 days
Rabies	Dog, Cat	4 months
Bacterial Infection	Zebra	2 weeks
Fowl Cholera	Poultry	14 days
Fowl Typhoid	Poultry	28 days
African Swine Fever	Swine	40 days
New Castle Disease	Birds	21 days
Fowl Plaque	Wild Birds	21 days
Chlamydiosis	Pigeon	45 days
Aspergillosis	Psittacine birds	45 days
Rinder Pest	Cattle	21 days
CBPP	Bovine	180 days
Anaplasmosis	Ruminants	100 days
TB	Bovine	3 months with negative
Enzootic bovineleucosis	Bovine	4 months
H.S.	Cattle	28 days
IBR	Bovine	30 days
Swine Fever	Swine	6 weeks
Porcine Brucellosis	Swine	30 days
Swine Transmissible Gastroenteritis	Swine	28 days
Pox	Sheep Goat	30 days
Blue Tongue	Sheep	40 days
CCPP	Sheep	180 days

Dourine	Horse	28 days
Glanders	Horse	28 days
Salmonellosis	Pregnant mares	6 weeks
Equine Influenza	Equine	28 days
Japanese encephalitis	Domestic & wild pig	28 days
Contagious Equine Metritis	Equine	30 days

Percentage, ppm, and ppb Conversions		
ppm	**ppb**	**Percentage**
0.001	1	0.0000001
0.01	10	0.000001
0.1	100	0.00001
1	1,000	0.0001
10		0.001
100		0.01
1,000		0.1
10,000		1
Other useful conversions: 1 mg/kg = 1 ppm 1 g/ton = 1.1 ppm 100 g/ton = 110 ppm		

Serum Biochemical Reference Ranges

In Conventional (USA) Units	Units	Dog	Cat	Cow	Horse	Pig	Sheep	Goat	Rabbit	Ostrich
ALT	u/L	8.2-57	8.3-53	6.9-35	2.7-21	22-47	15-44	15-52	48-80	20
Amylase	u/L	270-1,462	371-1,193	41-98	47-188	44-88	140-270		167-315	
Alk phos†	u/L	10.6-101	12-65	18-153	70-227	41-176	27-156	61-283	4-16	32-98
AST	u/L	8.9-49	9.2-40	45-110	116-287	15-55	49-123	66-230	14-113	131-486
Creatine kinase	u/L	14-120	17-150	14-107	34-166	66-489	7.7-101	16-48	218-2,705	294
GGT†	u/L	1.0-9.7	1.8-12	4.9-26	2.7-22	31-52	20-44	20-50	0-14	2.1
LDH†	u/L	24-219	35-225	309-938	102-341	160-425	83-476	79-265	34-129	
SDH†	u/L	3.1-7.6	2.4-6.1	6.1-18	1.2-8.5	0.5-4.9	3.5-21	9.3-21		
Bicarbonate	mEq/L	18-25	16-22	21-29	22-29	18-27	20-27		16-38	
Bilirubin	mg/dL	0.1-0.6	0.1-0.5	0.0-0.8	0.3-3.0	0.0-0.5	0.0-0.5	0.1-0.2	0-0.7	
Calcium	mg/dL	8.7-11.8	7.9-10.9	8.4-11.0	10.4-13.4	9.3-11.5	9.3-11.7	9.0-11.6	5.6-12.5	10.7-14
Chloride	mEq/L	102-117	108-130	96-109	97-110	97-106	101-113	100-112	92-112	100
Cholesterol	mg/dL	116-254	71-161	62-193	71-142	81-134	44-90	65-136	10-80	

Creatinine	mg/dL	0.5-1.6	0.5-1.9	0.6-1.8	0.9-2.0	0.8-2.3	0.9-2.0	0.7-1.5	0.5-2.5	0.1-0.4
Glucose	mg/dL	62-108	61-124	42-75	62-114	66-116	44-81	48-76	75-155	245
Magnesium	mg/dL	1.7-2.7	1.9-2.8	1.7-3.0	1.8-2.7	2.3-3.5	2.0-2.7	2.1-2.9		
Phosphorus	mg/dL	2.9-6.2	4.0-7.3	4.3-7.8	2.3-5.4	5.5-9.3	4.0-7.3	3.7-9.7	4.0-6.9	4.0-9.9
Potassium	mEq/L	3.8-5.6	3.8-5.3	4.0-5.8	2.8-4.7	4.4-6.5	4.3-6.3	3.8-5.7	3.6-6.9	3.0
Protein Albumin Globulin	g/dL g/dL g/dL	5.5-7.5 2.6-4.0 2.1-3.7	5.7-8.0 2.4-3.8 2.4-4.7	6.2-8.2 2.8-3.9 2.9-4.9	5.7-7.9 2.5-3.8 2.4-4.6	5.8-8.3 2.3-4.0 3.9-6.0	5.9-7.8 2.7-3.7 3.2-5.0	6.1-7.5 2.3- 3.6 2.7-4.4	5.4-8.3 2.4-4.6 1.5-2.8	3.8 1.8 2.0
Sodium	mEq/L	140-154	146-159	135-148	133-147	139-153	142-160	137-152	131-155	147
Urea nitrogen	mg/dL	8.8-26	15-31	7.8-25	10.4-25	8.2-25	10-26	13.26	13-29	1.1
Bicarbonate	mmol/L	18-25	16-22	21-29	22-29	18-27	20-27		16-38	
Bilirubin	mmol/L	0.9-10.6	1.2-7.9	0.7-14	5.4-51	0.3-8.2	0.7-8.6	1.7-4.3	0-12	
Calcium	mmol/L	2.2-3.0	2.0-2.7	2.1-2.8	2.6-3.3	2.3-2.9	2.3-2.9	2.3-2.9	1.4-3.1	2.7-3.5
Chloride	mmol/L	102-117	108-130	96-109	97-110	97-106	101-113	100-112	92-112	100
Cholesterol	mmol/L	3.0-6.6	1.8-4.2	1.6-5.0	1.8-3.7	2.1-3.5	1.1-2.3	1.7-3.5	0.3-2.1	
Creatinine	mmol/L	44-138	49-165	56-162	77-175	70-208	76-174	60-135	44-221	8.8-35
Glucose	mmol/L	3.4-6.0	3.4-6.9	2.3-4.1	3.5-6.3	3.7-6.4	2.4-4.5	2.7-4.2	4.1-8.5	14
Magnesium	mmol/L	0.7-1.1	0.8-1.2	0.7-1.2	0.7-1.1	0.9-1.4	0.8-1.1	0.9-1.2		
Phosphorus	mmol/L	1.0-2.0	1.3-2.4	1.4-2.5	0.7-1.7	1.8-3.0	1.3-2.4	1.2-3.1	1.3-2.2	1.3-3.2
Potassium	mmol/L	3.8-5.6	3.8-5.3	4.0-5.8	2.8-4.7	4.4-6.5	4.3-6.3	3.8-5.7	3.6-6.9	3.0
Protein Albumin Globulin	g/L g/L g/L	55-75 26-40 21-37	57-80 24-38 24-47	62-82 28-39 29-49	57-79 25-38 24-46	58-83 23-40 39-60	59-78 27-37 32-50	61-75 23- 36 27-44	54-83 24- 46 15-28	38 18 20
Sodium	mmol/L	140-154	146-159	135-148	133-147	139-153	142-160	137-152	131-155	147
Urea nitrogen	mmol/L	3.1-9.2	5.5-11.1	2.8-8.8	3.7-8.8	2.9-8.8	3.7-9.3	4.5-9.2	4.6-10.4	0.4

Note : †Alk phos = alkaline phosphatase; GGT = gamma glutamyltransferase; LDH = lactate dehydrogenase; SDH = sorbitol dehydrogenase

Ref. Veterinary Clinical Pathology, Veterinary Practice Publishing Co., 13(2), 1984

GUIDELINES FOR THERAPY OF DEHYDRATION*

Large Animals

Loss of Body Weight in %	Skinfold test in Seconds	Packed cell Volume in %	Total serum solids gms/dl.	Fluid required for replacement ml/kg B.W
4 – 6%	–	40 – 50	7 – 8	20 – 25 ml.
6 – 8%	2 – 4	50	8 – 9	30 – 50ml.
8 – 10%	6 – 10	55	9 – 10	50 – 80 ml.
10 – 12%	20 – 45	60	12	80 – 120 ml.

(In case of calves 35 % PCV is considered as normal, if it comes down to 40 % oral fluid therapy should be initiated. The clinician should resort to i/v fluid if PCV value is between 55-60 %. Cases where the PCV exceeds 60 % are often fatal) (Source : Veterinary Medicines Blood Handerson, 6th Ed. ELBS).

Dog

Body	Daily Turn Over of Water			Electrolytes needed/day Total mEq	
Wt Kg	Total Ml	ml/Kg	Ml/hr	Sodium	Potassium
1	140	140	6	4	3
10	752	75	31	23	15
20	1247	62	52	37	25
40	2068	52	86	62	41
100	4038	40	168	121	81